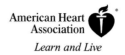

American Heart
Association
*Learn and Live*

# The AHA Clinical Series

SERIES EDITOR ELLIOTT ANTMAN

# Cardiogenic Shock

Judith Hochman would like to dedicate this book to Dr. Richard Fuchs, whose unwavering support (and editorial input) in this and other endeavors has been critical, and to Michael, Daniel, and Benjamin Hochman Fuchs, who inspire me to continue educating the next generations.

Magnus Ohman would like to dedicate this book to Elspeth, Elsa-Maria, Edward, and Henry. Although I hope you will never need to know about cardiogenic shock, your support of my endeavor to get the knowledge about serious heart conditions to the many cardiologists who care for these complex patients around the world is much appreciated.

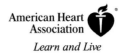

American Heart
Association
*Learn and Live*

## The AHA Clinical Series

SERIES EDITOR ELLIOTT ANTMAN

# Cardiogenic Shock

EDITED BY

## Judith S. Hochman, MD, FACC, FAHA

Harold Snyder Family Professor of Cardiology
Co-Director, NYU-HHC Clinical and Translational Science Institute
Clinical Chief, Leon Charney Division of Cardiology
Director, Cardiovascular Clinical Research Center
New York University School of Medicine
New York, New York
USA

## E. Magnus Ohman, MD, FRCPI, FESC, FACC, FSCAI

Professor of Medicine
Associate Director, Duke Heart Center
Director, Program for Advanced Coronary Disease
Duke Clinical Research Institute
Duke University Medical Center
Durham, North Carolina
USA

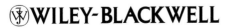

## WILEY-BLACKWELL

A John Wiley & Sons, Ltd., Publication

This edition first published 2009, © 2009 American Heart Association
American Heart Association National Center, 7272 Greenville Avenue, Dallas, TX 75231, USA
For further information on the American Heart Association:
www.americanheart.org

Blackwell Publishing was acquired by John Wiley & Sons in February 2007. Blackwell's publishing program has been
merged with Wiley's global Scientific, Technical and Medical business to form Wiley-Blackwell.

*Registered office:* John Wiley & Sons Ltd, The Atrium, Southern Gate, Chichester, West Sussex, PO19 8SQ, UK

*Editorial offices:* 9600 Garsington Road, Oxford, OX4 2DQ, UK
The Atrium, Southern Gate, Chichester, West Sussex, PO19 8SQ, UK
111 River Street, Hoboken, NJ 07030-5774, USA

For details of our global editorial offices, for customer services and for information about how to apply for permission
to reuse the copyright material in this book please see our website at www.wiley.com/wiley-blackwell

The right of the author to be identified as the author of this work has been asserted in accordance with the Copyright,
Designs and Patents Act 1988.

Wiley also publishes its books in a variety of electronic formats. Some content that appears in print may not be
available in electronic books.

Designations used by companies to distinguish their products are often claimed as trademarks. All brand names and
product names used in this book are trade names, service marks, trademarks or registered trademarks of their
respective owners. The publisher is not associated with any product or vendor mentioned in this book. This
publication is designed to provide accurate and authoritative information in regard to the subject matter covered. It is
sold on the understanding that the publisher is not engaged in rendering professional services. If professional advice
or other expert assistance is required, the services of a competent professional should be sought.

The contents of this work are intended to further general scientific research, understanding, and discussion only and
are not intended and should not be relied upon as recommending or promoting a specific method, diagnosis, or
treatment by physicians for any particular patient. The publisher and the author make no representations or
warranties with respect to the accuracy or completeness of the contents of this work and specifically disclaim all
warranties, including without limitation any implied warranties of fitness for a particular purpose. In view of ongoing
research, equipment modifications, changes in governmental regulations, and the constant flow of information
relating to the use of medicines, equipment, and devices, the reader is urged to review and evaluate the information
provided in the package insert or instructions for each medicine, equipment, or device for, among other things, any
changes in the instructions or indication of usage and for added warnings and precautions. Readers should consult
with a specialist where appropriate. The fact that an organization or Website is referred to in this work as a citation
and/or a potential source of further information does not mean that the author or the publisher endorses the
information the organization or Website may provide or recommendations it may make. Further, readers should be
aware that Internet Websites listed in this work may have changed or disappeared between when this work was
written and when it is read. No warranty may be created or extended by any promotional statements for this work.
Neither the publisher nor the author shall be liable for any damages arising herefrom.

*Library of Congress Cataloging-in-Publication Data*

Cardiogenic shock / edited by Judith S. Hochman, E. Magnus Ohman.
    p. ; cm. – (AHA clinical series)
    Includes bibliographical references.
    ISBN 978-1-4051-7926-3
    1. Cardiogenic shock.   I. Hochman, Judith S., 1951-  II. Ohman, Magnus.   III. American Heart Association.
IV. Series: AHA clinical series. [DNLM: 1. Shock, Cardiogenic. WG 300 C267471 2009]
    RC685.C18C368 2009
    616.1'207575–dc22                                    2008052028

A catalogue record for this book is available from the British Library.

Set in 9/12 pt Palatino by Aptara® Inc., New Delhi, India
Printed & bound in Singapore by Fabulous Printers Pte Ltd

1   2009

# Contents

# Contributors

## Editors

### Judith S. Hochman, MD, FACC, FAHA
Harold Snyder Family Professor of Cardiology
Co-Director, NYU-HHC Clinical and Translational Science Institute
Clinical Chief, Leon Charney Division of Cardiology
Director, Cardiovascular Clinical Research Center
New York University School of Medicine
New York, New York
USA

### E. Magnus Ohman, MD, FRCPI, FESC, FACC, FSCAI
Professor of Medicine
Associate Director, Duke Heart Center
Director, Program for Advanced Coronary Disease
Duke Clinical Research Institute
Duke University Medical Center
Durham, North Carolina
USA

## Contributors

### Kellan E. Ashley, MD
Chief Fellow, Cardiovascular Medicine
Heart and Vascular Institute
Cleveland Clinic Foundation
Cleveland, Ohio
USA

### Eric R. Bates, MD, FACC, FAHA
Professor of Internal Medicine
Division of Cardiovascular Diseases
Department of Internal Medicine
University of Michigan
Ann Arbor, Michigan
USA

## Christopher E. Buller, MD, FRCPC, FACC
Professor of Medicine
University of British Columbia
Head, Division of Cardiology
Vancouver General Hospital
Vancouver, British Columbia
Canada

## Vladimir Dzavik, MD, FRCPC, FAHA, FSCAI
Professor of Medicine, University of Toronto
Director, Cardiac Cath Lab and Interventional Cardiology
Peter Munk Cardiac Center, University Health Network
Toronto, Ontario
Canada

## Alexander Geppert, MD
Professor of Medicine
Director, Intensive Care Unit
3rd Department of Medicine with Cardiology and Emergency Medicine
Wilhelminen Hospital Vienna
Vienna
Austria

## Fredric Ginsberg, MD, FACC
Assistant Professor of Medicine
Robert Wood Johnson Medical School at Camden
University of Medicine and Dentistry of New Jersey
Camden, New Jersey
USA

## James A. Goldstein, MD, FACC
Director, Cardiovascular Research and Education
William Beaumont Hospital
Royal Oak, Michigan
USA

## David Hasdai, MD
Associate Professor
Sackler Faculty of Medicine
Tel Aviv University
Director, Cardiac Intensive Care Unit
Department of Cardiology
Rabin Medical Center
Petah Tikva
Israel

## Steven M. Hollenberg, MD, FACC
Professor of Medicine
Robert Wood Johnson Medical School/UMDNJ
Division of Cardiovascular Disease and Critical Care Medicine
Cooper University Hospital
Camden, New Jersey
USA

## David R. Holmes, Jr., MD, FACC
Professor of Medicine and Consultant
Cardiovascular Disease
Mayo Clinic
Rochester, Minnesota
USA

## Zaza Iakobishvili, MD, PhD
Intensive Cardiac Care Unit
Department of Cardiology
Rabin Medical Center
Petah Tikva
Israel

## Jason N. Katz, MD
Cardiology and Critical Care Fellow
Division of Cardiovascular Medicine
Division of Pulmonary, Allergy, & Critical Care Medicine
Duke University Medical Center
Durham, North Carolina
USA

## Venu Menon, MD, FACC, FAHA
Director, Coronary Care Unit
Cleveland Clinic Foundation
Cleveland, Ohio
USA

## Carmelo A. Milano, MD
Associate Professor of Medicine
Division of Cardiothoracic Surgery
Duke University School of Medicine
Durham, North Carolina
USA

## Arashk Motiei, MD
Senior Associate Consultant
Division of Cardiology
Mayo Clinic
Rochester, Minnesota
USA

## Joseph E. Parrillo, MD, FACC
Professor of Medicine
Robert Wood Johnson Medical School at Camden
University of Medicine and Dentistry of New Jersey
Chief, Department of Medicine
Edward D. Viner, MD Chair, Department of Medicine
Director, Cooper Heart Institute
Cooper University Hospital
Camden, New Jersey
USA

## Harmony R. Reynolds, MD, FACC, FASC
Assistant Professor of Medicine
Leon H. Charney Division of Cardiology
Cardiovascular Clinical Research Center
New York University School of Medicine
New York, New York
USA

## Joseph G. Rogers, MD
Associate Professor of Medicine
Medical Director, Cardiac Transplant and Mechanical Circulatory Support Program
Director, Duke Heart Failure Program
Division of Cardiovascular Medicine
Duke University School of Medicine
Durham, North Carolina
USA

## Michael H. Sketch, Jr., MD
Professor of Medicine
Division of Cardiology
Duke University Medical Center
Durham, North Carolina
USA

## John G. Webb, MD
McLeod Professor of Heart Valve Intervention
Division of Cardiology
University of British Columbia
Director, Cardiac Catheterization
St. Paul's Hospital
Vancouver, British Columbia
Canada

## Harvey D. White, MB, ChB, DSc, FRACP, FACC, FESC, FAHA, FHKCC (Hon), FCSANZ, FRSNZ
Professor of Medicine
Director of Coronary Care and Green Lane Cardiovascular Research Unit
Green Lane Cardiovascular Service
Auckland City Hospital
Auckland
New Zealand

## Cheuk-Kit Wong, MD, FCSANZ
Associate Professor and Consultant Physician in Cardiology
Dunedin School of Medicine
University of Otago
Dunedin
New Zealand

# Preface

When patients arrive at the hospital *in extremis*, physicians and health care providers face extraordinary challenges. It is our hope that this book on cardiogenic shock will provide a practical evidence-based approach to optimally managing patients with this complex disease as well as a historical perspective. Whereas there has been great progress in recent years in the management of acute myocardial infarction, the progress in cardiogenic shock has been more limited. Nevertheless, over the last decade, we have seen improvements in outcome based on the adoption of practices derived from pivotal randomized trial evidence and important observations from many dedicated researchers around the world.

We are indebted to the contributors to this book on cardiogenic shock. We believe they are among the most outstanding clinicians and researchers in their areas. They have provided outstanding reviews and succinct advice for the clinical setting, designing this volume to be a resource at your side.

We hope that you will use the principles and recommendations outlined in this book judiciously in your approach to treating patients with cardiogenic shock. The recommendations are intended to be consistent with the evidence and with the American Heart Association/American College of Cardiology guidelines. Increased compliance with guideline-recommended care has been demonstrated in the setting of acute coronary syndromes to result in improved outcomes.

We are also indebted to many other people that helped us in crafting this book: Penny Hodgson, whose tireless editorial work kept the book on track and helped to assure that the chapters had consistent formatting; Dr. Elliott Antman for his helpful comments and vision for this book; Betty Summers for her help collating comments and finding obscure articles that we remembered but could not easily locate; and Anna Yick for her help collating edits and checking facts.

Finally, we would like to thank our families for their generous support and encouragement.

Judith S. Hochman, MD

E. Magnus Ohman, MD

# Foreword

The strategic driving force behind the American Heart Association's mission of reducing disability and death from cardiovascular diseases and stroke is to change practice by providing information and solutions to health care professionals. The pillars of this strategy are Knowledge Discovery, Knowledge Processing, and Knowledge Transfer. The books in the AHA Clinical Series, of which *Cardiogenic Shock is* included, focus on high-interest, cutting-edge topics in cardiovascular medicine. This book series is a critical tool that supports the AHA mission of promoting healthy behavior and improved care of patients. Cardiology is a rapidly changing field, and practitioners need data to guide their clinical decision-making. The AHA Clinical Series serves this need by providing the latest information on the physiology, diagnosis, and management of a broad spectrum of conditions encountered in daily practice.

Rose Marie Robertson, MD, FAHA
Chief Science Officer, American Heart Association

Elliott Antman, MD, FAHA
Director, Samuel A. Levine Cardiac Unit,
Brigham and Women's Hospital

# Chapter 1

# Diagnosis, epidemiology, and risk factors

Zaza Iakobishvili, Harmony R. Reynolds, and David Hasdai

## Definitions and diagnosis

### Definitions

Cardiogenic shock is a state of decreased cardiac output and systemic perfusion in the presence of adequate intravascular volume, resulting in tissue hypoxia [1]. As early as 1912, Herrick described the clinical features of cardiogenic shock in patients with severe coronary artery disease: a weak, rapid pulse; feeble cardiac tones; pulmonary rales; dyspnea; and cyanosis [2]. The term cardiogenic shock is believed to have been originated in 1942 by Stead [3]. He described a series of two patients who had what he called "shock of cardiac origin." Later, the expression was rephrased as "cardiogenic shock."

The severity of shock can range from mild to severe, and practical definitions use somewhat arbitrary criteria. An essential feature of cardiogenic shock is systemic hypoperfusion, typically with hypotension; however, there is great variability in the severity of hypotension that defines shock, with the most common cut-off points for systolic blood pressure being <90 mm Hg or <80 mm Hg [4,5]. Patients with shock typically have signs of systemic hypoperfusion, including altered mental state, cool skin, and/or oliguria. Rales, indicating pulmonary edema, may or may not be present. Neither auscultation nor chest radiograph detects pulmonary edema in 30% of patients with cardiogenic shock [6]. The method used to measure blood pressure may also be important. Brachial cuff pressure measurements are often inaccurate in states of shock. Arterial blood pressure is more accurately monitored using intra-arterial cannulas; thus, this method is commonly advocated to ensure precise measurement.

*Cardiogenic Shock*. Edited by Judith S. Hochman and E. Magnus Ohman.
© 2009 American Heart Association, ISBN: 978-1-4051-7926-3

There is a subset of severe left ventricular (LV) failure patients who have "nonhypotensive cardiogenic shock" [7]. By definition, these patients have the clinical signs of peripheral hypoperfusion described above (with preserved systolic blood pressure measurements >90 mm Hg without vasopressor support). This occurs most often among patients with large anterior wall myocardial infarction (MI) and is associated with substantial in-hospital mortality, albeit lower than that of patients with classic cardiogenic shock. Thus, a diagnosis of cardiogenic shock may be made in patients with systemic hypoperfusion and blood pressure measurements of >90 mm Hg in several circumstances: (1) if medications and/or support devices are required to maintain normal hemodynamic parameters; (2) in the presence of systemic hypoperfusion with low cardiac output, with blood pressure maintained by marked vasoconstriction; and (3) if mean systemic pressure is ≥30 mm Hg lower than baseline in cases of preexisting hypertension.

In 1967, Killip and Kimball [8] proposed a crude clinical classification of hemodynamic status based on 250 patients with acute myocardial infarction (MI). This classification has withstood the test of time and is still in widespread use (Table 1.1). As the shock state persists, hypoperfusion of both the myocardium and peripheral tissues will induce anaerobic metabolism in these tissues and may result in lactic acidosis. Hyperlactatemia is considered a hallmark of hypoperfusion [9,10] and may supplement the clinical examination and blood pressure measurement when findings are inconclusive regarding shock status. The accumulation of lactic acid may cause mitochondrial swelling and degeneration, inducing glycogen depletion, which in turn may impair myocardial function and inhibit glycolysis, leading to irreversible ischemic damage. Serum lactate level is an important prognostic factor in cardiogenic shock [11]; in one multivariate analysis, a lactate level >6.5 mmol/L in cardiogenic shock patients was a very strong independent predictor of in-hospital mortality [odds ratio (OR) 295, $P < 0.01$] even after adjustment for age, sex, hypertension, and diabetes history [10].

Table 1.1 Clinical classification of hemodynamic status of acute MI patients.

| Class | Definition |
| --- | --- |
| I | No clinical signs of heart failure |
| II | Basilar rales and/or $S_3$ gallop, and/or elevated jugular venous pressure |
| III | Frank pulmonary edema |
| IV | Cardiogenic shock |

## Hemodynamics for diagnosis of cardiogenic shock

Along with metabolic parameters, hemodynamic data are very useful for diagnosis and prognostic assessment in cardiogenic shock patients. One of the earliest attempts to use hemodynamic evaluation to determine prognosis and to guide therapy found that all cardiogenic shock patients with LV filling pressure of >15 mm Hg and cardiac index <2.3 L/min died despite medical therapy [9]. The measurements with greatest prognostic value in addition to demographic and clinical variables appear to be cardiac output [12] and those measurements that incorporate cardiac output with systolic blood pressure, including stroke work [13] or cardiac power [14].

There is some variability in the definition of cardiogenic shock as used in clinical trials [7,12,14–17]. Most studies define shock as a state with systolic blood pressure of <90 mm Hg for at least 1 hour that is (1) not responsive to fluid administration alone; (2) secondary to cardiac dysfunction; and (3) associated with signs of hypoperfusion or a cardiac index of <2.2 L/min/m$^2$ and pulmonary artery wedge pressure (PAWP) >18 mm Hg. Hypotension that improves (increase in systolic blood pressure to >90 mm Hg) within 1 hour following administration of inotropic/vasopressor agents is often included in studies of cardiogenic shock, as is death within 1 hour of onset of hypotension when other criteria for cardiogenic shock are met. Some studies have specified invasive hemodynamic diagnostic criteria for cardiogenic shock, such as severely decreased cardiac output measurements derived from right heart catheterization. In most of these studies, cardiac index measurements of ≤2.2 L/min/m$^2$ were regarded as supporting the diagnosis of cardiogenic shock in the presence of other signs. Other investigators [15], however, regarded measurements of ≤1.8 L/min/m$^2$ as indicative of cardiogenic shock. An important consideration is whether the values were recorded on inotropic/vasopressor or circulatory device support; a 2.2–2.5 L/min/m$^2$ cut point is reasonable for those on support and 1.8–2.2 L/min/m$^2$ for those whose measurements are made off support [16].

The widespread availability of noninvasive means of assessing cardiac function, such as echocardiography, has reduced the use of right heart catheterization. Echocardiography with Doppler imaging has become a readily available modality for bedside hemodynamic assessment and for the evaluation of cardiac function, valvular status, and mechanical complications of acute coronary syndrome (ACS) [18]. Its use has steadily increased over the years, and currently it is performed frequently among ACS patients in many institutions.

In an analysis from Euro Heart Survey ACS, 68% of patients with cardiogenic shock underwent an echocardiographic evaluation [18]. Right heart catheterization was performed in just 111 of 549 patients with cardiogenic shock (20.2%) [18]. Noninvasively derived hemodynamic parameters, such as left atrial pressure approximated by transmitral flow patterns and cardiac output computed by echocardiography (derived stroke volume multiplied by heart rate), can advance the timely management of cardiogenic shock patients, obviating the need for right heart catheterization. The restrictive pattern of transmitral flow, defined as E wave deceleration time <140 ms, has positive predictive value of 80% for PAWP ≥20 mm Hg [19]. However, deceleration time >140 ms did not exclude an elevated PAWP. Transesophageal examination may be used in difficult cases to obtain hemodynamic information and to exclude mechanical causes of LV failure.

There are possible pitfalls in interpreting hemodynamic data. For example, cardiac output measurements may be above normal in patients for whom the underlying cause of cardiogenic shock is ventricular septal defect, and PAWP may be unexpectedly high in patients with right ventricular (RV) infarction because of leftward shift of the intraventricular septum (reversed Bernheim effect) or concomitant LV systolic dysfunction. Additionally, by the time right heart catheterization is performed, the patient with shock typically is already receiving supportive pharmacological treatment that can alter hemodynamic measurements. For example, treatment with a positive inotropic agent may improve a patient's subsequent cardiac output measurements, and treatment with diuretics may decrease subsequent PAWP measurements.

The caveats listed above illustrate the difficulty of diagnosing cardiogenic shock by means of numerical and laboratory values in isolation. Accordingly, shock is primarily diagnosed based on clinical findings supported by measured hemodynamic values (Table 1.2). Clinical evidence of a reduction in cardiac output with systemic hypoperfusion despite adequate filling pressures must be present for a diagnosis of cardiogenic shock. When right heart catheterization is performed, hemodynamics values should confirm low output and high filling pressures. If right heart catheterization is not planned, the combination of clinical examination, chest radiography, and echocardiography must clearly demonstrate systemic hypoperfusion, low cardiac output, and elevation of left atrial/pulmonary artery pressure and/or right atrial pressure. If the diagnosis is in any way unclear, right heart catheterization should be performed.

# Epidemiology

## Etiologies

Cardiogenic shock can occur as a result of a wide variety of cardiac disorders, including ACS, valvular disease, myocardial and/or pericardial disease, congenital lesions (in both children and adults), or mechanical injuries to the heart (Table 1.3; Chapter 8). Due to the great prevalence of coronary artery disease, cardiogenic shock as a complication of ACS is the predominant etiology.

Determining the etiology of cardiogenic shock in the individual patient may be challenging. The history and clinical examination may provide information on the etiology of cardiogenic shock in an individual patient, but there is quite a bit of overlap between syndromes; for example, chest pain is a cardinal feature of acute MI, myocarditis, and pericardial tamponade, and there may be overlap

**Table 1.2** Characteristic hemodynamic patterns usually observed in MI with and without hemodynamic instability and non-cardiogenic shock states

| | RA | RVS | RVD | PAS | PAD | PAW | CI | SVR |
|---|---|---|---|---|---|---|---|---|
| Normal values | <6 | <25 | 0–12 | <25 | 0–12 | <6–12 | ≥2.5 | (800–1600) |
| MI without pulmonary edema‡ | — | — | — | — | — | ~13 (5,18) | ~2.7 (2.2–4.3) | — |
| Pulmonary edema | ↔↑ | ↔↑ | ↔↑ | ↑ | ↑ | ↑ | ↔↓ | ↑ |
| **Cardiogenic shock** | | | | | | | | |
| LV failure | ↔↑ | ↔↑ | ↔↑ | ↔↑ | ↑ | ↑ | ↓ | ↔↑ |
| RV failure† | ↑ | ↓↔↑* | ↑ | ↓↔↑* | ↔↓↑* | ↓↔↑* | ↓ | ↑ |
| Cardiac tamponade | ↑ | ↔↑ | ↑ | ↔↑ | ↔↑ | ↔↑ | ↓ | ↑ |
| Acute mitral regurgitation | ↔↑ | ↑ | ↔↑ | ↔↑ | ↑ | ↔↑ | ↔↓ | ↔↑ |
| Ventricular septal rupture | ↑ | ↔↑ | ↑ | ↔↑ | ↔↑ | ↔↑ | ↑ PBF ↓ SBF | ↔↑ |
| Hypovolemic shock | ↓ | ↔↓ | ↔↓ | ↓ | ↓ | ↓ | ↓ | ↑ |
| Septic shock | ↓ | ↔↓ | ↔↓ | ↓ | ↓ | ↓ | ↑ | ↓ |

There is significant patient-to-patient variation. Pressures in RA, right atrium; RVS/D, right ventricular systolic/diastolic; PAS/D, pulmonary artery systolic/diastolic; PAW, pulmonary artery wedge are in mm Hg. CI, cardiac index (L/min/m$^2$); SVR, systemic vascular resistance (dynes/sec/cm$^5$); MI, myocardial infarction; P/SBF, pulmonary/systemic blood flow.

†"Isolated" or predominant RV failure. PAW, RVS and PA pressures may rise in RV failure after volume loading due to RV dilation, right-to-left shift of the interventricular septum, resulting in impaired LV filling. When biventricular failure is present, the patterns are similar to those shown for LV failure.

‡Forrester and colleagues classified nonreperfused MI patients into four hemodynamic subsets (*N Engl J Med* 1976;295:1356–62). PAWP and CI in clinically stable subset 1 patients are shown. Values in parentheses represent range.

Reprinted with permission from Hochman JS and Ingbar D, Cardiogenic Shock and Pulmonary Edema in Fauci AS, Braunwald E, Kasper DL et al., Harrison's Principles of Internal Medicine 17th Edition, McGraw-Hill Medical, 2008.

**Table 1.3** Differential diagnosis of suspected cardiogenic shock in the setting of acute MI

A. Myocardial Dysfunction
  – Predominant left ventricle
  – Predominant right ventricle
  – Both ventricles

B. Mechanical Complications
  – Ventricular septal rupture
  – Papillary muscle rupture
  – Free wall rupture and cardiac tamponade

C. Procedural Complications
  – Unsuspected coronary perforation
  – Unsuspected coronary dissection
  – Blood loss: access site, retroperitoneal

D. Significant Valvular Disease
  – Aortic stenosis
  – Mitral regurgitation
  – Mitral stenosis
  – Aortic regurgitation

E. Hypovolemia
  – Dehydration
  – Excessive diuresis
  – Hemorrhage

F. Mimicking Conditions
  – Acute aortic syndrome: aortic dissection or perforation
  – Acute pulmonary embolism
  – Pneumothorax
  – Adverse drug reaction: anaphylaxis
  – Septic shock with myocardial depression

G. Dynamic outflow obstruction
  – Hypertrophic cardiomyopathy
  – Takotsubo cardiomyopathy

H. Iatrogenic
  – Medications affecting hemodynamics (excess negative inotropy, vasodilation, diuresis)
  – Procedural complication
  – Hemorrhage

in the description of pain among these syndromes. The timing of symptoms may provide a clue to the occurrence of mechanical complications if, for example, chest pain recurs days after an initial episode and that recurrence is associated with shock. The absence of this pattern is not of diagnostic value, however, and mechanical complications may occur early in the course of MI.

The physical examination may provide diagnostic clues as well, particularly in the form of a new murmur as a herald of ventricular septal or papillary muscle rupture or acute mitral or aortic valve disease. Unfortunately, worsening of valvular heart disease may be accompanied by softening of an existing murmur, and, of course, murmurs are not a reliable indicator of valvular disease or rupture. However, the presence of a murmur in a patient with cardiogenic shock should prompt rapid echocardiographic evaluation.

### Electrocardiography

The electrocardiogram (ECG) may be helpful in the diagnosis of a particular etiology of shock. When ST-segment elevation acute MI (STEMI) causes LV failure, the degree and severity of the ECG abnormality should be concordant with the severity of the clinical condition. Modest ECG abnormalities should prompt consideration of other etiologies (Table 1.3). When marked ST elevations are present in several precordial leads, anterior MI is the most likely diagnosis and LV pump failure is the most likely cause of shock. A first inferior STEMI is less likely to cause shock; if inferior STEMI were the cause of shock, marked ST elevation with reciprocal ST depression, denoting extensive injury, would be expected on the ECG. RV infarction may complicate inferior MI as well; RV leads should be placed in cases of inferior MI with hypotension to search for right-sided ST elevation. Another possible finding of RV infarction is precordial ST elevation, which is largest in degree in V1-V2 and becomes smaller as one moves across the precordium. The absence of reciprocal changes or signs of RV infarction in the case of inferior MI with shock should prompt a search for complicating factors, such as myocardial or papillary muscle rupture. It should also be noted that ST elevation is not definitive evidence of STEMI; regional ST elevation may also be seen in acute myocarditis. Diffuse and marked ST depressions, most notable in V4-V6, indicate diffuse ischemia due to left main or severe triple vessel disease. Left bundle branch block may be seen as a reflection of a large STEMI, non–STEMI (NSTEMI) with prior infarcts, or underlying conditions associated with LV hypertrophy (e.g., aortic stenosis). Finally, a normal ECG in the presence of profound shock, particularly in the setting of arrhythmias, should lead to consideration of myocarditis.

### ACS as a cause of shock

Cardiogenic shock complicating ACS is not confined to the typical setting of large ST-segment elevation anterior wall infarction. Although shock occurs more frequently in the setting of ST-segment elevation (4.2–7.2% in fibrinolytic trials, 8.5–14.2% in the registries), it also occurs, albeit less commonly (2.1–2.6%), in ACS patients without ST-segment elevation, even without positive cardiac biomarkers [20–23]. Shock typically results from severe LV dysfunction but may also occur when LV function is well preserved. In the international **SH**ould we emergently revascularize **O**ccluded **C**oronaries for cardiogenic shoc**K**? (SHOCK) trial registry of 1190 patients with cardiogenic shock, the predominant cause of shock was LV failure (78.5%), whereas isolated RV shock occurred in only 2.8% of patients. Mechanical complications of acute MI were observed among the remaining patients: severe mitral regurgitation (MR; 6.9%), ventricular septal rupture (3.9%), and tamponade (1.4%) [24].

Data on the incidence of shock are derived from large population-based analyses as well as from subset analyses of randomized clinical trials examining effects of different treatment modalities in the various forms of ACS. Due to differences in the definition of cardiogenic shock and criteria for including patients, the reported incidence of cardiogenic shock complicating ACS varies among studies. For example, an incidence of cardiogenic shock during hospitalization of 2.6% was reported among 3465 patients with acute MI in the prethrombolysis era, a low figure that reflects exclusion of patients with signs of heart failure upon presentation [25]. In comparison, cardiogenic shock was present in 6.7% of 6676 consecutive acute MI patients managed noninvasively in the Trandolapril Cardiac Evaluation (TRACE) registry, which included STEMI and NSTEMI cases [26].

### ST–segment-elevation ACS and cardiogenic shock

Classically, cardiogenic shock has been considered a direct consequence of STEMI, most commonly caused by LV dysfunction resulting from continued ischemia and cell death. In three large international fibrinolytic therapy trials for STEMI, the incidence of shock ranged from 4.2% to 7.2% (Fig. 1.1) [12,27,28]. However, the reported incidence of cardiogenic shock among STEMI patients receiving fibrinolytic therapy may be biased, because patients with shock are often *not* enrolled in multicenter, randomized trials. Zeymer and colleagues reported a 14.2% incidence of cardiogenic shock in 9422 patients in an 80-hospital primary percutaneous coronary intervention (PCI) German registry [29].

Until recently, the incidence of cardiogenic shock among STEMI patients appeared to be quite stable, despite increasing use of early reperfusion therapy including primary PCI. Goldberg and colleagues [5] evaluated trends in the incidence of cardiogenic shock complicating STEMI in a single community from 1975 to 1997. The overall annual incidence for this period was 7.1% and ranged from 4.5% to 8.6%. In a large observational study [30] from the National Registry of Myocardial Infarction (NRMI-2, -3, -4), which analyzed data from 1.97 million acute STEMI patients hospitalized in the United States between 1994 and 2004, the incidence of cardiogenic shock was 8.6% overall and was quite stable over the study period. In the Euro Heart Survey of Acute Coronary Syndromes,

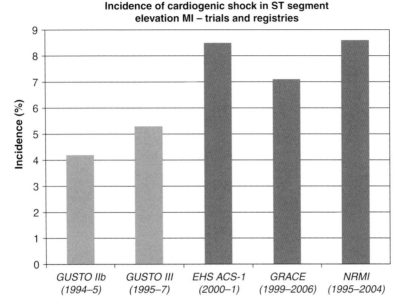

**Fig. 1.1** Incidence of cardiogenic shock in ST-segment elevation MI trials and registries [20,22,28,30,68]. The incidence of shock among patients in GUSTO IIb and III is lower, likely reflecting use of fibrinolytic therapy in all patients in the setting of these clinical trials as opposed to the registry patients. Differing incidences of shock in the registries may be related to different patient populations and/or slight differences in definitions of shock. In addition, the incidence of shock was found to be lower over time in the GRACE registry, which enrolled patients through 2006. Lighter boxes denote clinical trials; darker boxes denote registries. EHS ACS, Euro Heart Survey Acute Coronary Syndromes; GRACE, Global Registry of Acute Coronary Events; GUSTO, Global Utilization of Streptokinase and Tissue Plasminogen Activator for Occluded Coronary Arteries; NRMI, National Registry of Myocardial Infarction.

the incidence of shock was 8.5% in the STEMI group [31], and a recent report from the Global Registry of Acute Coronary Events (GRACE), which recruits patients with ACS in almost 100 hospitals in 14 countries (Argentina, Australia, Austria, Belgium, Brazil, Canada, France, Germany, Italy, New Zealand, Poland, Spain, the United Kingdom, and the United States), suggests a reduction in the incidence of cardiogenic shock after STEMI [20]. In this registry, the incidence of cardiogenic shock in the STEMI group was 7.1% in 1999, subsequently decreasing significantly to 4.7% in 2005 ($P = 0.02$) [20].

## Non–ST-elevation ACS and cardiogenic shock
In the setting of non–ST-elevation ACS (NSTE ACS), data regarding the incidence of cardiogenic shock are relatively limited. This has important

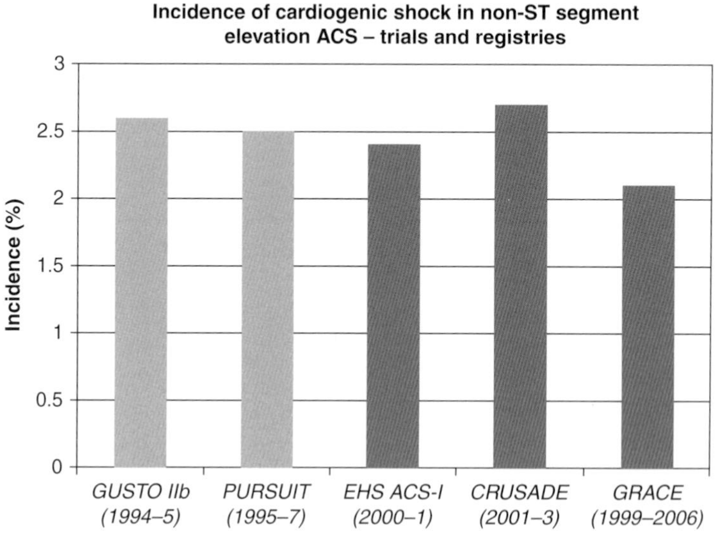

**Incidence of cardiogenic shock in non-ST segment elevation ACS – trials and registries**

**Fig. 1.2** Incidence of cardiogenic shock in non–ST-segment elevation acute coronary syndrome trials and registries [20–23,28]. The incidence of shock is uniformly lower among patients with NSTE ACS as compared with STEMI (compare with Fig. 1), most notably in the GUSTO IIb trial and the Euro Heart Survey and GRACE registry, which are also included in Fig. 1.1. These studies include patients with unstable angina, in which cardiogenic shock is known to occur. Lighter boxes denote clinical trials; darker boxes denote registries. CRUSADE, Can Rapid risk stratification of Unstable angina patients Suppress ADverse outcomes with Early implementation of the ACC/AHA guidelines; EHS ACS, Euro Heart Survey Acute Coronary Syndromes; GRACE, Global Registry of Acute Coronary Events; GUSTO, Global Utilization of Streptokinase and Tissue Plasminogen Activator for Occluded Coronary Arteries; PURSUIT, Platelet Glycoprotein IIb/IIIa in Unstable Angina: Receptor Suppression Using Integrilin Therapy.

implications, as the incidence of NSTE ACS appears to be increasing significantly as more sensitive cardiac markers are used [20]. In the Global Use of Strategies to Open Occluded Coronary Arteries (GUSTO IIb) trial [28], one of the largest clinical trials hitherto conducted, cardiogenic shock was predefined as a subset for analysis. Among 7986 patients with NSTE ACS, cardiogenic shock occurred in 2.6% of cases (Fig. 1.2). This was about half the incidence observed in the subgroup with ST-elevation acute coronary syndromes (STEACS) in the same trial [OR 0.50, 95% confidence interval (CI) 0.413, 0.612; $P < 0.001$]. The subset of patients with cardiogenic shock was also analyzed in the Platelet glycoprotein IIb/IIIa in Unstable angina: Receptor Suppression Using Integrilin Therapy (PURSUIT) trial of patients with NSTE ACS [21]. Of 9449 patients, 237 (2.5%) developed shock after enrollment. In another large survey (the Euro Heart

Survey of Acute Coronary Syndromes), the incidence of cardiogenic shock among patients admitted with NSTE ACS was 2.4% (of whom three quarters developed it during hospitalization) [22,31]. As more cases that were previously categorized as unstable angina are confirmed as NSTEMI with use of sensitive troponin assays, the incidence, but not the total number of patients, should continue to decline. In the GRACE registry, the incidence of shock among patients with NSTE ACS decreased significantly over a 6-year period, from 2.1% to 1.8% ($P = 0.01$) [20]. However, the CRUSADE (Can Rapid Risk Stratification of Unstable Angina Patients Suppress Adverse Outcomes With Early Implementation of the ACC/AHA Guidelines) quality improvement initiative evaluated care patterns and outcomes for 17,926 high-risk NSTE ACS patients (as determined by positive cardiac markers and/or ischemic electrocardiographic changes) at 248 United States hospitals with catheterization and revascularization facilities between March 2000 and September 2002, and found an incidence of cardiogenic shock that was remarkably consistent with all prior reports (2.6%) [23].

## RV infarction and cardiogenic shock

RV infarction is a distinct entity within the spectrum of cardiogenic shock. Most patients with RV infarction were not included in randomized trials; thus, detailed data regarding the frequency of shock among these patients are lacking. In the SHOCK registry, the proportion of patients with shock complicating MI who had shock due to "isolated" RV failure was 2.8% [24]. In contrast, RV infarction was a relatively common cause of shock among patients with STEMI, accounting for about 16% of cases in a single-center registry of STEMI [32]. Similarly, at Rabin Medical Center, RV infarction accounted for 19.6% of all cases of shock complicating STEMI [33].

## Time to development of cardiogenic shock in ACS

There is an apparent discrepancy, probably due to selection bias, between reports from randomized trials and population-based analyses regarding the timing of shock development. In randomized trials, approximately 90% of patients with shock developed it after study enrollment; only approximately 10% had shock upon arrival at the hospital. However, in a population-based study of unselected acute MI patients, 56% of shock patients had shock upon arrival [34]. In the SHOCK registry and trial, 26% of nontransferred patients were diagnosed with shock upon hospital arrival [35].

In the prethrombolysis era, Leor and colleagues [25] reported that shock developed at a median of 2 days after admission (range 3 hours to 16 days) in patients admitted without heart failure. Hands and colleagues [36] reported that cardiogenic shock developed after hospitalization in 60 (7.1%) of 845 patients presenting with acute MI. Half of patients who did not have shock upon admission developed shock within the first 24 hours.

In large fibrinolytic trials, the median time to the occurrence of shock among patients with persistent ST-segment elevation who developed shock in hospital was 10 or 11 hours [27,28,37], with most experiencing shock within the first 48 hours after enrollment. Shock occurred later, after symptom onset, in patients without ST-segment elevation compared with those with ST-segment elevation and is often associated with reinfarction in these cases. In GUSTO IIb, NSTE ACS patients developed shock a median of 76.2 hours after enrollment, in contrast to STEMI patients for whom the median time to onset was 9.6 hours [28]. In the SHOCK registry [38], time from acute MI onset to shock onset was also different: 8.9 hours for NSTE ACS patients versus 5.9 hours for STEMI patients. In the PURSUIT database of NSTE ACS, shock most commonly developed >48 hours after enrollment (median 94.0 hours) [21].

These data indicate that the window of opportunity for attempting to avert development of shock in STEMI is very short-lived; patients must be identified and measures should be taken within hours of presentation, including avoidance of measures that induce shock (Fig. 1.3). Very early reperfusion, which is the only therapy that prevents the development of shock in STEMI, is of paramount importance. The fact that cardiogenic shock develops later in NSTE ACS should not be interpreted as reflecting a more benign phenomenon; when it does occur, mortality is not lower than that seen among patients with STEMI complicated by shock (72.5% vs. 63.0% in the GUSTO IIb population, respectively, $P = $ NS) [28]. Recognition of the risk factors for shock and prevention of reinfarction post NSTEMI are important.

The finding that cardiogenic shock complicates unstable angina or NSTEMI extends the current shock paradigm in two respects: (1) ACS with or without ST-segment elevation can be complicated by cardiogenic shock; and (2) myocardial ischemia alone (without infarction) can be complicated by cardiogenic shock. The difference in time to development of shock between patients with versus those without ST elevation suggests variation in the underlying mechanisms of the condition. Moreover, it may reflect differences in the baseline clinical and demographic characteristics, differences in antecedent cardiac function, and differences in the extent and nature of the coronary artery disease. It may also reflect the difference in the pathogenesis of the acute event, an abrupt closure of the coronary artery in STEMI versus a gradual and more diffuse compromise in coronary blood flow without total occlusion of the artery in NSTE ACS.

# Risk factors

## Risk of development of cardiogenic shock

Timely recognition of a high-risk group of ACS patients prone to developing cardiogenic shock can be used as the central strategy for improving survival by avoiding measures that lead to iatrogenic shock (see below) and providing adequate therapeutic measures that can halt the deterioration that leads to this devastating condition.

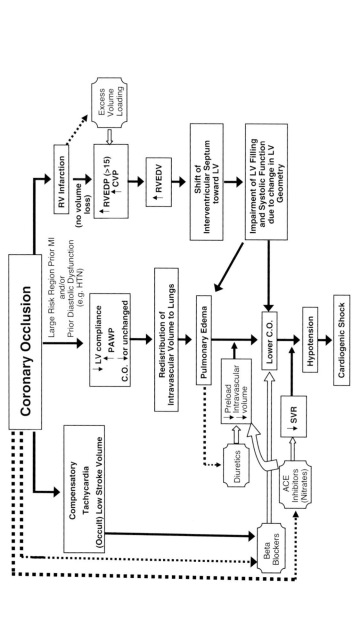

**Fig. 1.3 Iatrogenic shock [69].** The pathophysiology of iatrogenic shock that results from different scenarios of MI and pulmonary edema treatment is depicted. Acute pulmonary edema is a state of redistribution of intravascular volume into extracellular space in the lungs. When hemodynamic stability is tenuous, the additional decrease in plasma volume caused by diuretics in patients without prior HF may induce shock. Tachycardia is often compensatory for lower SV but is not appreciated as such. Treatment with beta-blockade lowers HR and SV, leading to frank shock. Decompensation may also occur when patients who are reliant on compensatory vasoconstriction are treated with ACE-inhibitors, particularly intravenously and early. Nitrates would be expected to have a similar effect but did not in the only systematic study, which used oral, low-dose treatment [63]. Volume expansion may be deleterious when used to excess or when RV filling pressure is already elevated because the RV may become volume overloaded with shift of the septum causing impairment in LV filling and contraction. (Reprinted with permission from Reynolds HR, Hochman JS. *Circulation* 2008;117(5):686–97.)

Certain demographic and clinical parameters are strongly associated with the development of shock. Leor and colleagues [25] reported that independent predictors for in-hospital shock were older age, female sex, prior angina, prior stroke, and peripheral vascular disease. Hands and colleagues [36] reported that the risk factors for developing cardiogenic shock were age >65 years, an LV ejection fraction <35%, larger infarct size (as estimated by serial cardiac marker measurements), prior MI, and diabetes mellitus. In these earlier studies, parameters from physical examination were not included in the analyses.

In an analysis of the GUSTO-I dataset [39] that included patients after fibrinolytic therapy, older age was the variable most strongly associated with the occurrence of shock; for every 10-year increase in age, the risk of developing shock was greater by 47%. Simple parameters derived from physical examination, such as systolic blood pressure, heart rate, and Killip class, among patients who did not present with cardiogenic shock were strong predictors for its subsequent development. The patient's age, combined with these physical parameters, provided 85% of the information needed to predict shock in this model.

Risk factors for cardiogenic shock have also been identified among patients with NSTE ACS in a retrospective analysis of the PURSUIT trial database [21]. In this trial, shock patients who received eptifibatide had a 50% reduction of 30-day mortality (58.5% vs. 73.5% for placebo; OR 0.51; 95% CI 0.28, 0.94; $P = 0.03$). Based on the scoring system developed for this analysis, cardiogenic shock was predicted primarily by age, the presence of ST depression in the initial ECG, and physical findings. Thus, despite the many differences between patients with or without persistent ST-segment elevation who develop shock, the baseline demographic and clinical variables associated with the development of the condition are similar.

The admission ECG along with relevant anamnestic and hemodynamic parameters can provide important information for quick risk stratification of acute MI patients. Retrospective analysis of the GUSTO-I clinical trial database aimed to determine the ability of initial ECG to predict all-cause mortality at 30 days following STEMI. After performing multivariable analysis, the sum of the absolute ST-segment deviation (both ST elevation and ST depression), heart rate, QRS duration, and ECG evidence of prior infarction (Q waves) appeared to be the strongest ECG predictors of mortality [40].

Bundle branch block on admission is relatively rare but carries important prognostic information. In the GUSTO-I trial, of all the 26,003 North American patients, 420 (1.6%) had left ($n = 131$) or right ($n = 289$) bundle branch block. These patients had higher 30-day mortality rates than matched control subjects (18% vs. 11%, $P = 0.003$, OR 1.8) and were more likely to experience cardiogenic shock (19% vs. 11%, $P = 0.008$, OR 1.78) [41].

Impaired fasting glucose, a state that precedes the development of diabetes mellitus, appears to increase the risk of shock in ACS patients. In the French RICO registry [42], 381 (38%) patients had diabetes mellitus, 145 (15%) had impaired fasting glucose, and 473 (47%) had normal fasting glucose. The rate of mortality in the group with impaired fasting glucose was twice that observed in the normal fasting glucose group (8% vs. 4%, $P = 0.049$). A significant increase in rates of cardiogenic shock (12% vs. 6%, $P = 0.011$) and ventricular arrhythmia (15% vs. 9%, $P = 0.035$) was observed in the impaired fasting glucose versus the normal fasting glucose group. After adjustment for confounding factors (age, sex, anterior location, and LV ejection fraction), impaired fasting glucose was a strong independent predictive factor for cardiogenic shock ($P = 0.005$).

Women may have a higher incidence of cardiogenic shock than men. Data from the SHOCK registry [43] indicated a higher prevalence of mechanical complications as the cause of shock in women; severe MR occurred in 11.4% of women versus 7.1% of men with shock ($P = 0.01$), and ventricular septal rupture developed in 7.7% of women versus 3.5% of men with shock ($P = 0.003$). Women also tend to be older and have higher rates of prior hypertension and diabetes mellitus, and lower ejection fractions, than men with shock.

## Outcomes in cardiogenic shock

The contemporary in-hospital mortality rate for cardiogenic shock remains extremely high at about 50–60% for all age groups. Patients with mechanical complications have even higher mortality rates, particularly without surgical intervention. Those with ventricular septal rupture have the highest mortality: 87% in the SHOCK Registry [24]. Papillary muscle rupture had a similarly high mortality before the era of surgical intervention, but with prompt surgical intervention, mortality is approximately 30% [44]. Surgical techniques for repair of free wall rupture are evolving with short-term survival approaching the survival after repair of papillary muscle rupture [45].

In the SHOCK trial registry examining cardiogenic shock caused by RV infarction, mortality was unexpectedly high in patients with predominant RV shock and similar to patients with predominantly LV failure shock—despite the younger age, lower rate of anterior MI, and higher prevalence of single-vessel coronary disease among RV compared with LV shock patients and their similar benefit from revascularization [46].

## Predictors of death in cardiogenic shock once shock has developed

### Demographics and hemodynamics

Older age has been associated with mortality in a number of trials and registries [12,29,47,48]. The apparent lack of survival benefit of early revascularization for the elderly in the SHOCK trial was found to be related to a chance imbalance in ejection fraction among elderly patients. Higher mortality rates among Hispanic and African American patients in the SHOCK registry ($P = 0.05$) did not persist after adjustment for patient characteristics and use of revascularization ($P = 0.26$) [49], with all race/ethnicity subgroups benefiting equally [50]. Female sex was independently associated with outcome in one large registry (ACC-NCDR) [48]. Taking all of the evidence into account, female sex does not seem to be an independent predictor of poor outcome [29,43,51,52], although it should be noted that two larger registries did not report the independent effect of sex on outcome [5,30].

Diabetic patients with ACS complicated by cardiogenic shock had a higher risk profile than nondiabetic patients. In-hospital survival of diabetic patients in the SHOCK registry, however, was only marginally lower than that of non-diabetic patients after adjusting for risk factors [53].

The extent of LV injury that causes cardiogenic shock is generally large, and although ST elevation is the more common finding, mortality rates do not differ significantly by ST-segment status on the ECG [21,28,38].

Hemodynamic variables reflect the severity of the shock syndrome and have prognostic value. The hemodynamic measurements with greatest prognostic value appear to be cardiac output [12] or those measurements that incorporate cardiac output with systolic blood pressure, including stroke work [13] or cardiac power [14]. In the SHOCK trial, the strongest association with in-hospital mortality was found for cardiac power. Cardiac power was calculated as mean arterial pressure × cardiac output/451 [14]. Also in SHOCK, the presence of cardiogenic shock on admission appeared to be an independent predictor of in-hospital mortality as compared with cardiogenic shock that developed during hospitalization (68% vs. 49%, $P = 0.039$), reflecting more deranged hemodynamics in those with shock at the time of admission [35].

### Angiographic and echocardiographic predictors

Angiography in patients with cardiogenic shock most often demonstrates multivessel coronary disease (left main stenosis in 23% of patients, 3-vessel disease in 64% of patients, 2-vessel disease in 22% of patients, and 1-vessel disease in 14% of patients) [47]. In the SHOCK trial, angiography also revealed high rates of the left anterior descending coronary artery as the predominant culprit, as well as reduced coronary flow and complex lesion types [54]. Compensatory hyperkinesis is a favorable response, which develops in myocardial segments that are not involved in acute MI; this response helps maintain cardiac output. Failure to develop such a response, because of previous infarction, high-grade coronary stenosis, or metabolic abnormalities that develop remote from a large infarct zone, is an important risk factor for cardiogenic shock and death.

In a SHOCK trial substudy, 175 echocardiograms were performed within 24 hours of randomization to the early revascularization (ERV) or initial medical stabilization groups [55]. Median LV ejection fraction was 28%. MR of at least moderate degree was seen in 39% of patients; severe MR was an exclusion criterion for the trial. Short- and long-term mortality were independently associated with initial LV systolic function (EF) and mitral regurgitation (MR) as assessed by echocardiography. LV volumes were not independently associated with death. The benefit of ERV was seen across the spectrum of baseline ejection fraction and MR (in a population that excluded shock due to severe MR).

## Risk models for shock mortality

The large database of the American College of Cardiology–National Cardiovascular Data Registry (ACC-NCDR) [48] identified 483 patients who underwent PCI for cardiogenic shock secondary to acute MI among 326,369 consecutive PCI procedures, performed at 243 institutions between January 1, 1998, and September 1, 2002. Female sex, advanced age, baseline renal insufficiency (creatinine > 2.0 mg/dL), and total occlusion of the left anterior descending artery were identified as independent predictors of in-hospital mortality.

Although useful, this model does not address patients who were not selected for PCI or the benefit of PCI in patients at different levels of risk. A risk model using data from the SHOCK trial and registry has been developed and allows good discrimination of risk with and without use of early revascularization [56]. Two stages of risk assessment were identified: with and without invasive hemodynamic measurements. The model without invasive hemodynamics includes age, systolic blood pressure, anoxic brain injury, end-organ hypoperfusion, shock on admission, creatinine ≥1.9, prior CABG, and non-inferior location of MI. If EF was available, it replaced non-inferior MI as a marker of risk. In the model that includes invasive hemodynamics, older age, lower LV ejection fraction, anoxic brain damage, end-organ hypoperfusion, and lower stroke work are independent predictors of death. The addition of invasive hemodynamics reduced the number of terms in the model but added only modestly to risk discrimination.

Both of these risk models from the SHOCK trial and registry demonstrated better survival among patients undergoing emergency revascularization regardless of risk category.

## Improvement in survival of cardiogenic shock over time

The outcome of cardiogenic shock seems to have improved slightly during a 23-year period with the greatest improvement in mortality during the 1990s [5]. From 1975 through 1990, the in-hospital mortality from cardiogenic shock averaged 77%, declining to 61% between 1993 and 1995 and further to 59% in 1997. Revascularization was strongly associated with survival [5] in this community-based sample. The SHOCK trial established the usefulness of an aggressive approach to cardiogenic shock patients [47,57]. Emergent coronary revascularization became the standard of care for cardiogenic shock due to pump failure and is highly recommended by American Heart Association and American College of Cardiology guidelines for the treatment of unstable angina and non-ST elevation as well as ST-elevation MI [58,59].

Implementation of the guideline recommendation for emergency revascular-ization in patients with acute MI and shock appears to have caused an additional decline in in-hospital mortality from 60% in 1995 to 48% by 2004 among patients in the US National Registry of Myocardial Infarction [30]. In the last decade, the in-hospital mortality rate in large "real-world" registries is remarkably consistent at 50–60%. In the Global Registry of Acute Coronary Events (GRACE), which enrolled patients between 1999 and 2001, the in-hospital mortality rate for cardiogenic shock patients was 59% [52]. In the Euro Heart Survey of ACS, the in-hospital mortality rate for cardiogenic shock was 52% in a period span-ning 2000–2001 [22]. In-hospital mortality was 59.4% in 1998–2002 in the large database of the ACC-NCDR [48].

### Iatrogenic shock

Medications often used in the early management of ACS, such as beta-blockers, angiotensin converting enzyme inhibitors, and morphine all exert a profound effect on systemic hemodynamics, and thus have been associated with the development of shock (Fig. 1.4) [60–62]. In the Clopidogrel and Metoprolol in Myocardial Infarction Trial (COMMIT) [60], cardiogenic shock was a secondary outcome. Unexpectedly, this mega-trial found no reduction in 30-day, all-cause mortality with the early use of IV followed by oral beta blockers. This was largely due to an increased risk of cardiogenic shock, especially during the first day, which offset a reduction in reinfarction and ventricular fibrillation. Therefore, in patients with high risk for the development of cardiogenic shock, early use of beta-blocking agents is a newly recognized iatrogenic risk factor. Variables that were determined to be independently associated with excess risk of cardiogenic

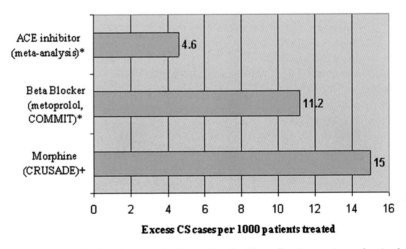

**Fig. 1.4** Excess risk of cardiogenic shock associated with medication use in randomized trials* and registry+.

shock were older age (>70 years), female sex, higher Killip class (>Class I), later time from symptom onset, definite ECG abnormalities, lower blood pressure (<120 mm Hg systolic), higher heart rate (>110 beats per minute), and previous hypertension.

The COMMIT findings demonstrate that early, IV beta blockade is contraindicated in patients with basilar rales or S3 gallop or pulmonary edema (Killip Class II–III). In contrast, it is strongly recommended to initiate low-dose oral beta-blockers prior to discharge with a gradual titration regimen, as used for chronic heart failure patients, for patients with MI and LV dysfunction.

As has been shown previously, medications that are beneficial in the long term after MI may be deleterious in some patients in the short term. A very large meta-analysis of early use of angiotensin-converting enzyme inhibition found an excess of cardiogenic shock of 4.6 patients per 1000 treated. In this study, older age, lower blood pressure, and higher heart rate at presentation were associated with the development of cardiogenic shock [62]. Interestingly, nitrate use was not associated with excess risk of cardiogenic shock in a randomized trial [63]. Given the widespread use of these medications, their potential deleterious effect is significant, and thus these agents should be used vigilantly in patients at risk.

In certain cases, depletion of intravascular volume with diuretics may also contribute to the development of shock (Fig. 1.3). The underlying mechanism entails decreased LV compliance caused by ischemia, and consequent redistribution of intravascular volume into the lungs leading to depletion of systemic intravascular volume. The administration of diuretics in this state may further deplete systemic intravascular volume, resulting in shock. Thus, when pulmonary edema complicates ACS, treatment with low-dose diuretics in conjunction with low-dose nitrate and positioning of the patient is preferable.

Conversely, volume loading may also cause shock in the case of RV infarction. In this clinical setting, the classical teaching is that RV pressure and thus cardiac output is maintained by volume supplementation. In fact, RV diastolic pressure is often high in the course of RV infarction, and excess fluid administration may lead to movement of the interventricular septum into the left ventricle, compromising LV systolic and diastolic function [64]. Invasive measurement or noninvasive estimation of right atrial pressure should be performed in cases of RV infarction with shock; the optimal range in most patients is 10–15 mm Hg, but there is variability among patients and the best range must be identified for the individual patient.

### Long-term outcome

Available data regarding long-term outcome of patients with cardiogenic shock and acute MI show that, by far, the largest mortality risk is in the early period after infarction. In the SHOCK trial population, the 6-year survival rates for hospital survivors was 62.4% versus 44.4% for the early revascularization and initial medical stabilization groups, respectively, with annualized death rates of 8.3% versus 14.3% and, for the 1-year survivors, 8.0% versus 10.7% [65]. Assignment to early revascularization was the only independent predictor of 1-year survival [66]. Singh and colleagues showed that, among patients with cardiogenic shock who survived 30 days after fibrinolytic treatment of STEMI in the GUSTO-I trial, annual mortality rates over the ensuing 15 years were 2% to 4%. These mortality rates approximate those of patients without shock [67]. Furthermore, patients who survive cardiogenic shock usually have good functional status, with up to 80% completely asymptomatic and most in functional class I or II [66].

Therefore, an aggressive approach to diagnosis and early treatment of cardiogenic shock is strongly recommended in all candidates.

# References

1. Hasdai D. *Cardiogenic Shock: Diagnosis and Treatment*. Totowa, NJ: Humana Press, 2002.
2. Herrick JB. Landmark article (*JAMA* 1912). Clinical features of sudden obstruction of the coronary arteries. *JAMA* 1983;250(13):1757–65.
3. Stead EAJ, Ebert RV. Shock syndrome produced by failure of the heart. *Arch Intern Med* 1942;69:369.
4. Goldberg RJ, Gore JM, Alpert JS, et al. Cardiogenic shock after acute myocardial infarction. Incidence and mortality from a community-wide perspective, 1975 to 1988. *N Engl J Med* 1991;325(16):1117–22.
5. Goldberg RJ, Samad NA, Yarzebski J, Gurwitz J, Bigelow C, Gore JM. Temporal trends in cardiogenic shock complicating acute myocardial infarction. *N Engl J Med* 1999;340(15):1162–8.
6. Menon V, White H, LeJemtel T, Webb JG, Sleeper LA, Hochman JS. The clinical profile of patients with suspected cardiogenic shock due to predominant left ventricular failure: a report from the SHOCK Trial Registry. SHould we emergently revascularize Occluded Coronaries in cardiogenic shocK? *J Am Coll Cardiol* 2000;36(3 Suppl A): 1071–6.
7. Menon V, Slater JN, White HD, Sleeper LA, Cocke T, Hochman JS. Acute myocardial infarction complicated by systemic hypoperfusion without hypotension: report of the SHOCK trial registry. *Am J Med* 2000;108(5):374–80.
8. Killip T 3rd, Kimball JT. Treatment of myocardial infarction in a coronary care unit. A two year experience with 250 patients. *Am J Cardiol* 1967;20(4):457-64.
9. Ratshin RA, Rackley CE, Russell RO Jr. Hemodynamic evaluation of left ventricular function in shock complicating myocardial infarction. *Circulation* 1972;45(1):127–39.
10. Valente S, Lazzeri C, Vecchio S, et al. Predictors of in-hospital mortality after percutaneous coronary intervention for cardiogenic shock. *Int J Cardiol* 2007;114(2):176–82.
11. Afifi AA, Chang PC, Liu VY, da Luz PL, Weil MH, Shubin H. Prognostic indexes in acute myocardial infarction complicated by shock. *Am J Cardiol* 1974;33(7):826–32.
12. Hasdai D, Holmes DR Jr, Califf RM, et al. Cardiogenic shock complicating acute myocardial infarction: predictors of death. GUSTO Investigators. Global Utilization of Streptokinase and Tissue-Plasminogen Activator for Occluded Coronary Arteries. *Am Heart J* 1999;138(1 Pt 1):21–31.

13. Swan HJ, Forrester JS, Diamond G, Chatterjee K, Parmley WW. Hemodynamic spectrum of myocardial infarction and cardiogenic shock. A conceptual model. *Circulation* 1972;45(5):1097–110.

14. Fincke R, Hochman JS, Lowe AM, et al. Cardiac power is the strongest hemodynamic correlate of mortality in cardiogenic shock: a report from the SHOCK trial registry. *J Am Coll Cardiol* 2004;44(2):340–8.

15. Antman EM. ST-elevation myocardial infaction: Management. In: Zipes DP, Libby P, Bonow RO, Braunwald E, eds. *Braunwald's Heart Disease A Textbook of Cardiovascular Medicine* (7th Edition). Philadelphia: Elsevier Saunders, 2005:1167–226.

16. Dzavik V, Cotter G, Reynolds HR, et al. Effect of nitric oxide synthase inhibition on haemodynamics and outcome of patients with persistent cardiogenic shock complicating acute myocardial infarction: a phase II dose-ranging study. *Eur Heart J* 2007;28(9):1109–16.

17. Hasdai D, Lev EI, Behar S, et al. Acute coronary syndromes in patients with pre-existing moderate to severe valvular disease of the heart: lessons from the Euro-Heart Survey of acute coronary syndromes. *Eur Heart J* 2003;24(7):623–9.

18. Porter A, Iakobishvili Z, Haim M, et al. Balloon-floating right heart catheter monitoring for acute coronary syndromes complicated by heart failure–discordance between guidelines and reality. *Cardiology* 2005;104(4):186–90.

19. Reynolds HR, Anand SK, Fox JM, et al. Restrictive physiology in cardiogenic shock: observations from echocardiography. *Am Heart J* 2006;151(4):890, e899–15.

20. Fox KA, Steg PG, Eagle KA, et al. Decline in rates of death and heart failure in acute coronary syndromes, 1999-2006. *JAMA* 2007;297(17):1892–900.

21. Hasdai D, Harrington RA, Hochman JS, et al. Platelet glycoprotein IIb/IIIa blockade and outcome of cardiogenic shock complicating acute coronary syndromes without persistent ST-segment elevation. *J Am Coll Cardiol* 2000;36(3):685–92.

22. Iakobishvili Z, Behar S, Boyko V, Battler A, Hasdai D. Does current treatment of cardiogenic shock complicating the acute coronary syndromes comply with guidelines? *Am Heart J* 2005;149(1):98–103.

23. Bhatt DL, Roe MT, Peterson ED, et al. Utilization of early invasive management strategies for high-risk patients with non-ST-segment elevation acute coronary syndromes: results from the CRUSADE Quality Improvement Initiative. *JAMA* 2004;292(17):2096–104.

24. Hochman JS, Buller CE, Sleeper LA, et al. Cardiogenic shock complicating acute myocardial infarction–etiologies, management and outcome: a report from the SHOCK Trial Registry. SHould we emergently revascularize Occluded Coronaries for cardiogenic shocK? *J Am Coll Cardiol* 2000;36(3 Suppl A):1063–70.

25. Leor J, Goldbourt U, Reicher-Reiss H, et al. Cardiogenic shock complicating acute myocardial infarction in patients without heart failure on admission: incidence, risk factors, and outcome. SPRINT Study Group. *Am J Med* 1993;94(3):265–73.

26. Lindholm MG, Kober L, Boesgaard S, Torp-Pedersen C, Aldershvile J. Cardiogenic shock complicating acute myocardial infarction; prognostic impact of early and late shock development. *Eur Heart J* 2003;24(3):258–65.

27. Holmes DR Jr, Bates ER, Kleiman NS, et al. Contemporary reperfusion therapy for cardiogenic shock: the GUSTO-I trial experience. The GUSTO-I Investigators. Global Utilization of Streptokinase and Tissue Plasminogen Activator for Occluded Coronary Arteries. *J Am Coll Cardiol* 1995;26(3):668–74.

28. Holmes DR Jr, Berger PB, Hochman JS, et al. Cardiogenic shock in patients with acute ischemic syndromes with and without ST-segment elevation. *Circulation* 1999;100(20):2067–73.

29. Zeymer U, Vogt A, Zahn R, et al. Predictors of in-hospital mortality in 1333 patients with acute myocardial infarction complicated by cardiogenic shock treated with primary percutaneous coronary intervention (PCI); Results of the primary PCI registry of the Arbeitsgemeinschaft Leitende Kardiologische Krankenhausarzte (ALKK). *Eur Heart J* 2004;25(4):322–8.

30. Babaev A, Frederick PD, Pasta DJ, Every N, Sichrovsky T, Hochman JS. Trends in management and outcomes of patients with acute myocardial infarction complicated by cardiogenic shock. *JAMA* 2005;294(4):448–54.

31. Hasdai D, Behar S, Wallentin L, et al. A prospective survey of the characteristics, treatments and outcomes of patients with acute coronary syndromes in Europe and the Mediterranean basin; the Euro Heart Survey of Acute Coronary Syndromes (Euro Heart Survey ACS). *Eur Heart J* 2002;23(15):1190–201.

32. Brodie BR, Stuckey TD, Hansen C, Bradshaw BH, Downey WE, Pulsipher MW. Comparison of late survival in patients with cardiogenic shock due to right ventricular infarction versus left ventricular pump failure following primary percutaneous coronary intervention for ST-elevation acute myocardial infarction. *Am J Cardiol* 2007;99(4):431-5.

33. Fuchs S, Brosh D, Hasdai D, Teplitsky I, Iakobishvili Z, Rehavia E, Battler A, Kornowski R, Assali A. Predominant right compared to left ventricular involvement in patients with ST elevation myocardial infarction complicated by cardiogenic shock— a contemporary perspective. The 52nd Annual conference of the Israel Heart Society book of abstracts, 2005, p. 35.

34. Barbash IM, Hasdai D, Behar S, et al: Usefulness of pre- versus postadmission cardiogenic shock during acute myocardial infarction in predicting survival. *Am J Cardiol* 2001;87(10):1200–3, A1207.

35. Jeger RV, Harkness SM, Ramanathan K, et al. Emergency revascularization in patients with cardiogenic shock on admission: a report from the SHOCK trial and registry. *Eur Heart J* 2006;27(6):664–70.

36. Hands ME, Rutherford JD, Muller JE, et al. The in-hospital development of cardiogenic shock after myocardial infarction: incidence, predictors of occurrence, outcome and prognostic factors. The MILIS Study Group. *J Am Coll Cardiol* 1989;14(1):40–6, discussion 47–8.

37. A comparison of recombinant hirudin with heparin for the treatment of acute coronary syndromes. The Global Use of Strategies to Open Occluded Coronary Arteries (GUSTO) IIb investigators. *N Engl J Med* 1996;335(11):775–82.

38. Jacobs AK, French JK, Col J, et al. Cardiogenic shock with non-ST-segment elevation myocardial infarction: a report from the SHOCK Trial Registry. SHould we emergently revascularize Occluded coronaries for Cardiogenic shocK? *J Am Coll Cardiol* 2000;36 (3 Suppl A):1091–6.

39. Hasdai D, Califf RM, Thompson TD, et al. Predictors of cardiogenic shock after thrombolytic therapy for acute myocardial infarction. *J Am Coll Cardiol* 2000;35(1): 136–43.

40. Hathaway WR, Peterson ED, Wagner GS, et al. Prognostic significance of the initial electrocardiogram in patients with acute myocardial infarction. GUSTO-I

Investigators. Global Utilization of Streptokinase and t-PA for Occluded Coronary Arteries. *JAMA* 1998;279(5):387–91.

41. Sgarbossa EB, Pinski SL, Topol EJ, et al. Acute myocardial infarction and complete bundle branch block at hospital admission: clinical characteristics and outcome in the thrombolytic era. GUSTO-I Investigators. Global Utilization of Streptokinase and t-PA [tissue-type plasminogen activator] for Occluded Coronary Arteries. *J Am Coll Cardiol* 1998;31(1):105–10.

42. Zeller M, Cottin Y, Brindisi MC, et al. Impaired fasting glucose and cardiogenic shock in patients with acute myocardial infarction. *Eur Heart J* 2004;25(4):308–12.

43. Wong SC, Sleeper LA, Monrad ES, et al. Absence of gender differences in clinical outcomes in patients with cardiogenic shock complicating acute myocardial infarction. A report from the SHOCK Trial Registry. *J Am Coll Cardiol* 2001;38(5): 1395–401.

44. Nishimura RA, Schaff HV, Gersh BJ, Holmes DR Jr, Tajik AJ. Early repair of mechanical complications after acute myocardial infarction. *JAMA* 1986;256(1):47–50.

45. Canovas SJ, Lim E, Dalmau MJ, et al. Midterm clinical and echocardiographic results with patch glue repair of left ventricular free wall rupture. *Circulation* 2003;108 (Suppl 1):II237–40.

46. Jacobs AK, Leopold JA, Bates E, et al. Cardiogenic shock caused by right ventricular infarction: a report from the SHOCK registry. *J Am Coll Cardiol* 2003;41(8):1273–9.

47. Hochman JS, Sleeper LA, Webb JG, et al. Early revascularization in acute myocardial infarction complicated by cardiogenic shock. SHOCK Investigators. Should We Emergently Revascularize Occluded Coronaries for Cardiogenic Shock. *N Engl J Med* 1999;341(9):625–34.

48. Klein LW, Shaw RE, Krone RJ, et al. Mortality after emergent percutaneous coronary intervention in cardiogenic shock secondary to acute myocardial infarction and usefulness of a mortality prediction model. *Am J Cardiol* 2005;96(1):35–41.

49. Palmeri ST, Lowe AM, Sleeper LA, Saucedo JF, Desvigne-Nickens P, Hochman JS. Racial and ethnic differences in the treatment and outcome of cardiogenic shock following acute myocardial infarction. *Am J Cardiol* 2005;96(8):1042–9.

50. Ortolani P, Marzocchi A, Marrozzini C, et al. Clinical comparison of "normal-hours" vs "off-hours" percutaneous coronary interventions for ST-elevation myocardial infarction. *Am Heart J* 2007;154(2):366–72.

51. Antoniucci D, Migliorini A, Moschi G, et al. Does gender affect the clinical outcome of patients with acute myocardial infarction complicated by cardiogenic shock who undergo percutaneous coronary intervention? *Catheter Cardiovasc Interv* 2003;59(4):423–8.

52. Dauerman HL, Goldberg RJ, White K, et al. Revascularization, stenting, and outcomes of patients with acute myocardial infarction complicated by cardiogenic shock. *Am J Cardiol* 2002;90(8):838–42.

53. Shindler DM, Palmeri ST, Antonelli TA, et al. Diabetes mellitus in cardiogenic shock complicating acute myocardial infarction: a report from the SHOCK Trial Registry. SHould we emergently revascularize Occluded Coronaries for cardiogenic shocK? *J Am Coll Cardiol* 2000;36(3 Suppl A):1097–103.

54. Sanborn TA, Sleeper LA, Webb JG, et al. Correlates of one-year survival inpatients with cardiogenic shock complicating acute myocardial infarction: angiographic findings from the SHOCK trial. *J Am Coll Cardiol* 2003;42(8):1373–9.

55. Picard MH, Davidoff R, Sleeper LA, et al. Echocardiographic predictors of survival and response to early revascularization in cardiogenic shock. *Circulation* 2003;107(2):279–84.

56. Sleeper LA, Jacobs AK, LeJemtel TH, Webb JG, Hochman JS. A mortality model and severity scoring system for cardiogenic shock complicating acute myocardial infarction. *Circulation* 2000;102(18):3840, II-3795.

57. Hochman JS, Sleeper LA, White HD, et al. One-year survival following early revascularization for cardiogenic shock. *JAMA* 2001;285(2):190–2.

58. Anderson JL, Adams CD, Antman EM, et al. ACC/AHA 2007 guidelines for the management of patients with unstable angina/non ST-elevation myocardial infarction: a report of the American College of Cardiology/American Heart Association Task Force on Practice Guidelines (Writing Committee to Revise the 2002 Guidelines for the Management of Patients With Unstable Angina/Non ST-Elevation Myocardial Infarction): developed in collaboration with the American College of Emergency Physicians, the Society for Cardiovascular Angiography and Interventions, and the Society of Thoracic Surgeons: endorsed by the American Association of Cardiovascular and Pulmonary Rehabilitation and the Society for Academic Emergency Medicine. *Circulation* 2007;116(7):e148–304.

59. Antman EM, Anbe DT, Armstrong PW, et al. ACC/AHA guidelines for the management of patients with ST-elevation myocardial infarction–executive summary: a report of the American College of Cardiology/American Heart Association Task Force on Practice Guidelines (Writing Committee to Revise the 1999 Guidelines for the Management of Patients With Acute Myocardial Infarction). *Circulation* 2004;110(5):588–636.

60. Chen ZM, Pan HC, Chen YP, et al. Early intravenous then oral metoprolol in 45,852 patients with acute myocardial infarction: randomised placebo-controlled trial. *Lancet* 2005;366(9497):1622–32.

61. Meine TJ, Roe MT, Chen AY, et al. Association of intravenous morphine use and outcomes in acute coronary syndromes: results from the CRUSADE Quality Improvement Initiative. *Am Heart J* 2005;149(6):1043–9.

62. ACE-IMICG. Indications for ACE inhibitors in the early treatment of acute myocardial infarction: systematic overview of individual data from 100,000 patients in randomized trials. ACE Inhibitor Myocardial Infarction Collaborative Group. *Circulation* 1998;97(22):2202–12.

63. ISIS-4: a randomised factorial trial assessing early oral captopril, oral mononitrate, and intravenous magnesium sulphate in 58,050 patients with suspected acute myocardial infarction. ISIS-4 (Fourth International Study of Infarct Survival) Collaborative Group. *Lancet* 1995;345(8951):669–85.

64. Brookes C, Ravn H, White P, Moeldrup U, Oldershaw P, Redington A. Acute right ventricular dilatation in response to ischemia significantly impairs left ventricular systolic performance. *Circulation* 1999;100(7):761–7.

65. Hochman JS, Sleeper LA, Webb JG, et al. Early revascularization and long-term survival in cardiogenic shock complicating acute myocardial infarction. *JAMA* 2006;295(21):2511–5.

66. Sleeper LA, Ramanathan K, Picard MH, et al. Functional status and quality of life after emergency revascularization for cardiogenic shock complicating acute myocardial infarction. *J Am Coll Cardiol* 2005;46(2):266–73.

67. Singh M, White J, Hasdai D, et al. Long-term outcome and its predictors among patients with ST-segment elevation myocardial infarction complicated by shock: insights from the GUSTO-I trial. *J Am Coll Cardiol* 2007;50(18):1752–8.
68. Hasdai D, Holmes DR Jr, Topol EJ, et al. Frequency and clinical outcome of cardiogenic shock during acute myocardial infarction among patients receiving reteplase or alteplase. Results from GUSTO-III. Global Use of Strategies to Open Occluded Coronary Arteries. *Eur Heart J* 1999;20(2):128–35.
69. Reynolds HR, Hochman JS. Cardiogenic shock: current concepts and improving outcomes. *Circulation* 2008;117(5):686–97.
70. Hochman JS, Ingbar D. Cardiogenic shock and pulmonary edema. In: Wiener CM, ed. *Harrison's Principles of Internal Medicine* (17th Edition). New York: McGraw-Hill, 2008:1702–7.

# Chapter 2

# Pathophysiology

Steven M. Hollenberg

## Introduction

The predominant cause of cardiogenic shock is left ventricular (LV) failure in the setting of acute myocardial infarction [1]. Cardiogenic shock usually results from an extensive acute infarction, although a smaller infarction in a patient with previously compromised LV function may also precipitate shock. Cardiogenic shock can also be caused by mechanical complications of infarction, such as acute mitral regurgitation, rupture of the interventricular septum, rupture of the free wall, or by large right ventricular (RV) infarctions. The distribution of causes of cardiogenic shock complicating acute myocardial infarction in the prospective SHOCK trial registry [1] is shown in Fig. 2.1. LV failure accounted for 79% of cases, with mechanical causes comprising 12% and isolated RV infarction comprising 3%. Causes such as coexistent severe valvular heart disease, excess dosing of beta-blocker or calcium channel blocker therapy, severe dilated cardiomyopathy, recent hemorrhage, or cardiac catheterization laboratory complications accounted for the remaining 7% [1]. Other important etiologies of cardiogenic shock include end-stage cardiomyopathy, prolonged cardiopulmonary bypass, valvular disease, myocardial contusion, sepsis with unusually profound myocardial depression, fulminant myocarditis, and apical ballooning [1,2]. Concurrent conditions, such as hemorrhage or infection, may also contribute to shock.

Regardless of the initiating cause, the primary inciting factor in cardiogenic shock is the heart's inability to deliver cardiac output sufficient to maintain adequate perfusion. Accordingly, this chapter will start with consideration of systemic hemodynamic abnormalities in cardiogenic shock, with an emphasis

*Cardiogenic Shock.* Edited by Judith S. Hochman and E. Magnus Ohman.
© 2009 American Heart Association, ISBN: 978-1-4051-7926-3

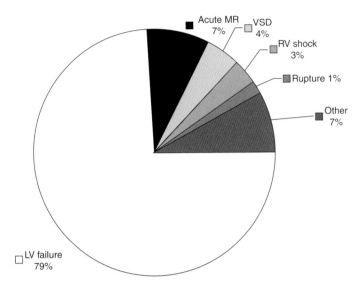

**Fig. 2.1** Causes of cardiogenic shock in patients with myocardial infarction in the SHOCK registry ($N = 1190$) and trial cohort ($N = 232$ enrolled concurrently to the registry). (Adapted from Hochman, et al. *J Am Coll Cardiol* 2000;36:1063–1070). Six patients fell into more than 1 category. Abbreviations: LV, left ventricular; RV, right ventricular; MR, mitral regurgitation; VSD, ventricular septal defect. (Total percentage is slightly more than 100% due to rounding off.)

on how those abnormalities may initiate a self-sustaining vicious cycle in which myocardial dysfunction begets ischemia, which further worsens myocardial dysfunction. We will also consider the vascular consequences of abnormal hemodynamics in shock, which include adaptive mechanisms that cause vasoconstriction in an attempt to maintain blood pressure, mechanisms that may increase afterload, and, conversely, situations in which abnormal vasodilation contributes to hypotension in cardiogenic shock.

We will then discuss myocardial pathology, including mechanisms of expansion of myocardial infarction, consequences of remote ischemia, diastolic abnormalities, and the contribution of valvular dysfunction. We will also consider cellular pathophysiology in cardiogenic shock. Finally, mechanisms of reversible myocardial dysfunction will be discussed, since the potential for reversibility provides the rationale for both reperfusion and supportive therapies in cardiogenic shock.

## Systemic effects

### Classic paradigm

Cardiac dysfunction in patients with cardiogenic shock is usually initiated by an extensive myocardial infarction, although a smaller infarction in a patient with

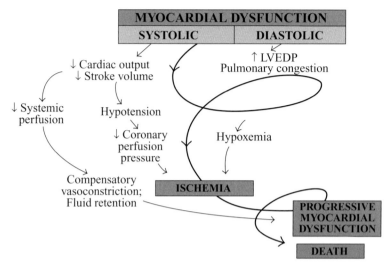

**Fig. 2.2** The "downward spiral" in cardiogenic shock. Stroke volume and cardiac output fall with LV dysfunction, producing hypotension and tachycardia that reduce coronary blood flow. Increasing ventricular diastolic pressure reduces coronary blood flow, and increased wall stress elevates myocardial oxygen requirements. All of these factors combine to worsen ischemia. The falling cardiac output also compromises systemic perfusion. Compensatory mechanisms include sympathetic stimulation and fluid retention to increase preload. These mechanisms can actually worsen cardiogenic shock by increasing myocardial oxygen demand and afterload. Thus, a vicious cycle can be established. Abbreviations: LVEDP, left ventricular end diastolic pressure. (Reprinted with permission from Hollenberg et al, *Ann Intern Med* 1999;31:47–59.)

previously compromised LV function may also precipitate shock. Myocardial dysfunction resulting from ischemia worsens that ischemia, creating a downward spiral (Fig. 2.2) [2]. When a critical mass of LV myocardium becomes ischemic or necrotic and fails to pump, stroke volume and cardiac output decrease. Myocardial perfusion, which depends on the pressure gradient between the coronary arterial system and the left ventricle, and on the duration of diastole, is compromised by hypotension and tachycardia, thereby exacerbating ischemia. The increased ventricular diastolic pressures caused by pump failure further reduce coronary perfusion pressure, and the additional wall stress elevates myocardial oxygen requirements, further worsening ischemia.

LV dysfunction increases left atrial (LA) pressure, and ischemia increases diastolic stiffness, increasing LA pressure. This in turn may result in pulmonary congestion and consequent hypoxia, which can exacerbate myocardial ischemia as well as impair RV performance. Fluid retention and impaired diastolic filling caused by tachycardia and ischemia may result in pulmonary congestion and hypoxia.

When myocardial function is depressed, several compensatory mechanisms designed to increase cardiac output are activated, including sympathetic stimulation to increase heart rate and contractility and activation of the renin/angiotensin/aldosterone system, which leads to renal fluid retention and increased preload. These compensatory mechanisms may become maladaptive and can actually worsen the situation when cardiogenic shock develops. Increased heart rate and contractility increase myocardial oxygen demand and exacerbate ischemia. Natriuretic peptides are also released in response to increases in wall stress [3]. These molecules have vasodilatory effects, although the extent to which they offset vasoconstrictive influences in the setting of cardiogenic shock is uncertain.

The vascular response to impaired cardiac output is vasoconstriction to maintain systemic blood pressure and coronary perfusion pressure. However, this increases myocardial afterload and may further impair cardiac performance and increase myocardial oxygen demand. This increased demand, in the face of inadequate perfusion, worsens ischemia and begins a vicious cycle that may end in death if not interrupted (Fig. 2.2); the interruption of this cycle of myocardial dysfunction and ischemia forms the basis of therapeutic regimens for cardiogenic shock. Impaired systemic perfusion can also lead to lactic acidosis, which further compromises systolic performance.

### Effects of inflammation on hemodynamics

Recent data suggest that not all patients fit into this classic paradigm. In the SHOCK trial, the average systemic vascular resistance (SVR) was not elevated and the range of values was wide, suggesting that compensatory vasoconstriction is not universal. Supporting this notion is the fact that the mean ejection fraction in the SHOCK trial was only moderately decreased (30%), indicating that mechanisms other than pump failure were at work [4,5]. In the SHOCK trial, some patients had fever and elevated white blood cell counts along with decreased SVR, suggesting a systemic inflammatory response syndrome [6]. This has led to an expansion of the classic paradigm to include the possibility that inflammatory responses contribute to vasodilation and myocardial dysfunction, leading clinically to persistence of shock (Fig. 2.3) [7].

The heart releases cytokines after myocardial infarction [8], which can activate inducible nitric oxide synthase (iNOS), leading to vasodilation and worsening hypotension [9]. High levels of nitric oxide resulting from iNOS expression are associated with LV dysfunction [10]. Under the right conditions, nitric oxide can also combine with superoxide to form peroxynitrite, a toxic radical that can impair myocardial contractility [11]. Recent findings suggest that nitric oxide synthase and arginase may be elevated in cardiogenic shock and that levels of endogenous nitric oxide inhibitors correlate with hemodynamic dysfunction and excess mortality [12].

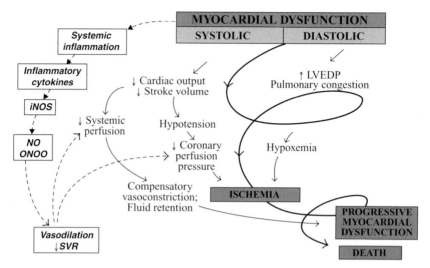

**Fig. 2.3** Expansion of the pathophysiologic paradigm of cardiogenic shock to include the potential contribution of inflammatory mediators. Abbreviations: LVEDP, left ventricular end diastolic pressure; NO, nitric oxide; iNOS, inducible nitric oxide synthase; ONOO⁻, peroxynitrite; SVR, systemic vascular resistance. (Reprinted with permission from Hochman, *Circulation* 2003;107:2998–3003.)

Circulating inflammatory mediators, including interleukin-6 (IL-6) and tumor necrosis factor, are also increased in cardiogenic shock, and IL-6 levels correlate with organ failure and excess mortality [13]. Interestingly, inflammatory mediators may cause BNP release [3] and so elevated BNP levels in cardiogenic shock may be markers not only of hemodynamic decompensation but also of the degree of inflammation. These immune-activated mechanisms that result in inappropriate vasodilation and myocardial dysfunction appear to be common to a number of different forms of shock [3,14].

In addition to abnormalities in the macrocirculation, there may be microcirculatory abnormalities as well. Orthogonal polarization spectral imaging, a technique that allows direct observation of microcirculatory flow, has been used to demonstrate decreased small-vessel perfusion in the sublingual circulation in patients with cardiogenic shock [15]. Both the proportion of vessels with absent flow and the proportion of vessels with intermittent flow were increased in shock. The perturbations in microvascular flow seen in patients with cardiogenic shock are qualitatively and quantitatively similar to those observed in patients with septic shock [16,17]. Inflammatory cascades activated in both septic and cardiogenic shock may have similar effects on the microcirculation, potentially mediated by the effects of iNOS, oxidative stress, and peroxynitrite described above. Microcirculatory abnormalities, particularly those leading to regional heterogeneity in blood flow, play an important role in the pathogenesis of organ failure.

## Myocardial pathology

Acute myocardial infarction is a dynamic process that evolves over hours. There is a central zone of infarction, surrounded by a border zone of jeopardized ischemic myocardium that may be salvageable by reperfusion. If reperfusion is not established, a "wavefront" of necrosis proceeds outward from the central core [18]. The amount of myocardial necrosis is an important predictor of the propensity to develop cardiogenic shock. An autopsy study reported by Page and colleagues of 34 patients dying after myocardial infarction found that, of the 20 patients who had cardiogenic shock, 19 had necrosis of 40% or more of the LV mass, whereas 13 of the 14 patients who died without shock had infarctions less than 35% of LV mass [19]. Similar findings were reported by Alonso and colleagues, with an average of 51% of the LV necrosed in patients dying with cardiogenic shock, compared with 23% average necrosis in patients dying suddenly with arrhythmias [20]. These studies led to the concept that pump failure ensues after a critical mass of LV myocardium is lost.

Loss of myocardium is not necessarily confined to the initial infarction period, however. Progressive myocardial necrosis has been frequently observed in clinical and pathologic studies of patients with cardiogenic shock [19,21]. This is consistent with epidemiologic observations that indicate that the majority of hospital patients develop shock over a period of hours to days after initial presentation [1,22]. Patients who develop shock after admission often have evidence of infarct extension, which represents additional myocardial necrosis after the initial insult. Infarct extension can result from reocclusion of a transiently patent infarct artery, propagation of intracoronary thrombus, or a combination of decreased coronary perfusion pressure and increased myocardial oxygen demand [23,24]. Myocytes at the border zone of an infarction are more susceptible to additional ischemic episodes; therefore, these adjacent segments are at particular risk [25]. This marginal extension has been termed "piecemeal necrosis" and appears pathologically as foci of necrosis more recent than the original infarction [26]. Reinfarction is not only a cause of cardiogenic shock, but is also associated with high mortality; in one series almost one-fourth of patients with early reinfarction after fibrinolytic therapy developed cardiogenic shock [27].

Infarct expansion is conceptually distinct and refers to expansion and thinning of the infarct area in the first hours to days of acute myocardial infarction as myocytes slip past each other. Infarct expansion is an early form of pathologic remodeling that can distort both regional and global ventricular geometry and lead to increased wall stress [26]. Infarct expansion causes enlargement of the left ventricle, which initially serves as a compensatory mechanism to maintain stroke volume. However, this increases wall stress, which in turn imposes additional mechanical strain on myocytes, potentially causing further slippage. Infarct expansion is seen most dramatically after extensive anterior myocardial infarction and is often an important contributor to late development of cardiogenic shock [24,26]. Despite the conceptual distinction between infarct expansion and infarct extension, there is a gray area in which infarcts may enlarge by a combination of both mechanisms. Localized increases in wall stress resulting from infarct expansion can increase oxygen demand and compromise viability of marginally perfused myocytes in border zones. In addition, regional increases in wall stress can active matrix metalloproteases, contributing to thinning and stretching of the infarct area, and can also lead to nonischemic infarct extension by inducing myocyte apoptosis in border areas [28].

## Remote ischemia
Pump failure in cardiogenic shock need not result only from infarcted myocardium; myocardial ischemia can contribute significantly to systolic dysfunction. Ischemia remote from the infarct zone may be particularly important in this respect [29,30]. Patients with cardiogenic shock usually have multivessel coronary artery disease [1,21], with limited vasodilator reserve, impaired autoregulation, and consequent pressure-dependent coronary flow in several perfusion territories [31]. Hypotension can thus limit coronary perfusion pressure, thereby impairing the contractility of noninfarcted myocardium in patients with shock [32]. In addition, secondary effects of hypoperfusion, such as hypoxia, acidosis, and metabolic derangements, can further impair contractility of uninfarcted muscle. This can limit hyperkinesis of uninvolved segments, an important compensatory mechanism typically seen early after myocardial infarction [29,30].

## Diastolic function
Myocardial diastolic function is also impaired in patients with cardiogenic shock. Myocardial ischemia decreases compliance, increasing LV filling pressure at a given end-diastolic volume [33]. Greater LV diastolic pressures increase myocardial oxygen demand and decrease coronary perfusion pressure, further exacerbating ischemia and ventricular dysfunction. Elevation of LV pressures can lead to pulmonary edema and hypoxemia (Fig. 2.2).

## Valvular abnormalities
In addition to abnormalities in myocardial performance, valvular abnormalities, particularly mitral regurgitation, can contribute to increased pulmonary congestion (see Chapter 7). Rupture of a papillary muscle or adjacent chordae tendinae, through release of metalloproteases, is a mechanical complication of myocardial infarction that is well known to precipitate cardiogenic shock. Its presentation is dramatic, with rapid onset of pulmonary edema and shock. Papillary muscle rupture, however, is relatively uncommon. A much more common and

more important contributor to myocardial dysfunction is ischemic mitral regurgitation.

The classic view of ischemic mitral regurgitation is that it results from dysfunction of the papillary muscles. This view has been challenged by animal experiments demonstrating that inducing papillary muscle dysfunction does not cause either prolapse of the mitral valve leaflets or mitral regurgitation [34]; mitral regurgitation occurred in this model only when global LV dysfunction with ventricular dilation was present [34]. Ischemic mitral regurgitation appears to result primarily from changes in LV geometry that cause displacement of the papillary muscles so that they no longer effectively close the mitral valve in systole [35]. As such, ischemic mitral regurgitation is a dynamic process and may change over time, which has implications for its correction [35]. With respect to the development of cardiogenic shock, postinfarction remodeling may cause ischemic mitral regurgitation, precipitating the development of shock and/or contributing to its severity.

# Cellular pathology

## Myocardial energy metabolism

The heart normally extracts virtually all of the oxygen supplied by coronary flow; thus, its ability to compensate for decreases in flow by increasing oxygen extraction is extremely limited. Under normal aerobic conditions, cardiac metabolism of fatty acids supplies 60–90% of the energy required for the synthesis of adenosine triphosphate (ATP); the rest comes from oxidation of pyruvate formed by glycolysis. Approximately two-thirds of ATP used by the heart goes to contractile shortening; the remaining one-third is used by sarcolemmal, sarcoplasmic reticulum, and mitochondrial ion pumps [36]. With sudden occlusion of a major branch of a coronary artery, oxidative phosphorylation in mitochondria is shut off, and ATP formation is consequently reduced. Myocardial metabolism shifts from aerobic to anaerobic glycolysis within seconds, and the reduced aerobic ATP formation stimulates an increase in myocardial glucose uptake and glycogen breakdown. During ischemic conditions, there is production of lactate from pyruvate, which leads to a rise in tissue lactate and $H^+$, resulting in lower intracellular pH and a reduction in contractile function [36].

## Cellular ion pumps

With prolonged myocardial cellular hypoxia, ATP and intracellular energy reserves are depleted, and active energy-dependent ion transport pumps eventually fail. Cellular homeostasis is ordinarily maintained by active cation pumps (most prominently sodium ATPase, calcium ATPase, sodium–potassium ATPase, sodium–calcium ATPase, and sodium–hydrogen ATPase) that counterbalance flow along electrochemical gradients. In the absence of active pump fluxes, transmembrane movements of sodium, calcium, potassium, and hydrogen are determined by these electrochemical gradients [37]. Sodium flows down its concentration gradient into the cell, and the resulting increase in cellular osmolarity brings water with it by osmosis. Calcium, chloride, and hydrogen leak inward as well, whereas potassium and magnesium leak out [38].

## Myocyte necrosis

Increased cellular osmolarity causes microscopically identifiable swelling of the cytoplasmic space and cellular organelles, as well as formation of plasma membrane blebs. If inward sodium leakage continues unabated, the swollen myocytes develop holes and ultimately rupture, eliciting an inflammatory response. This process is most commonly referred to as *necrosis*, although *oncosis* is a more precise term [38].

Failure of cellular energy metabolism can also lead to activation of intracellular lysosomes, organelles involved in the cellular digestive machinery. Lysosomes contain acid phosphatases, which are normally latent because lysosomal pH is tightly regulated by energy-dependent proton pumps [38]. When ATP is depleted, failure of both the lysosomal and sarcoplasmic ion pumps can lead to acidosis with activation of acid hydrolases in the lysosomes, including proteases, phospholipases, glucosidases, and endonucleases [38]. Failure of calcium pumps with consequently increased intracellular calcium also increases activity of calcium-dependent enzymes, including proteases, phospholipase $A_2$, and endonucleases. Accumulation of hydrolytic products, such as amino acids, free fatty acids, and other metabolites, within lysosomes creates an osmotic load that can lead to swelling and eventually to rupture. When lysosomes rupture, proteases and other enzymes are released into the cytosol. These proteases can degrade histones in the nucleosomes and thus render unprotected DNA susceptible to cleavage by endonucleases. The process of pathological autodigestion can spread throughout the cell, with devastating consequences [37].

Thus, the classic pathological signature of necrotic cell death includes mitochondrial swelling, accumulation of denatured proteins and chromatin in the cytoplasm, lysosomal breakdown, and fracture of the mitochondria, nuclear envelope, and plasma membrane [37]. Contraction bands in cardiac myofibrils are also usually observed.

## Apoptosis

Accumulating evidence indicates that apoptosis (programmed cell death) may also contribute to myocyte loss in myocardial infarction [25,39]. Although myonecrosis clearly outweighs apoptosis in the core of an infarcted area, evidence for apoptosis has been found consistently in the border zone of infarcts after ischemia and reperfusion and sporadically in areas remote from the ischemia area [25,39].

Apoptosis, a term derived from a Greek word that describes the falling of petals from a flower, is a mode of cell death distinct from necrosis. Whereas necrosis is characterized by swelling of the cell and mitochondria, loss of membrane integrity, and an intense subsequent inflammatory process, apoptosis is associated with shrinkage of the cell, little or no swelling of mitochondria, and an initially intact membrane. Apoptotic cells are engulfed by phagocytes with only a minimal inflammatory response. Apoptosis is mediated by activation of a unique class of aspartate-specific proteases termed caspases, and, importantly, is energy-dependent. Apoptosis can be initiated either through an external pathway involving stimulation of cell surface death receptors or by an internal pathway initiated by mitochondrial repolarization [40].

There are a number of potential triggers of apoptosis, but the ones most likely to be operative in border zones of acutely infarcting myocardium are oxidative stress in the setting of ischemia/reperfusion, stretching of myocytes, and activation of inflammatory cascades [39]. During ischemia and reperfusion, reactive oxygen species, increased calcium levels, and free fatty acids present in the cytoplasm decrease the mitochondrial transmembrane potential. This change in membrane potential can lead to release of cytochrome C into the cytoplasm, which activates caspases and can initiate apoptosis. In addition, once a critical drop in mitochondrial transmembrane potential has occurred, large channels called mitochondrial permeability transition pores are formed, fully dissipating the transmembrane gradient and thus uncoupling electron transport from ATP synthesis. Formation of these pores is considered a "point of no return," after which cell death is inevitable [39].

Although there has been debate about the relative magnitude of necrotic and apoptotic cell loss in myocardial infarction, and concerns about technical aspects of distinguishing the two in this setting, data suggest that approximately 10% of cells in the border zone are apoptotic [25]. Because apoptosis requires energy, it would not be expected in the central anoxic zone but rather along the tenuously perfused border zones. Myocyte stretching due to acute remodeling as described above, in addition to ischemia, may also stimulate apoptosis. In addition, reperfusion is clearly desirable in order to limit the area of necrosis, but its benefits may be attenuated by ischemia–reperfusion-induced apoptosis in border zones, extending the area of infarction. The time course of apoptotic cell death after infarction is very difficult to determine, but some data suggest that apoptosis begins within hours of an acute insult, with the result that apoptosis could potentially contribute to clinical deterioration with development of cardiogenic shock after acute infarction [25]. Ongoing apoptosis could also be an important factor in late remodeling after acute infarction as well.

What is most important about the notion that apoptotic cell death contributes to myocyte loss in acute infarction, however, is that apoptosis is a potential therapeutic target. Inhibitors of apoptosis have been found to attenuate myocardial injury in animal models of postischemic reperfusion [40]. Such inhibitors may also have therapeutic potential for myocyte salvage after large infarctions, but both a deeper understanding of the magnitude and mechanisms of apoptosis after infarction as well as appropriate clinical trials will be needed [39].

## Reversible myocardial dysfunction

A key to understanding the pathophysiology and treatment of cardiogenic shock is the realization that areas of myocardium can be nonfunctional, yet viable, and can contribute importantly to the development of cardiogenic shock after myocardial infarction. This reversible dysfunction is usually described as resulting from one of two phenomena (stunning and hibernation), but recent findings have blurred their distinction considerably.

### Myocardial stunning

Myocardial stunning is postischemic dysfunction that persists despite restoration of normal blood flow. Because normally perfused myocardium is viable, myocardial performance is expected to recover completely [41]. Myocardial stunning was originally defined in canine models, in which 15 minutes of ischemia followed by reperfusion led to prolonged contractile dysfunction that required hours or even days for full return of function [42]. Stunning can also be observed after more prolonged periods of ischemia. Documentation of stunning in clinical practice is challenging because it is necessary to demonstrate depressed but reversible regional dysfunction in an area with normal or near-normal blood flow. Stunning is more commonly inferred from a delay in improvement in myocardial performance after revascularization [43]. Stunning has been invoked in a number of clinical situations, including after stress testing in patients with severe coronary artery disease, in which some patients can be shown to have persistent wall motion abnormalities, and after cardiopulmonary bypass [41,43]. Bolli and colleagues studied post-bypass stunning by leaving an ultrasonic probe on the epicardial surface for 2–3 days in 31 patients following bypass surgery; LV wall thickening fell after surgery, reached a nadir at 2–6 hours, and subsequently improved, usually returning to baseline by 24–48 hours [44]. Direct evidence for myocardial stunning in humans has been obtained by demonstrating normal perfusion using positron emission tomography (PET) scanning with $^{13}$N-ammonia to measure myocardial blood flow in patients with persistent wall motion abnormalities demonstrated by echocardiography following angioplasty for unstable angina [45]. Myocardial stunning in cardiogenic shock might result from global ischemia during cardiac arrest or following restoration of coronary blood flow by revascularization after total occlusion in acute infarction.

The pathogenesis of stunning has not been established conclusively but is likely a multifactorial process involving a number of cellular perturbations and the interaction of several pathogenetic mechanisms. Early experiments in animal models employing 15-minute coronary occlusions indicated that oxygen-derived free radicals, particularly hydroxyl ($\bullet$OH), but also superoxide ($\bullet O_2^-$), hydrogen peroxide ($H_2O_2$), and potentially peroxynitrite ($ONOO^-$), are liberated during the first few minutes of reperfusion, indicating that stunning is at least in part a form of reperfusion injury [42,46]. Free radical scavengers are protective, but only when given very early (within 1 minute of initiation of reperfusion in some models); even then, protection is not complete [41]. This suggests that some of the derangements that produce stunning occur during ischemia rather than after reperfusion and that other mechanisms are involved as well. Data from isolated cardiac myocytes suggest that circulating myocardial depressant substances may contribute to contractile dysfunction in myocardial stunning [47].

Another line of investigation has implicated perturbation of calcium homeostasis in myocardial stunning. Reperfusion can lead to cellular calcium overload. During ischemia, energy depletion impairs outward sodium pumps and intracellular sodium increases, but sodium–calcium exchange is inhibited by concomitant acidosis. With reperfusion, the acidosis reverses more quickly than the sodium overload, and the reactivated sodium–calcium exchange causes transient calcium overload [48]; reactive oxygen species may contribute to calcium overload as well [49]. Such overload can activate calcium-dependent proteases, termed calpains.

Although calcium transients are normal in stunned myocardial cells, responsiveness of the contractile apparatus to calcium is decreased. Evidence suggests that calcium responsiveness is decreased by degradation of myofilaments by proteases [50]. This notion is an attractive explanation of the transient nature of myocardial dysfunction in stunning, as slow recovery would occur with resynthesis of new myofilaments [49].

The free radical and calcium hypotheses are not mutually exclusive. Free radical generation, calcium overload, and decreased myofilament calcium responsiveness may well be different facets of the pathogenesis of stunning. Stunned myocardium retains contractile reserve and will respond to inotropic stimulation.

## Reperfusion injury

Myocardial reperfusion is required for survival of ischemic myocardium, but reperfusion may itself lead to additional myocardial injury beyond that generated by ischemia alone. The clinical manifestations of ischemia–reperfusion can include myocardial stunning as described above, but may also encompass endothelial dysfunction, microvascular injury, and the no-reflow phenomenon.

Coronary endothelial dysfunction after ischemia and reperfusion has been demonstrated in animal models [51] and also in clinical settings, such as following cardiac transplantation [52]. This dysfunction is characterized not only by alterations of vasomotor tone, with a loss of vasodilatory responses and an increased production of vasoconstrictors, but also by activation of platelets and neutrophils, both of which can promote inflammation as well as generation of a prothrombotic phenotype. Activated neutrophils release cytotoxic and chemotactic substances, such as cytokines, proteases, leukotrienes, and free radicals.

Microvascular dysfunction after ischemia/reperfusion results from a combination of endothelial dysfunction, microvascular obstruction, edema, and oxidative stress. Microvascular obstruction may occur because of embolization of platelets downstream, either spontaneously or following percutaneous intervention, formation of in situ thrombus in small vessels, plugging of capillaries by neutrophils or swollen injured endothelial cells, or, more likely, a combination of these mechanisms. Activated neutrophils release oxygen free radicals, proteases, and other inflammatory mediators that further amplify infiltration of neutrophils into jeopardized areas of myocardium [53]. Activated platelets release vasoconstrictive substances that can exacerbate microcirculatory spasm and can also recruit and activate neutrophils [53]. Microcirculatory edema may occur simply as a consequence of ischemia, with failure of ion pumps and osmotic stress, but may also be worsened by inflammatory mediators.

When microvascular dysfunction is sufficiently severe, microcirculatory perfusion is compromised despite adequate coronary artery revascularization, a phenomenon termed "no-reflow." No-reflow has been detected by nuclear scintigraphy, myocardial contrast echocardiography, magnetic resonance imaging, and PET [51,53,54] and is associated with incomplete resolution of ST elevation, increased troponin release, and adverse clinical outcomes, including a higher risk of death or myocardial reinfarction [54]. No-reflow may also predispose patients to late complications, such as septal or free wall rupture [51].

How best to treat patients with no-reflow remains uncertain. Nitroglycerin is often ineffective in the presence of severe endothelial damage. Other vasodilators, such as verapamil, diltiazem, nicardipine, nitroprusside, and adenosine, can produce improvement in corrected TIMI frame counts and TIMI flow scores, but have not yet been shown unequivocally to improve clinical outcomes [54]. Clinical trials of therapies to reduce reperfusion injury (including anti inflammatory agents, complement activation inhibitors, adhesion molecule antibodies, magnesium, and glucose/insulin/potassium) have similarly failed to show improved outcomes [54]. Other therapies show promise but await testing in randomized clinical trials.

## Myocardial hibernation

Hibernating myocardium is a term originally coined to denote myocardial segments with persistently impaired function at rest due to severely reduced coronary blood flow; inherent in this definition of hibernating myocardium is the notion that function can be normalized by improving blood flow [42,55]. Hibernation is viewed as an adaptive response that reduces myocardial contractile function in an area of hypoperfusion so as to restore equilibrium between flow and function, thus minimizing the potential for ischemia or necrosis. Myocardial cells remain viable, with decreased calcium transients and force generation; when flow is restored, calcium transients and force generation normalize [56].

Patients with viable yet dysfunctional myocardium can be identified by a number of methods. Indices of regional wall motion, systolic wall thickening, and regional coronary blood flow are of limited utility because, by definition, hibernating myocardium has reduced systolic function and perfusion. Methods that reflect intact cellular metabolic processes, cell membrane integrity, or myocardial inotropic reserve are more accurate at detecting viable myocardium. Such methods include nuclear imaging, usually with 4-hour redistribution imaging or late reinjection, dobutamine stress echocardiography, and PET scanning to detect metabolic activity [57]. Of these, PET scanning is the most sensitive. Ischemic myocardium uses glucose preferentially as a metabolic substrate, and such utilization can be detected by uptake of [$^{18}$F]-fluorodeoxyglucose (FDG). In conjunction with myocardial perfusion imaging with $^{13}$N-ammonia, regions with enhanced FDG uptake relative to perfusion can be identified [58].

Although increasing myocardial oxygen demand might be expected to worsen ischemia in hibernating myocardium, it has been shown that such segments retain inotropic reserve and will respond to low doses of dobutamine. Demonstration of such inotropic reserve by dobutamine echocardiography has a positive accuracy of 86% and a negative accuracy of 80% in predicting functional outcome after revascularization, similar to results achieved with thallium reinjection [57].

Regardless of the technique used to identify hibernating myocardium, it is clear that revascularization can lead to improved segmental and overall myocardial function [59], which in turn translates into improved prognosis [57]. In the context of cardiogenic shock, it is also important to recognize that hibernating segments retain some contractile reserve and will respond to low doses of inotropic agents, as long as those agents do not induce further ischemia. Hibernation remote from the area of infarction may also be important, as increased contractility in noninfarcted areas represents an important compensatory response [26,60].

Although hibernation is conceptually different from myocardial stunning, recent investigations have challenged the clear distinction between the two conditions. Although ischemic myocardial segments adapt function to perfusion over the short term without developing infarction, this tenuous balance cannot be maintained for long without at least some necrosis [61]. In fact, in the presence of severe stenosis, increases in myocardial oxygen demand can precipitate deterioration in metabolism and lactate release. It is now clear that repetitive episodes of myocardial stunning can occur in areas of viable myocardium subtended by a critical coronary stenosis, and that such episodes can recapitulate the hibernation phenotype, complicating the distinction between myocardial stunning and hibernation [41,55,62].

Regardless of the degree of overlap, the therapeutic implications of myocardial stunning and hibernation make their consideration vital in patients with cardiogenic shock. As previously noted, contractile function of hibernating myocardium improves with revascularization, and stunned myocardium retains inotropic reserve and can respond to inotropic stimulation [41]. In addition, the fact that the severity of the antecedent ischemic insult determines the intensity of stunning [41] provides one rationale for reestablishing patency of occluded coronary arteries in patients with cardiogenic shock. Finally, the notion that some myocardial tissue may recover function emphasizes the importance of measures to support hemodynamics and thus minimize myocardial necrosis in patients with shock.

## Conclusions

The pathophysiology of cardiogenic shock is complex and differs from patient to patient. Only a minority of patients present with shock, with most developing it within the first hours of a myocardial infarction. This suggests the potential for prompt intervention to prevent the development of shock. In particular, the vicious cycle in which ischemia leads to myocardial dysfunction and compensatory mechanisms that in turn worsen ischemia provides a powerful rationale for early and aggressive revascularization in patients with cardiogenic shock. Other mechanisms, however, may lead to inappropriate vasodilation, and addressing those mechanisms may have therapeutic potential. In addition, microcirculatory abnormalities may play an important role in mediating hypoperfusion in shock, and the potential regional heterogeneity of those perturbations should be addressed by innovative diagnostic and therapeutic strategies.

In the center of the infarct area, oncolytic cell death predominates, but apoptosis may play a role in border zones. Because apoptosis causes a much less dramatic inflammatory response but requires energy, this suggests that restoration of blood flow to tenuous areas at the margin of the infarct zone might not only save cells but also decrease acute infarct remodeling. In addition, inhibition of apoptosis might represent a promising therapeutic target.

Finally, areas of nonfunctional yet viable myocardium can contribute importantly to the development of cardiogenic shock after myocardial infarction. In this context, the distinctions among stunning, reperfusion injury, and hibernation are less important than the realization that the pathophysiology of these overlapping conditions provides a powerful rationale not only for reperfusion therapy, but also for supportive therapies aimed at optimizing hemodynamics in the early course of cardiogenic shock, since recovery of function may be achieved.

# References

1. Hochman JS, Buller CE, Sleeper LA, Boland J, Dzavik V, Sanborn TA, Godfrey E, White H, Lim J, LeJemtel T, for the SHOCK Study Group. Cardiogenic Shock Complicating Acute Myocardial Infarction-Etiologies, Management and Outcome; Overall Findings of the SHOCK Trial Registry. *J Am Coll Cardiol* 2000;36:1063–1070.

2. Hollenberg SM, Kavinsky CJ, Parrillo JE. Cardiogenic shock. *Ann Intern Med* 1999;131:47–59.

3. Rudiger A, Gasser S, Fischler M, et al. Comparable increase of B-type natriuretic peptide and amino-terminal pro-B-type natriuretic peptide levels in patients with severe sepsis, septic shock, and acute heart failure. *Crit Care Med* 2006;34:2140–4.

4. Hochman JS, Sleeper LA, Webb JG, et al. Early revascularization in acute myocardial infarction complicated by cardiogenic shock. *N Engl J Med* 1999;341:625–34.

5. Picard MH, Davidoff R, Sleeper LA, et al. Echocardiographic predictors of survival and response to early revascularization in cardiogenic shock. *Circulation* 2003;107:279–84.

6. Kohsaka S, Menon V, Lowe AM, et al. Systemic inflammatory response syndrome after acute myocardial infarction complicated by cardiogenic shock. *Arch Intern Med* 2005;165:1643–50.

7. Hochman JS. Cardiogenic shock complicating acute myocardial infarction: expanding the paradigm. *Circulation* 2003;107:2998–3002.

8. Neumann FJ, Ott I, Gawaz M, et al. Cardiac release of cytokines and inflammatory responses in acute myocardial infarction. *Circulation* 1995;92:748–55.

9. Shah AM. Inducible nitric oxide synthase and cardiovascular disease. *Cardiovasc Res* 2000;45:148–55.

10. Feng Q, Lu X, Jones DL, et al. Increased inducible nitric oxide synthase expression contributes to myocardial dysfunction and higher mortality after myocardial infarction in mice. *Circulation* 2001;104:700–4.

11. Ferdinandy P, Danial H, Ambrus I, et al. Peroxynitrite is a major contributor to cytokine-induced myocardial contractile failure. *Circ Res* 2000;87:241–7.

12. Nicholls SJ, Wang Z, Koeth R, et al. Metabolic profiling of arginine and nitric oxide pathways predicts hemodynamic abnormalities and mortality in patients with cardiogenic shock after acute myocardial infarction. *Circulation* 2007;116:2315–24.

13. Geppert A, Dorninger A, Delle-Karth G, et al. Plasma concentrations of interleukin-6, organ failure, vasopressor support, and successful coronary revascularization in predicting 30-day mortality of patients with cardiogenic shock complicating acute myocardial infarction. *Crit Care Med* 2006;34:2035–42.

14. Geppert A, Steiner A, Zorn G, et al. Multiple organ failure in patients with cardiogenic shock is associated with high plasma levels of interleukin-6. *Crit Care Med* 2002;30:1987–94.

15. De Backer D, Creteur J, Dubois MJ, et al. Microvascular alterations in patients with acute severe heart failure and cardiogenic shock. *Am Heart J* 2004;147:91–9.

16. De Backer D, Creteur J, Preiser JC, et al. Microvascular blood flow is altered in patients with sepsis. *Am J Respir Crit Care Med* 2002;166:98–104.

17. Trzeciak S, Dellinger RP, Parrillo JE, et al. Early microcirculatory perfusion derangements in patients with severe sepsis and septic shock: relationship to hemodynamics, oxygen transport, and survival. *Ann Emerg Med* 2007;49:88–98, e1–2.

18. Reimer KA, Lowe JE, Rasmussen MM, et al. The wavefront phenomenon of ischemic cell death. 1. Myocardial infarct size vs duration of coronary occlusion in dogs. *Circulation* 1977;56:786–94.

19. Page DL, Caulfield JB, Kaster JA, et al. Myocardial changes associated with cardiogenic shock. *N Engl J Med* 1971;285:133–7.

20. Alonso DR, Scheidt S, Post M, et al. Pathophysiology of cardiogenic shock. Quantification of myocardial necrosis, clinical, pathologic and electrocardiographic correlations. *Circulation* 1973;48:588–96.

21. Califf RM, Bengtson JR. Cardiogenic shock. *N Engl J Med* 1994;330:1724–30.

22. Holmes DR Jr, Bates ER, Kleiman NS, et al. Contemporary reperfusion therapy for cardiogenic shock: the GUSTO-I trial experience. The GUSTO-I Investigators. Global Utilization of Streptokinase and Tissue Plasminogen Activator for Occluded Coronary Arteries. *J Am Coll Cardiol* 1995;26:668–74.

23. Leor J, Goldbourt U, Reicher-Reiss H, et al. Cardiogenic shock complicating acute myocardial infarction in patients without heart failure on admission: incidence, risk factors, and outcome. SPRINT Study Group. *Am J Med* 1993;94:265–73.

24. Hands ME, Rutherford JD, Muller JE, et al. The in-hospital development of cardiogenic shock after myocardial infarction: incidence, predictors of occurrence, outcome and prognostic factors. The MILIS Study Group. *J Am Coll Cardiol* 1989;14:40–6.

25. Olivetti G, Quaini F, Sala R, et al. Acute myocardial infarction in humans is associated with activation of programmed myocyte cell death in the surviving portion of the heart. *J Mol Cell Cardiol* 1994;28:2005–16.

26. Weisman HF, Healy B. Myocardial infarct expansion, infarct extension, and reinfarction: pathophysiologic concepts. *Prog Cardiovasc Dis* 1987;30:73–110.

27. Ohman EM, Topol EJ, Califf RM, et al. An analysis of the cause of early mortality after administration of thrombolytic therapy. The Thrombolysis Angioplasty in Myocardial Infarction Study Group. *Coron Artery Dis* 1993;4:957–64.

28. Ratcliffe MB. Non-ischemic infarct extension. A new type of infarct enlargement and a potential therapeutic target. *J Am Coll Cardiol* 2002;40:1168–71.

29. Widimsky P, Gregor P, Cervenka V, et al. Severe diffuse hypokinesis of the remote myocardium–the main cause of cardiogenic shock? An echocardiographic study of 75 patients with extremely large myocardial infarctions. *Cor Vasa* 1988;30:27–34.

30. Grines CL, Topol EJ, Califf RM, et al. Prognostic implications and predictors of enhanced regional wall motion of the noninfarct zone after thrombolysis and angioplasty therapy of acute myocardial infarction. The TAMI Study Groups. *Circulation* 1989;80:245–53.

31. McGhie AI, Golstein RA. Pathogenesis and management of acute heart failure and cardiogenic shock: role of inotropic therapy. *Chest* 1992;102:626S–32S.

32. Webb JG. Interventional management of cardiogenic shock. *Can J Cardiol* 1998;14: 233–44.

33. Harizi RC, Bianco JA, Alpert JS. Diastolic function of the heart in clinical cardiology. *Arch Intern Med* 1988;148:99–109.

34. Kaul S, Spotnitz WD, Glasheen WP, et al. Mechanism of ischemic mitral regurgitation. An experimental evaluation. *Circulation* 1991;84:2167–80.

35. Levine RA, Schwammenthal E. Ischemic mitral regurgitation on the threshold of a solution: from paradoxes to unifying concepts. *Circulation* 2005;112:745–58.

36. Stanley WC. Myocardial energy metabolism during ischemia and the mechanisms of metabolic therapies. *J Cardiovasc Pharmacol Ther* 2004;9 (Suppl 1):S31–45.

37. Hollenberg SM, Parrillo JE. Shock. In: Fauci AS, Braunwald E, Isselbacher KJ, et al, eds. *Harrison's Principles of Internal Medicine* (14th edition). New York: McGraw-Hill, 1997:214–22.

38. Okuda M. A multidisciplinary overview of cardiogenic shock. *Shock* 2006;25: 557–70.

39. Bartling B, Holtz J, Darmer D. Contribution of myocyte apoptosis to myocardial infarction? *Basic Res Cardiol* 1998;93:71–84.

40. Scarabelli TM, Knight R, Stephanou A, et al. Clinical implications of apoptosis in ischemic myocardium. *Curr Probl Cardiol* 2006;31:181–264.

41. Bolli R. Basic and clinical aspects of myocardial stunning. *Prog Cardiovasc Dis* 1998;40:477–516.

42. Kloner RA, Jennings RB. Consequences of brief ischemia: stunning, preconditioning, and their clinical implications: part 1. *Circulation* 2001;104:2981–9.

43. Ballantyne CM, Verani MS, Short HD, et al. Delayed recovery of severely "stunned" myocardium with the support of a left ventricular assist device after coronary artery bypass graft surgery. *J Am Coll Cardiol* 1987;10:710–2.

44. Bolli R, Hartley CJ, Chelly JE, et al. An accurate nontraumatic ultrasonic method to monitor myocardial wall thickening in patients undergoing cardial surgery. *J Am Coll Cardiol* 1990;15:1055–65.

45. Gerber BL, Wijns W, Vanoverschelde JL, et al. Myocardial perfusion and oxygen consumption in reperfused noninfarcted dysfunctional myocardium after unstable angina: direct evidence for myocardial stunning in humans. *J Am Coll Cardiol* 1999;34:1939–46.

46. Jeroudi MO, Hartley CJ, Bolli R. Myocardial reperfusion injury: role of oxygen radicals and potential therapy with antioxidants. *Am J Cardiol* 1994;73:2B–7B.

47. Brar R, Kumar A, Schaer GL, et al. Release of soluble myocardial depressant activity by reperfused myocardium (abstract). *J Am Coll Cardiol* 1996;27:386A.

48. Atar D, Gao WD, Marban E. Alterations of excitation-contraction coupling in stunned myocardium and in failing myocardium. *J Mol Cell Cardiol* 1995;27:783–91.

49. Bolli R, Marban E. Molecular and cellular mechanisms of myocardial stunning. *Physiol Rev* 1999;79:609–34.

50. Gao WD, Liu Y, Mellgren R, et al. Intrinsic myofilament alterations underlying the decreased contractility of stunned myocardium. A consequence of Ca2+-dependent proteolysis? *Circ Res* 1996;78:455–65.

51. Moens AL, Claeys MJ, Timmermans JP, et al. Myocardial ischemia/reperfusion-injury, a clinical view on a complex pathophysiological process. *Int J Cardiol* 2005;100:179–90.

52. Hollenberg SM, Klein LW, Parrillo JE, et al. Coronary endothelial dysfunction after heart transplantation predicts allograft vasculopathy and cardiac death. *Circulation* 2001;104:3091–6.

53. Michaels AD, Gibson CM, Barron HV. Microvascular dysfunction in acute myocardial infarction: focus on the roles of platelet and inflammatory mediators in the no-reflow phenomenon. *Am J Cardiol* 2000;85:50B–60B.

54. Gibson CM. Has my patient achieved adequate myocardial reperfusion? *Circulation* 2003;108:504–7.

55. Wijns W, Vatner SF, Camici PG. Hibernating myocardium. *N Engl J Med* 1998;339: 173–81.

56. Marban E. Myocardial stunning and hibernation. The physiology behind the colloquialisms. *Circulation* 1991;83:681–8.

57. Bonow RO. The hibernating myocardium: implications for management of congestive heart failure. *Am J Cardiol* 1995;75:17A–25A.

58. Pagano D, Bonser RS, Townend JN, et al. Predictive value of dobutamine echocardiography and positron emission tomography in identifying hibernating myocardium in patients with postischaemic heart failure. *Heart* 1998;79:281–8.

59. Topol EJ, Weiss JL, Guzman PA, et al. Immediate improvement of dysfunctional myocardial segments after coronary revascularization: detection by intraoperative transesophageal echocardiography. *J Am Coll Cardiol* 1984;4:1123–34.

60. Harrison JK, Califf RM, Woodlief LH, et al. Systolic left ventricular function after reperfusion therapy for acute myocardial infarction. Analysis of determinants of improvement. The TAMI Study Group. *Circulation* 1993;87:1531–41.

61. Canty JM Jr, Fallavollita JA. Hibernating myocardium. *J Nucl Cardiol* 2005;12: 104–19.

62. Kim SJ, Peppas A, Hong SK, et al. Persistent stunning induces myocardial hibernation and protection: flow/function and metabolic mechanisms. *Circ Res* 2003;92: 1233–9.

# Chapter 3

# General management: pharmacotherapy and mechanical ventilation

Alexander Geppert and Vladimír Džavík

## Introduction

Pharmacotherapy is a key component of the management of patients with acute myocardial infarction (MI) complicated by cardiogenic shock. While almost none of the pharmaceutical agents commonly utilized to treat patients in cardiogenic shock have been studied in trials with adequate power to test their effect on mortality, many are nonetheless considered essential to achieve rapid hemodynamic stabilization and allow implementation of therapies to reverse the process that has led to the shock state. Such therapies include reperfusion of the infarct-related artery to improve myocardial function by myocardial salvage, if shock occurs early after coronary occlusion or on the basis of improved flow to ischemic peri-infarct zones, and by preventing coronary reocclusion. Ventilation strategies in cardiogenic shock have also been poorly studied and are often implemented late in the cardiac intensive care setting. This chapter reviews the evidence behind the use of common pharmaceutical agents utilized in the setting of pump failure and mechanical complications and discusses appropriate ventilation strategies. The management of other conditions that cause shock, such as hypertrophic cardiomyopathy and critical valvular disease, is addressed in Chapters 7 and 8.

The main goal of vasoactive drug therapy in cardiogenic shock is to optimize perfusion while minimizing toxicity, since all inotropic and vasopressor agents cause significant toxicity at higher doses. In several cardiogenic shock risk models, vasopressor use (number of agents, specific agent used, and higher dosages) has been associated with excess mortality [1–3]. This may reflect severity of the underlying shock state and/or toxicity. The European Guidelines for treatment

*Cardiogenic Shock.* Edited by Judith S. Hochman and E. Magnus Ohman.
© 2009 American Heart Association, ISBN: 978-1-4051-7926-3

of acute heart failure recommend close monitoring of mixed venous saturation, a marker of tissue oxygenation and a parameter easily monitored continuously, although modulation of a low mixed oxygen saturation by vasoactive therapy to prevent organ failure has not been validated by randomized studies.

Invasive hemodynamic monitoring (arterial line, cardiac output monitoring) is recommended to guide and monitor the effects of the therapy, although the goals to be reached have not been consensually defined. It is unclear whether efforts should be directed at increasing the cardiac output or targeting a particular mean arterial blood pressure. We recommend that the administration and titration of vasoactive therapy and volume manipulation be guided by indices of organ perfusion (e.g. urine output) while maintaining adequate oxygenation.

## Inotrope and vasopressor therapy

In spite of the paucity of randomized trial evidence of a therapeutic benefit, pharmacologic support with inotropic and vasopressor agents remains a mainstay of therapy of patients with acute MI complicated by cardiogenic shock, as recommended by the American Heart Association (AHA)/American College of Cardiology (ACC) guidelines for the management of patients with ST-elevation MI [4] and the ESC/ESICM guidelines for the management of patients with acute heart failure [5]. The AHA/ACC guidelines differentiate between low-output syndrome without shock and a low-output syndrome with shock. In the former it is recommended to begin with an inotrope, e.g. dobutamine; in the latter it is recommended to start with dopamine or, if the systolic blood pressure is below 70 mm Hg, with norepinephrine. In clinical practice, patients are, therefore, usually treated with a combination of inotropes and vasopressors. Vasopressors are contraindicated in patients with nonhypotensive forms of cardiogenic shock; mechanical complications of acute MI that might have been the cause of shock should be treated appropriately. Mechanical reperfusion should be undertaken based on the results of the SHOCK trial, and intra-aortic balloon counterpulsation should be initiated in the absence of specific contraindications. The initial hemodynamic stabilization using catecholamines, often in combination, is nevertheless of paramount importance because improvement of organ perfusion and prevention of multiple organ failure are essential for survival (see Table 3.1). From a physiological perspective, inotropic agents shift the starling relationship (between preload and stroke volume-cardiac output) to a higher plateau (increased contractility). The choice and amount of inotropes/vasopressors given in cardiogenic shock might vary substantially among hospitals and the agents used may have different actions on organ perfusion. Dopamine is the preferred primary vasopressor agent in some, and norepinephrine in others [3]. In general, the lowest possible doses of inotropic and pressor agents should be utilized to adequately support vital tissue perfusion while limiting adverse consequences, some of which may not be immediately apparent. For example, administration of dopamine leads to activation

**Table 3.1** Inotropic and vasopressor therapy in cardiogenic shock.

| Indication | Agent | Dosage | Comments |
| --- | --- | --- | --- |
| Shock secondary to predominant left ventricular dysfunction; shock secondary to mechanical complication: severe acute mitral regurgitation, ventricular septal rupture | Dopamine | 3–15 µg/kg/min | First-line agent Avoid doses >15 µg/kg/min Consider adding second agent |
| | Dobutamine | 3–15 µg/kg/min | Second-line agent Consider especially if SVR, PVR elevated |
| | Norepinephrine | 0.01–3.0 µg/kg/min | Second-line agent if dopamine ≥10 µg/kg/min is insufficient May be utilized as first-line agent, especially if hypotension is profound (systolic <70 mm Hg) |
| | Epinephrine | 0.01–1.00 µg/kg/min | Utilized commonly in surgical settings as first- or second-line therapy Experimentally, deleterious effects compared to norepinehrine |
| | Vasopressin | 0.01–0.10 IU/min | Consider using for more longstanding shock with decreased catecholamine sensitivity May improve catecholamine sensitivity |
| | Levosimendan | Bolus dose of 6–12 µg/kg followed by 0.05–0.2 µg/kg/min for 24 hours | Not available in North America Utilized as second-line agent in some European countries |
| | Phosphodiesterase inhibitors | | Avoid due to vasodilatory effect and potential for exacerbation of hypotension |
| Shock secondary to predominant right ventricular dysfunction | Dobutamine | 5–15 µg/kg/min | First-line agent Initiate once hydration status is adequate (PAWP ≥15 mm Hg) or if CVP is clearly elevated |

of proteolytic enzymes, pro-apoptotic signal cascades, mitochondrial damage, and eventual membrane disruption and necrosis due to further augmentation of already elevated levels of cytosolic $Ca^2$ in postischemic cardiac myocytes [6]. Moderate doses of combinations of medications may be more effective than maximal doses of any individual agent. The combination of dopamine and dobutamine at doses of approximately 7.5 µg/kg/min each can result in improved hemodynamics and fewer important adverse effects when compared to either agent administered individually at 15 µg/kg/min [7].

## Dobutamine

Acting via stimulation of $\beta_1$ and $\beta_2$ receptors, dobutamine is the inotropic agent of reference, but has limited effect on increasing arterial pressure. Quite to the contrary, the $\beta$-adrenergic effects of dobutamine cause peripheral vasodilation, although the vasodilating effects observed are usually smaller than those observed with some alternative inotropic drugs (see below). While the decrease in afterload can further increase cardiac output, a decrease in arterial blood pressure can result in myocardial ischemia by reducing coronary perfusion pressure. The use of dobutamine as a $\beta$-mimetic agent alone is therefore usually restricted to nonhypotensive forms of cardiogenic shock. Other potential adverse effects of $\beta$-adrenergic stimulation include an increase in myocardial infarct size [8], especially if dobutamine administration is followed by a substantial increase in heart rate and an increased incidence of arrhythmias. Concerns have also been raised regarding tolerance, loss of hemodynamic effect with prolonged use [9], and the need for increased dosages in the case of recent $\beta$-blocker therapy [10]. The therapy should usually begin with doses between 2 and 5 µg/kg/min without a loading dose and be titrated according to the desired effects. As the elimination half-life of dobutamine is very short, its effects are rapidly dissipated when the infusion ceases. An increase of dobutamine doses above 20 µg/kg/min is not recommended by the AHA [4] or by the ESC/ESICM [5] guidelines as untoward side effects of the drug will predominate. Therefore, if maximal doses of dobutamine do not produce the desired effect (an increase in cardiac output), dobutamine should be combined with alternative drugs, e.g. phosphodiesterase inhibitors (PDEIs). Levosimendan, not available for use in North America, is commonly utilized for this indication in other parts of the world.

## Dopamine

As an endogenous central neurotransmitter and immediate precursor to norepinephrine, dopamine acts on dopaminergic as well as adrenergic receptors, eliciting a variety of dose-dependent effects. At low doses up to 3 µg/kg/min, it stimulates dopaminergic $D_1$ postsynaptic receptors concentrated in the coronary, renal, mesenteric, and cerebral beds, as well as $D_2$ presynaptic receptors present in the vasculature and renal tissues, causing vasodilation and increasing blood flow to these tissues. Although dopamine is said to have natriuretic effects [11], a renal protective effect has not been shown [12]. At doses between

3 and 10 µg/kg/min, dopamine increases cardiac contractility and chronotropy by means of a mild effect on $\beta_1$-adrenergic receptors, resulting in a release of norepinephrine and reduction of reuptake in presynaptic sympathetic nerve terminals. A mild peripheral vasoconstrictive effect is also observed that, due to an effect on $\alpha_1$-adrenergic receptors, becomes pronounced and predominant at infusion rates beyond 10 µg/kg/min.

Dopamine is recommended as the first-line inotropic/vasopressor agent to be administered in true hypotensive cardiogenic shock [4]. The infusion should begin at 5 µg/kg/min and be rapidly up-titrated to achieve the desired effect on blood pressure. Doses beyond 12.5–15.0 µg/kg/min should be avoided and second-line inotropic/vasopressor therapy should be initiated in case of inadequate response to dopamine. The use of "renal dose" dopamine, either alone or in combination with other inotropic or vasopressor agents, to maintain or improve renal function has been largely abandoned following the results of a multicenter trial that failed to demonstrate clinically significant protection from renal dysfunction with continuous intravenous infusion of low-dose dopamine in critically ill patients at risk of renal failure [12]. Sakr et al. reported a significantly higher mortality in shock patients receiving dopamine (77% received doses >5 µg/kg/min) as compared to patients who received norepinephrine in the Sepsis Occurrence in Critically Ill Patients (SOAP) study, an observational study of more than 1000 patients with shock (40% with septic shock) in more than 190 European intensive care units (ICUs) [3]. ICU mortality was 42.9% in patients receiving dopamine compared with 35.7% in patients not receiving dopamine; dopamine use was an independent risk factor for mortality in a multivariable analysis [3]. However, it is not clear whether dopamine was responsible for this increase in mortality or whether it was simply a surrogate marker of more critically ill patients. Moreover, this association was not observed in nonseptic shock patients.

## Norepinephrine

Norepinephrine is the major endogenous neurotransmitter released by post-ganglionic adrenergic nerves. It behaves primarily as a vasoconstrictor but also as a mild inotrope, due to its effect on $\alpha_1$-adrenergic receptors and to a lesser extent on $\beta$-receptors. Its major effect is to increase systolic, diastolic, and pulse pressure, while its effect on cardiac output is negligible. As a result of the elevated diastolic pressure and an indirect effect on cardiac myocytes to release local vasodilators, coronary flow is also increased [13]. At least in the setting of septic shock, it has a more favorable effect on splanchnic circulation than epinephrine and may even exert a more favorable action in this regard than dopamine [14]. Prolonged administration can result in direct toxicity to cardiac myocytes [15].

Whether it is utilized as a second-line agent to stabilize patients in cardiogenic shock, as recommended by the AHA/ACC guidelines, or as first-line therapy, norepinephrine is administered as an infusion ranging from 0.01 to

3.0 µg/kg/min. The median dose administered in patients with persistent shock despite an open infarct artery and vasopressor support in the Tilarginine Acetate Injection in a Randomized International Study in Unstable MI Patients With Cardiogenic Shock (TRIUMPH) was 0.2 µg/kg/min [2]. In contrast to the SOAP findings [3], preliminary TRIUMPH results suggest that norepinephrine use was independently associated with excess mortality. As noted, this may reflect selection of this agent for patients with the most severe shock.

## Epinephrine

Also an endogenous catecholamine, epinephrine has a high affinity for $\beta_1$-, $\beta_2$-, and $\alpha_1$-adrenergic receptors present in cardiac and vascular smooth muscle, with $\beta$ effects being more pronounced at low doses and $\alpha_1$ effects at higher doses. The net effect of administration is an increase in arterial and venous pulmonary pressures. Epinephrine increases coronary blood flow by increasing the relative duration of diastole at higher heart rates and, similar to norepinephrine, by stimulating myocytes to release local vasodilators [16]. Prolonged administration at high doses can cause myocyte apoptosis and damage the arterial walls, causing focal regions of myocardial contraction band necrosis not unlike MI in appearance [17]. The doses of epinephrine in clinical use are similar to those of norepinephrine. In septic shock, international guidelines recommend the combination of dobutamine + norepinephrine over epinephrine. In fact, human and animal studies suggest some advantages of norepinephrine and dobutamine over epinephrine (less tachycardia, less disadvantageous effects on splanchnic circulation). However a multicenter trial [18] comparing the administration of dobutamine + norepinephrine to the administration of epinephrine in more than 300 patients with septic shock did not find a significant difference in efficacy and safety between epinephrine alone and norepinephrine + dobutamine. Similarly an Australian study (CAT study [19]) found no significant difference in the time to shock resolution with either epinephrine or norepinephrine (35.1 h IQR 13.8–70 h vs 40.0 IQR 14.5–120 h) in 280 patients who required vasopressors for any cause. There was no difference in the maximal daily dose to achieve the predefined mean arterial pressure goal and also no significant difference in 28-day and 90-day mortality between the subgroup of patients receiving epinephrine and those receiving norepinephrine (28-day mortality rates: 22.5% with epinephrine and 26.1% with norepinephrine $p = 0.48$). However, the use of epinephrine was associated with development of significant tachycardia and lactic acidosis, as well as increased insulin requirements in the first 24 hours. Of note epinephrine-induced lactic acidosis was not associated with loss of haemodynamic efficacy of the vasopressor.

## Phosphodiesterase inhibitors

Enoximone and milrinone are the two phosphodiesterase inhibitors (PDEIs) used in clinical practice. They act by decreasing the rate of intracellular cyclic adenosine monophosphate (cAMP) degradation, thus increasing the concentrations of cytosolic $Ca^{2+}$. As with dobutamine, the PDEIs increase cardiac contractility at the expense of increased myocardial oxygen consumption and their vasodilatory effects are stronger than those of dobutamine. However, as the inotropic effects of dobutamine and PDEI appear to be additive, the two agents can be combined in order to increase the desired inotropic effect. Because they do not involve the $\beta$-receptor directly, PDEIs can exert their effects even in the presence of $\beta$-blocker therapy [10].

The drugs are usually started with a bolus dose (25 µg/kg for milrinone and 250–750 µg/kg for enoximone) over 10–20 min followed by a continuous infusion of 0.25–0.75 µg/kg/min (milrinone) or 1.25–7.5 µg/kg/min (enoximone). Because their vasodilating effects can be problematic in hypotensive patients and patients needing vasopressor therapy, we recommend that the bolus dose be omitted in cardiogenic shock.

Another unwanted side effect of the PDEIs is their proarrhythmic potential, especially with prolonged use [20]. Furthermore, a post hoc analysis of the OPTIME-CHF study data revealed an increased rate of death and rehospitalization in the milrinone-treated patients with ischemic heart disease compared to placebo [21], which casts doubt regarding its use in patients with cardiogenic shock complicating acute MI. As with levosimendan, there has been no large study to date comparing the administration of PDEI with placebo or with dobutamine in cardiogenic shock. Preliminary results of a small study of 25 patients with cardiogenic shock showed that the hemodynamic effects of levosimendan and enoximone were comparable [22]. Although there was apparently a lower mortality rate in the levosimendan group, the small number of events renders the study prone to chance findings [23].

## Levosimendan

In contrast to the $\beta$-adrenergic drug dobutamine and PDEIs such as milrinone that act via a cAMP-mediated increase in intracellular $Ca^{2+}$ concentrations, levosimendan exerts its positive inotropic effects by $Ca^{2+}$ sensitization of myocardial myofilaments. Therefore, levosimendan may have a theoretical advantage of inducing less tachycardia, fewer arrhythmias, and lower oxygen consumption than dobutamine or the pure PDEIs like milrinone [24]. The metabolism of levosimendan furthermore produces a long-lasting active metabolite with similar $Ca^{2+}$ sensitization capacity as the parent compound, and to which are ascribed the long-lasting positive inotropic effects following administration of levosimendan. At high intracellular concentrations, levosimendan might also inhibit phosphodiesterase III [25,26], but this effect is not seen at the concentrations that are reached with the clinically recommended dosage. In addition, levosimendan seems to have anti-ischemic effects by opening mitochondrial $K_{ATP}$ channels [27]. By opening ATP-sensitive $K^+$ channels, levosimendan produces systemic and pulmonary vasodilation [24]. While the decrease in pulmonary resistance might improve right ventricular performance, the effects on the peripheral vasculature might be problematic in vasopressor-dependent patients.

Levosimendan is usually started with a bolus dose of 6–12 µg/kg followed by a continuous infusion of 0.1–0.2 µg/kg/min for 24 hours. Vasodilation with its drop in blood pressure can usually be prevented by avoiding a bolus dose or reducing the bolus dose to 6 µg/kg, by increasing preload (volume administration), or by increasing the vasopressor dose. In the large randomized studies of levosimendan in acute heart failure (e.g. SURVIVE [28], RUSSLAN [29], and LIDO [30]), patients with cardiogenic shock and patients on vasopressor support were excluded. There are no large randomized studies analyzing the effect of levosimendan administration instead of or in addition to dobutamine in patients with cardiogenic shock or on vasopressor support. Small observational studies [31–33] did not report severe adverse effects of levosimendan use in this setting and showed an increase in cardiac output and a decrease in cardiac filling pressures. A study of levosimendan administration in 25 patients with refractory cardiogenic shock following acute MI reported a 30% increase in cardiac output and in cardiac power output (the product of cardiac output and mean arterial blood pressure), demonstrating that the increase in cardiac output by levosimendan was not solely due to a reduction in afterload [34]. Adverse effects included the need to increase the vasopressor dose by about 30% and a parallel substantial increase in volume administration [34]. The effects of dobutamine (mean and maximum doses not specified) and levosimendan were compared in 22 patients with cardiogenic shock following percutaneous coronary intervention (PCI); levosimendan reached the predefined goal, an increase in cardiac power output by 30% more often than dobutamine [35]. Both drugs had similar effects on decreasing pulmonary artery wedge pressure. Whether a 30% increase in the vasopressor dose is also acceptable at high vasopressor doses without producing an excess in untoward side effects, e.g. on organ perfusion, remains to be determined. Although animal data suggest that levosimendan is superior in improving gut mucosal blood flow under resting conditions compared to dobutamine or milrinone, independent of its systemic effects [36,37], it remains to be seen whether this alternate inotrope can also improve organ perfusion in cardiogenic shock. Despite the theoretical promise, clinical trials of levosimendan in patients with severe heart failure have demonstrated disappointing results compared to dobutamine or placebo [28,38].

## Vasopressin

Interest in the possible utility of vasopressin in cardiogenic shock was spurred by observations of beneficial effects of the drug during cardiac arrest [39]. Vasopressin or 'antidiuretic hormone' is a nona-peptide, stored primarily in granules in the posterior pituitary gland and released in response to increased plasma osmolality, hypotension, pain, nausea, or hypoxia [40]. Synthesis by the heart in response to elevated cardiac wall stress [41] and by the adrenal gland in response to increased catecholamine secretion also occurs [42]. Its homeostatic effects on the circulation are through $V_{1a}$ receptors in vascular smooth muscle where it mediates pressor activity, and $V_{1b}$ receptors in the pituitary gland, as well as $V_2$ receptors in the renal collecting duct system by increasing water permeability and thus water reabsorption. Major biological effects include vasoconstriction, glyconeogenesis, platelet aggregation, and ACTH (adrenocorticotropic hormone) release. Coronary and cerebral vessels constrict more in direct response to vasopressin than to catecholamines in experimental and cardiac arrest settings. Vasopressin has a neutral or depressant effect on cardiac output [43,44] modulated by a dose-dependent increase in peripheral vascular resistance and resultant increase in reflexive vagal tone [45]. In addition, vasopressin increases vascular sensitivity to norepinephrine, resulting in further pressor augmentation, and may also directly promote vasoconstriction, through inhibition of ATP-activated potassium channels [46], attenuation of nitric oxide (NO) production [47], and reversal of adrenergic receptor downregulation [48]. Its pressor effects are maintained during hypoxic and acidotic conditions, common during shock of any etiology. While in the initial phases of shock, endogenous vasopressin levels are significantly elevated to help maintain end-organ perfusion [49]; as the shock state progresses, the levels fall precipitously, possibly due to loss of neurohypophyseal stores [50], autonomic dysfunction [51], and inhibition of vasopressin release by norepinephrine [52]. Loss of vascular tone, as well as worsening hypotension and end-organ perfusion, may ensue.

Administration of vasopressin may be particularly useful in norepinephrine-resistant shock [53] and may decrease the need for higher doses of norepinephrine, thus reducing cardiotoxicity and proarrhythmia [54]. It may also attenuate interleukin-induced generation of NO [55]. For the most part, information on clinical use of vasopressin in shock is derived from studies in noncardiogenic shock states. In a randomized study of 48 patients with catecholamine-resistant vasodilatory shock, a combined infusion of vasopressin (4 IU/hr) and norepinephrine was found to be superior to norepinephrine alone with respect to surrogate endpoints, its administration resulting in significantly lower heart rate, lower norepinephrine requirements, and a decrease in new tachyarrhythmias [54]. Gastrointestinal perfusion was also better preserved in the vasopressin group, this being an important observation due to concerns about the possibility of vasopressin causing splanchnic ischemia. The study was too small to adequately assess safety or clinical outcome superiority and addressed vasodilatory, not cardiogenic, shock. In an uncontrolled, retrospective study of vasopressin administration in postarrest vasoplegic shock, advanced cardiac failure could be reversed in more than 90% of patients who had been unresponsive to a combination including milrinone, epinephrine, and norepinephrine [56]. In the only study examining the effect of this agent in cardiogenic shock complicating acute MI, vasopressin (1–4 IU/hr) was found to increase mean arterial pressure, with no adverse effects on cardiac power index, cardiac index, or wedge pressure [57]. However, a rise in mean arterial pressure does not necessarily lead to improved outcome and there are insufficient mortality data to recommend routine use of vasopressin.

## The nitric oxide story

Patients with acute MI complicated by cardiogenic shock often have an elevated temperature and white blood cell count in the absence of sepsis. Furthermore, the mean left ventricular (LV) ejection fraction of patients in the SHOCK trial was 30%, while their mean systemic vascular resistance was well within the normal range, suggesting that factors other than pure LV dysfunction were in play [58]. The constellation of these observations was consistent with the contribution of a systemic inflammatory response syndrome to the genesis and persistence of cardiogenic shock. Furthermore, experimental evidence suggested that nonspecific inhibition of NO synthase can improve recovery of function in an ischemic/reperfused heart [59].

A nonrandomized single-center study of 11 patients with persistent cardiogenic shock despite percutaneous revascularization reported marked improvement in hemodynamics after administration of L-N-monomethyl arginine (L-NMMA), a nonselective inhibitor of NO synthase; eight of these patients survived to hospital discharge [60]. A follow-up, open-label, randomized pilot study of 30 patients suggested a dramatic reduction in 30-day mortality from 67% to 29% in the 15 patients randomized to L-nitroarginine-methylester (L-NAME), another nonselective NO synthase inhibitor [61]. A multicenter Phase II dose-ranging study of L-NMMA in 79 patients with persistent shock after PCI [62] found milder and less sustained improvement in mean arterial pressure than that observed in the single center studies by Cotter. These small studies formed the basis for TRIUMPH, a large multicenter trial with a planned patient sample of 658 patients, adequate in terms of power to test the effect of the therapy on mortality [2]. The trial was terminated due to futility at the recommendation of the data safety monitoring board after 398 patients were enrolled. While improvement in systolic blood pressure was significantly greater in the L-NMMA group at 2 hours after study drug administration, there was no difference in mortality between the study groups at 30 days or 6 months (Fig. 3.1). In spite of the failure of this therapy to improve outcome, a biological effect of NO synthase inhibition was demonstrated. Further investigation involving this mechanism may thus be worthwhile, whether it might involve different doses or duration of therapy (in SHOCK-2 and TRIUMPH total duration of study drug infusion was 5 hours) or more focused inhibition of inducible NO synthase.

## Diuresis

Use of intravenous low-to medium-dose bolus of loop diuretics constitutes standard, guideline-supported therapy in patients with fluid overload and

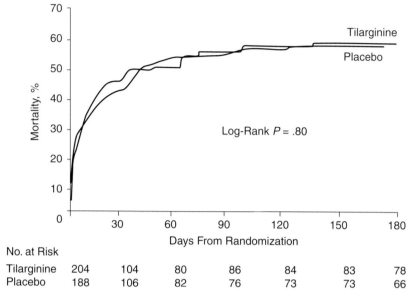

| No. at Risk | 30 | 60 | 90 | 120 | 150 | 180 |
|---|---|---|---|---|---|---|
| Tilarginine | 204 | 104 | 80 | 86 | 84 | 83 | 78 |
| Placebo | 188 | 106 | 82 | 76 | 73 | 73 | 66 |

**Fig. 3.1** Kaplan–Meier curve of mortality at 6 months in the TRIUMPH randomized trial of L-N-monomethyl arginine (Tilarginine) in patients with persistent cardiogenic shock in spite of establishment of infarct-related artery patency. Reprinted with permission from Alexander JH, Reynolds HR, Stebbins AL, et al. *JAMA* 2007;297:1657–66.

pulmonary congestion. In the setting of severe heart failure and cardiogenic shock, renal hypoperfusion also results in decrease in renal function. Indeed, acute renal failure is a frequent complication of cardiogenic shock. Management of 'fluid overload' in shock patients can be problematic. Loop diuretics have for decades been the mainstay of therapy to treat pulmonary edema and to augment urine output in the oliguric state. However, as with other pharmacotherapeutic modalities, there is a surprising paucity of data on what constitutes the optimal diuretic protocol, or for that matter, on whether in the presence of acute renal dysfunction loop diuretics alter outcome. A recent meta-analysis of trials of furosemide to treat acute renal failure of varied etiologies failed to show improvement in outcome [63]. Although diuretic therapy does not prevent or ameliorate acute renal failure, it does help to augment urine output. In this regard, several studies, not specifically in the cardiogenic shock setting, have compared continuous furosemide infusion with intermittent bolus therapy in critically ill patients. While no specific benefits with respect to kidney function have been observed, in general lower doses of furosemide are needed to maintain urine output when continuous infusion is utilized than when intermittent boluses are given. Infusion therapy is generally begun at 5 mg/hr and may be titrated as high as 20 mg/hr.

# Management of metabolic abnormalities

Patients in cardiogenic shock often develop metabolic derangements that further compromise organ function and outcome. Metabolic acidosis is a common abnormality, particularly in those with severe and prolonged cardiogenic shock. It is an anion gap acidosis that can be caused by both increased production and decreased clearance of lactic acid. An anion gap acidosis is a predictor of higher mortality in patients with acute MI even in the absence of cardiogenic shock [64]. In cardiogenic shock, the lactate excess has been shown to result primarily from an increase in lactate generation, in turn likely a result of increased production of glucose and a shift toward anaerobic glycolysis in the shock state [65]. Thus, acidosis in shock patients is generally accompanied by a marked hyperglycemic state [66]. While the acidotic state further compromises myocardial and organ function in general, the evidence supporting the use of sodium bicarbonate to correct it is weak [67]. The general principle in any acidotic patient is to correct the underlying cause, which in the case of cardiogenic shock means correcting the low-output state, to the extent possible, by means of revascularization and mechanical support of cardiac output.

Insofar as hyperglycemia is a major contributor to lactate in the shock state, lowering glucose toward the normal range with a carefully monitored insulin infusion is essential. Even in the absence of shock, hyperglycemia is associated with higher mortality in patients with acute MI, whether they are treated with pharmacologic reperfusion or percutaneous intervention. Furthermore, high levels of glucose exert a proinflammatory effect and increase oxidative stress. Insulin, on the other hand, when infused during acute MI has been shown to markedly reduce C-reactive protein in addition to reducing levels of plasminogen activator inhibitor-1 [68]. The majority of studies testing the effect of modulating glucose metabolism in the acute MI setting have used the combination of glucose–insulin–potassium (GIK). While earlier randomized studies specifically in diabetic patients with acute MI suggested benefit [69], more recent studies in diabetic as well as nondiabetic patients [70–73] failed to show any benefit of the GIK regimen in reducing mortality [71–74]. This may very well be due to the significantly higher glucose levels on study therapy in the group randomized to GIK. The large volume of fluid needed for the GIK protocol is also likely deleterious, especially for patients with any degree of heart failure [72,73]. Therefore, the GIK regimen cannot be recommended in the management of acute MI (Fig. 3.2). However, insulin administration to normalize abnormal blood glucose levels has numerous physiological benefits, including reduction of inflammation, reduction of infarct size [75], and improvement of platelet dysfunction [76]. Evidence suggests that insulin therapy decreases morbidity and mortality in critically ill patient populations in ICU settings, including those with cardiogenic shock [77]. Furthermore, in a recent observational study, patients with ST-elevation MI who presented with a serum glucose $\geq 11.0$ mmol/L had a significantly lower 30-day mortality if they were treated with an insulin regimen (Fig. 3.3) [78].

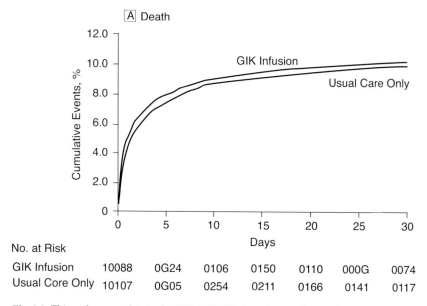

**Fig. 3.2** Thirty-day mortality in the CREATE-ECLA randomized trial of glucose–insulin–potassium in acute myocardial infarction. Reprinted with permission from Mehta SR, Yusuf S, Diaz R, et al. *JAMA* 2005;293:437–46.

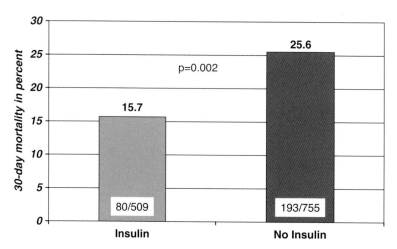

**Fig. 3.3** The relationship between insulin use and 30-day mortality in ST-elevation MI patients without known diabetes and a presenting blood glucose ≥11.0 mmol/L in the National Audit of Myocardial Infarction Project conducted in 201 hospitals in England and Wales.

Although specific data on optimal glucose targets in cardiogenic shock are not available, in a randomized trial in the surgical intensive care population on ventilatory support, lowering blood glucose with insulin infusion to the 80–110 mg/dL range lowered in-hospital mortality by 34% [79]. Although there were 39 instances of hypoglycemia among the 765 patients assigned to intensive insulin therapy, only 2 were symptomatic, and none were associated with serious sequelae. A follow-up study in patients in a medical ICU setting, however, failed to reproduce the beneficial effect of the intensive regimen [80]. Lowering blood glucose levels to 100–139 mg/dL with insulin infusion as in the Yale Protocol [81] may be more practical. Indeed, a recent trial of insulin in severe septic shock patients demonstrated that targeting to a mean blood glucose level of 112 mg/dL offers no clinical benefit over a strategy of targeting to a mean level of 151 mg/dL [82]. Thus, while randomized trials are still needed in the cardiogenic shock setting, the weight of evidence in heterogeneous critically ill populations points to a need for modest normalization of elevated blood glucose, carefully monitored insulin therapy, and potassium replacement when needed due to the known shifts that will occur.

## Arrhythmia management

Life-threatening ventricular tachyarrhythmias are a relatively common occurrence in patients in cardiogenic shock. Ventricular fibrillation or pulseless ventricular tachycardia should be treated with an unsynchronized electric shock of 200 J, to be followed immediately by a second shock of 200–300 J and subsequent shocks of 360 J in case the first ones are unsuccessful. An amiodarone bolus of 300 mg or 5 mg/kg should be administered intravenously if the arrhythmia does not respond or recurs [4]. A repeat shock should then be administered. Any acid–base and electrolyte abnormalities that might contribute to the arrhythmia should be promptly corrected. Specifically, serum potassium should be corrected to >4.0 mmol/L and magnesium to >2.0 mmol/L. Ischemia should be corrected with appropriate reperfusion and intra-aortic balloon counterpulsation therapy. Prophylactic antiarrhythmic therapy is not recommended.

Ventricular tachycardia causing hemodynamic instability (but not collapse) should be treated with a synchronized shock of 100 J followed by shocks at higher energy levels, following appropriate anesthesia or sedation with agents and doses that are associated with a lower risk of further reducing the blood pressure.

An amiodarone infusion beginning with 360 mg over 6 hours followed by 540 mg over the next 18 hours can be utilized following successful cardioversion. Further 150-mg boluses of amiodarone can be administered intravenously in case of recurrent ventricular tachycardia (or fibrillation) up to a total dose of 2.2 g in 24 hours. Lidocaine can also be utilized at doses of 75–100 mg IV per dose.

Atrial fibrillation resulting in further hemodynamic deterioration should be treated with synchronized direct current (DC) cardioversion at 200 J, again under appropriate anesthesia or conscious sedation. In case of recurrent or unresponsive atrial fibrillation, amiodarone therapy should be initiated as previously described. $\beta$-blockers and calcium channel blockers should be avoided due to their negative inotropic effects. Digoxin, which also has inotropic properties, may be used for rate control.

Symptomatic bradycardia that occurs in patients who are already receiving agents that are $\beta_1$-adrenergic agonists and who have not responded to a bolus dose of atropine 1–3 mg should be promptly treated with temporary transvenous pacing or, if this is not immediately available, transthoracic pacing. Atrioventricular synchrony may be important to maintain cardiac output, especially in patients with right ventricular infarction and shock. The effects of transvenous ventricular pacing are therefore difficult to predict.

## Sedation

Propofol, often utilized as the drug of choice in this setting, can profoundly exacerbate hypotension, in addition to having a delayed onset of action in the hypotensive patient with a low cardiac output. The sedative combination of fentanyl and a benzodiazepine such as midazolam is thus a more desirable combination for the patient with shock. The combination of ketamine and midazolam is an alternative combination utilized by anesthesiologists in this situation. Etomidate is no longer used for long term sedation since this causes long term adrenal suppression and increased mortality [83]. A single dose of etomidate has been reported to cause adrenal suppression for at least 24 hours in 50% of patients who received this drug for induction of anesthesia, but this usually resolves by 48 hours [84]. Therefore, the fact that etomidate is better tolerated during endotracheal intubation than propofol in terms of hemodynamics in patients with cardiogenic shock should be critically weighed against potential risks and alternative agents, such as midazolam. In a recently published randomized trial of dexmedetomidine vs. midazolam in a medical/surgical ICU population, the group randomized to dexmedetomidine had less delirium and shorter time to extubation than the group randomized to midazolam. However, dexmedetomidine-assigned patients were more than twice as likely to develop bradycardia. These effects could be even more pronounced in cardiogenic shock, thus, until the drug has been studied and shown to be safe in this setting, its use is not recommended [85].

## Reperfusion therapy

Fibrinolytic therapy is far less effective in achieving reperfusion in patients in cardiogenic shock than in normotensive ST-elevation MI patients [86]. Nonetheless, especially in the case of patients who present in cardiogenic shock, timely mechanical reperfusion therapy is unavailable to most. Thus, if a door-to-balloon time of more than 90 minutes is anticipated [58], the patient in shock should be treated with a fibrinolytic agent, particularly when the onset of symptoms was within the past 3 hours. All candidates for invasive care should be transferred emergently for cardiac catheterization; a fibrinolytic agent should be administered to those with ST-elevation MI and no mechanical complication who cannot undergo invasive care. IABP with fibrinolytic therapy may further improve outcomes (see Chapter 4).

## Anticoagulant and antiplatelet therapy

Unfractionated heparin rather than low-molecular-weight heparin as an adjunct to fibrinolytic therapy will facilitate subsequent invasive diagnosis and therapy. As patients may turn out to be candidates for emergent surgical revascularization, clopidogrel is not recommended prior to coronary angiography unless surgical revascularization is not an option. Once the need for surgery has been ruled out, clopidogrel 600 mg should be administered either orally or by nasogastric tube in the event that the patient is intubated. Glycoprotein IIb/IIIa inhibitor therapy increases the bleeding risk immediately after full-dose fibrinolytic therapy. If timely angiography and primary revascularization is anticipated, a glycoprotein IIb/IIIa inhibitor infusion should be initiated after an appropriate bolus either in the referring hospital or tertiary center. In the community hospital this is most likely to be one of the two small-molecule, short-acting agents, either eptifibatide or tirofiban. The ACC/AHA guidelines recommend that if based on the result of the coronary angiography, coronary artery bypass surgery is the revascularization strategy of choice, glycoprotein IIb/IIIa inhibition should be discontinued 4 hours prior to the surgical procedure, although in an emergent setting, the benefit-to-risk ratio is favorable for emergency surgery.

The direct antithrombin bivalirudin has not been studied in cardiogenic shock, but is indicated in patients with heparin-induced thrombocytopenia. In the absence of the latter, we preferentially recommend the use of heparin over bivalirudin until data are available on the safety of bivalirudin in the presence of intra-aortic balloon pump (IABP) support, an element of therapy in the majority of patients in cardiogenic shock.

## Initiation of secondary preventive agents

In general, the introduction of preventive pharmacotherapies is left to the convalescent phase in survivors of cardiogenic shock. A short-acting angiotensin-converting enzyme (ACE) inhibitor should be initiated at a very low dose agent when shock has resolved. For patients with residual severe LV dysfunction, tolerability of the first few ACE inhibitor doses (captopril 6.25 mg) can be improved by concurrent administration with inotropic or IABP support as it is being down-titrated before cessation. β-blockers should be initiated just prior to discharge with the very slow titration protocol used for chronic heart failure patients (ACC

AHA HF). Carvedilol is the preferred agent based on its vasodilatory properties. Aldosterone inhibitors should be utilized in those with an ejection fraction
<40%. Lipid-lowering therapy can be initiated at an earlier phase, at full doses
known to improve outcome in patients with acute coronary syndromes.

## Summary for clinical practice

In patients with a low-output syndrome but without hypotension, inotropic
therapy should start with the administration of dobutamine in a dosage of
2–5 μg/kg/min. Vasopressor therapy should be added, as needed if hypotension subsequently develops. In those with cardiogenic shock, dopamine beginning at doses from 5 to 10 μg/kg/min or norepinephrine beginning at doses
from 0.01–0.05 μg/kg/min (maximum dose 3 μg/kg/min) should be initiated,
recognizing that there are inadequate data to support the preferential use of
either agent. If dopamine is ineffective, norepinephrine should be substituted.
Preliminary data suggest that vasopressin may be useful in patients with prolonged shock who may have lost their catecholamine responsivity [87]. Addition
of dobutamine to a vasopressor can further increase cardiac output; however, in
the severely hypotensive patient, its ß effect may result in a fall in blood pressure.
It is useful to monitor the effects of the pharmacologic therapy by measuring
cardiac output and mixed venous oxygen saturation invasively, but titration of
inotropes and vasopressors should be determined by indices of organ perfusion (e.g. urine output) while maintaining adequate oxygenation. Levosimendan and PDEI are not first-line inotropic agents in cardiogenic shock as their
vasodilating properties (particularly bolus loading doses) result in hypotension and they require repeated monitoring of cardiac output, vascular resistance, and preload. As important as the use of inotrope and vasopressor therapy is for initial stabilization, correction of metabolic abnormalities, especially
hyperglycemia, is essential as is treatment of the underlying condition, i.e. coronary revascularization or repair of a mechanical complication.

## Mechanical ventilation in cardiogenic shock

### Effects of mechanical ventilation

The major objectives of mechanical ventilation in the setting of acute heart
failure and cardiogenic shock are to provide adequate oxygenation (oxygen saturation of 95–98% in order to ensure adequate tissue oxygenation [5]), to recruit
atelectatic lung regions, thereby decreasing shunting and improving lung compliance, to reduce the work of respiratory muscles, and finally to reduce preload
and afterload. The ESC/ESICM guidelines for management of acute heart failure emphasize the importance of maintaining adequate oxygen saturation to
maximize tissue oxygenation and prevent end-organ dysfunction and multiple
organ failure [5]. The task force on acute heart failure of the ESC, however,

also emphasized in its guidelines that "despite this intuitive approach to giving oxygen, there is little evidence available to suggest that giving increasing doses of oxygen results in an improved outcome. In fact, studies have demonstrated that hyperoxia can be associated with reduced coronary blood flow, reduced cardiac output, increased blood pressure, increased systemic vascular resistance, and a trend to higher mortality" [5,88]. Therefore, while the administration of increased concentrations of oxygen to hypoxemic patients is without question, it is unclear whether oxygen should be given to patients without evidence of hypoxemia. The minimum $FiO_2$ that results in adequate oxygen saturation (ideally 95–98% [5]) should be used when instituting mechanical ventilation in patients with cardiogenic shock.

Mechanical ventilation also leads to a reduction in respiratory muscle work and thus a reduction of oxygen consumption. Animal data suggest that 25% of the oxygen consumed in cardiogenic shock is utilized by the respiratory muscles. Accordingly, it has been shown that mechanical ventilation reduces arterial lactate levels [89].

A reduction of preload and afterload by implementation of positive end-expiratory pressure (PEEP) and positive intrathoracic pressure might improve gas exchange but has variable effects on hemodynamics. The effects of mechanical ventilation depend on the volume state of the patient. In hypovolemic patients, and in patients with right ventricular infarction, mechanical ventilation may decrease cardiac output with compensatory mechanisms like tachycardia and enhanced oxygen consumption due to the reduction in preload. Furthermore, by increasing intrathoracic pressure, the afterload for the right ventricle may increase, causing dilation of the right ventricle and a septal shift to the left, compromising LV inflow and LV mechanics. However, due to the decrease in afterload for the left ventricle, cardiac output may increase and thus mechanical ventilation may improve the function of a failing heart. The individual effects of mechanical ventilation on hemodynamics in an individual patient can, therefore, be difficult to predict.

### Indications for mechanical ventilation in acute heart failure

There is no universally accepted indication for mechanical ventilation for critically ill patients in general. Similarly, the decision to mechanically ventilate a patient in cardiogenic shock is individualized based on clinical assessment and on the chosen therapeutic plan. Pathophysiological indications for mechanical ventilation include hypoxemic as well as hypercapnic respiratory failure. If there are no other pulmonary (e.g. chronic obstructive pulmonary disease [COPD]) or cerebral diseases (e.g. stroke or hypoxic injury), hypercapnic respiratory failure is a late event in cardiogenic shock, usually resulting from progressive respiratory muscle weakness, caused by a combination of hypoxemia due to pulmonary edema and low cardiac output.

Guidelines recommend instituting invasive mechanical ventilation (with endotracheal intubation) in the case of acute heart failure–induced respiratory muscle fatigue [5] with hypercapnia, a confused state of mind and/or a decreased respiratory rate. They suggest that trials of oxygen therapy or non-invasive ventilation like continuous positive airway pressure (CPAP) or non-invasive positive pressure ventilation (NIPPV) to reverse hypoxemia. A trial of non-invasive ventilation can also be beneficial in hypercapnic respiratory failure. However, once patients exhibit a decreased respiratory rate (indicating progressive $CO_2$ narcosis), invasive mechanical ventilation should be instituted without delay, preferably via the orotracheal route. In unconscious patients, invasive mechanical ventilation should be instituted in order to prevent aspiration following gastric regurgitation. Another consideration is the need for immediate coronary intervention in a patient with pulmonary edema secondary to ST-elevation MI. Invasive mechanical ventilation in this setting assures adequate oxygenation, reduction in oxygen consumption, and stress relief for the patient via concomitantly instituted sedation and analgesia and, therefore, facilitates coronary intervention.

However, because the use of CPAP and NIPPV via face mask or helmet in acute cardiogenic pulmonary edema is associated with a significant reduction in the need for endotracheal intubation and invasive mechanical ventilation, the patient's clinical condition should be assessed early on for suitability for non-invasive mechanical ventilation (see Fig. 3.4). Several trials have examined the use of CPAP and NIPPV by face mask in patients with cardiogenic pulmonary edema, but none assessed the effects in patients with cardiogenic shock. CPAP [90] and NIPPV [91–94] improve oxygenation, decrease symptoms and signs of acute heart failure, decrease the need for endotracheal intubation, and may improve survival. Indeed, a meta-analysis suggested that the use of either CPAP or NIPPV resulted in a mortality reduction of about 50% (from 20 to 11%) [95] (Fig. 3.5). However, the 3CPO study compared therapy by oxygen mask to CPAP and NIPPV in a 1:1:1 randomization pattern in 1156 patients with cardiogenic pulmonary edema and demonstrated that non-invasive ventilation resulted in more rapid resolution of metabolic abnormalities and respiratory distress but did not improve survival at 7 or 30 days (oxygen mask 9.8% 7-day and 16.7% 30-day mortality vs. 9.5% and 15.4% in the non-invasively ventilated group, $p$ = not significant) [96]. This study also showed that NIPPV was not superior to CPAP when comparing the two modes of non-invasive ventilation directly in terms of mortality or intubation rate. Another meta-analysis suggested that the reduction in mortality is almost completely due to the beneficial effects observed in patients with COPD and not in patients with hypoxemic respiratory failure [97]. In addition, this study found that patients who were successfully managed with non-invasive ventilation had a mortality rate of 17%, compared to a mortality rate of 48% in patients who required intubation after failure of non-invasive ventilation. This high mortality rate in patients needing invasive ventilation after failure of non-invasive ventilation, which was higher than that of patients with intubation early on, reminds us that a delay in instituting invasive mechanical ventilation potentially carries a significant risk of death. Patients

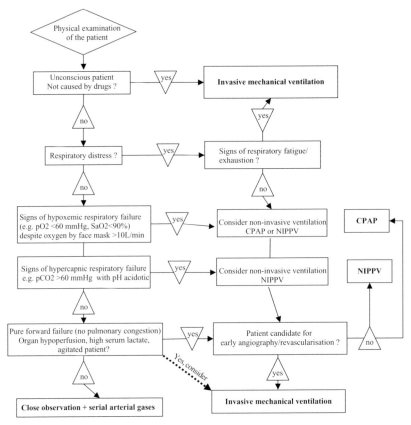

**Fig. 3.4** An algorithm for ventilation in cardiogenic shock. CPAP, continuous positive airway pressure; NIPPV, non-invasive positive pressure ventilation (augmented spontaneous ventilation, e.g. by face mask).

who are non-invasively ventilated therefore require close observation and repetitive blood gas analysis within the first hour in order to rapidly detect failure of non-invasive ventilation and thus institute adequate ventilatory support. Patients with cardiogenic shock in need of early coronary angiography and revascularization should probably be intubated early on, as a trial of non-invasive ventilation might further delay revascularization.

## Complications of invasive mechanical ventilation

Complications of invasive mechanical ventilation via endotracheal intubation include traumatic injury to the upper airway, to the lung itself (barotrauma due to excessive airway pressure), an increased risk of nosocomial, ventilator-associated pneumonia, especially with prolonged mechanical ventilation, and

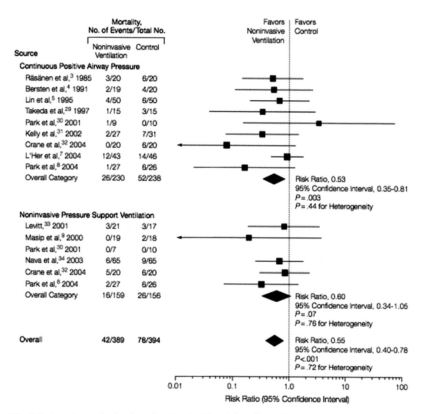

**Fig. 3.5** A meta-analysis of randomized trials of the effect of non-invasive ventilation on death in patients with acute cardiogenic pulmonary edema. (Reprinted with permission from Masip J, Roque M, Sanchez B, et al. *JAMA* 2005;294:3124–30.)

hemodynamic depression, especially with the use of high levels of PEEP. As noted previously, mechanical ventilation in hypovolemic patients or in preload-dependent situations, e.g. in patients with right ventricular infarction, might cause a reduction in preload and therefore a reduced cardiac output such that fluid administration and perhaps inotropic and vasopressor therapy may need to be temporarily increased.

## Mechanical ventilation in cardiogenic shock (see also algorithm presented in Fig. 3.4)

To date there are no large prospective randomized studies to guide us with respect to optimal timing of mechanical ventilation in patients with cardiogenic shock. Animal data suggest that artificial ventilation substantially decreases the severity of lactic acidosis and prolongs survival [89]. The mortality rate of patients with acute MI requiring invasive mechanical ventilation is high whether or not they present in cardiogenic shock [98]. It is higher in patients with a $PaO_2/FiO_2$ <200 on admission and related to an APACHE II score above 29, acute renal failure and a low initial LV ejection fraction. However, in 1999 a small study reported that patients with MI and cardiogenic shock refractory to pharmacotherapy (dobutamine and dopamine) and requiring IABP are more likely to survive when also treated with mechanical ventilation with PEEP (10 cm $H_2O$) [99]. The study was too small to elucidate potential mechanisms behind this observed survival benefit, and the large survival benefit could not be reproduced in observational studies [100]. However, in light of the above-elucidated mechanisms, it appears that mechanical ventilation in cardiogenic shock may have a number of advantages and that timely institution may save lives. Special attention is directed to the patient with cardiogenic shock and respiratory failure in need of coronary revascularization.

In all other patients with cardiogenic shock (e.g. those who are not candidates for immediate coronary intervention), respiratory failure should be managed similar to acute heart failure. Accordingly, invasive mechanical ventilation should be instituted in situations where non-invasive ventilation does not reverse hypoxemia, relieve respiratory distress (decrease work of breathing), provide adequate ventilation, and prevent respiratory muscle fatigue. This implies that non-invasive ventilatory support should be considered before proceeding to endotracheal intubation in all cardiogenic shock patients who are not candidates for coronary angiography/revascularization. The indication to mechanically ventilate patients with cardiogenic shock and pure low-output state and severe lactic acidosis, without pulmonary congestion, is also a controversial issue. In fact, the reduction in respiratory muscle work and therefore in respiratory muscle oxygen consumption might be beneficial in patients with severe lactic acidosis because of tissue hypoperfusion, redirecting oxygen from the respiratory muscles to other tissues. However, these patients with pure forward failure are most at risk for developing negative effects of mechanical ventilation—relative "hypovolemia" in previously hypervolemic patients, following administration of sedative and analgesic drugs and preload reduction. This can be partially circumvented by increasing volume administration immediately prior to intubation.

## Choice of ventilation modality

Unlike the situation in septic shock, no studies have compared different ventilator regimens in cardiogenic shock. Regarding non-invasive ventilation, the 3CPO study found no difference in mortality and intubation rate between patients who were treated via non-invasive ventilation either by CPAP or by NIPPV. Therefore in patients with cardiogenic pulmonary edema, NIPPV and CPAP seem to be equivalent. In general, however, if patients are hypercapnic and hypoxemic, NIPPV rather than CPAP should be used, as NIPPV might unload the respiratory muscles and support ventilation and $CO_2$ elimination more than CPAP might do.

If invasive mechanical ventilation is necessary, patients should probably be treated in a manner that is analogous to the situation in septic shock. High plateau pressures should be avoided in order to minimize the risk of baro-trauma, and ventilation should be started with tidal volumes of 6 mL/kg ideal body weight and then titrated according to clinical needs, provided that plateau/peak pressures can be kept below 30 mbar. PEEP should be instituted to optimize alveolar recruitment; however, high levels of PEEP should be avoided to minimize the risk of further deterioration of cardiovascular function.

Mechanical ventilation using tidal volumes of no more than 6 mL/kg pre-dicted body weight has been shown to reduce plasma levels of systemic inflammation and reduce mortality when compared to a tidal volume of 12 mL/kg predicted body weight in patients with acute respiratory distress syn-drome (ARDS) [101]. Because an international study in a mixed population of ICU patients with mechanical ventilation, including pulmonary edema, COPD exacerbation, congestive heart failure, and other etiologies, established a rela-tionship between high tidal volume and high plateau pressures and mortality [102], it appears prudent to institute this "protective ventilation strategy" even in patients without ARDS, until specific trials are available. Thus, patients with cardiogenic shock should also be ventilated using the principles of "protective ventilation" as soon as possible after the initial stabilization period following endotracheal intubation.

Reduction in tidal volume, by decreasing intrathoracic pressures, may also cause an increase in cardiac output via an increase of venous return and a reduction in right ventricular afterload. However, any detrimental effects of hypercapnia on cardiac output and organ function should be avoided as patients ventilated with low tidal volumes were found to have an increased need for hemodialysis [103]. Therefore it is suggested to keep the pH in a normal range, especially in the initial phases of shock in as much as acidosis results in diminished adrenergic responsivity. If in later phases of shock the principles of "permissive hypercapnia" are to be applied in order to prevent high plateau pressures then the pH should be maintained above 7.15–7.20 such as in the case of acute respiratory distress syndrome complicating critical illness [104]. Whether this threshold is similarly valid in patients with cardiogenic shock has, however, never been investigated. Reduction in tidal volume can cause dere-cruitment of alveoles and atelectasis necessitating an increase in PEEP and $FiO_2$ to assure adequate oxygenation. Consequently it may be necessary to increase fluid administration and vasopressor/inotropic therapy to counteract the neg-ative effects on cardiac output of higher PEEP levels. Obviously, this is likely to be better tolerated by patients with normal cardiac function than by patients in cardiogenic shock. In this context, a strategy of high PEEP/low $FiO_2$ (average PEEP level 13.2 ± 3.5 cm $H_2O$) to improve oxygenation in patients with a tidal volume of not more than 6 mL/kg was not more beneficial than a strategy of lower PEEP (average PEEP level 8.3 ± 3.2 cm $H_2O$) and higher $FiO_2$ in terms of mortality [105]. Given the potential negative effects of high PEEP levels on cardiovascular function, cardiogenic shock patients should not be ventilated with high levels of PEEP unless severe oxygenation failure necessitates maximum levels of $FiO_2$ and PEEP. Thus, hemodynamic as well as respiratory variables must be considered when reducing the tidal volume in an individual patient with cardiogenic shock.

## Controlled ventilation or spontaneous breathing?

Whenever possible, spontaneous ventilation should be supported by the respirator and spontaneous modes of ventilation are preferable to controlled modes of ventilation. Patients must be ventilated using a controlled mode of ventilation immediately after intubation, given the effects of sedatives, analgesics, and neuromuscular blocking agents used during intubation. In this situation the ventilator should be initially set to a PEEP of $\geq 5$, a tidal volume of 6mL/kg (provided that peak airway pressures are kept below 30 cm $H_2O$ and that respiratory acidosis does not occur), an $FiO_2$ of 100% with a respiratory rate of 12–15 per minute in order to provide adequate oxygenation and $CO_2$ elimination. Thereafter the settings should be adapted to individual needs according to the principles elucidated above.

Spontaneous forms of mechanical ventilation should be applied as soon as hemodynamic stability allows progressive reduction of sedating agents and awakening of the patient. Given that patient–respirator asynchrony and agitation of the patient may occur upon down-titration of sedation and have detrimental consequences in patients with cardiogenic shock, the positive effects of spontaneous modes of ventilation (redistribution of tidal volume, reduction of atelectatic regions in the dependent parts of the lungs) must be balanced against the negative effects. Nevertheless, mechanical ventilation should be discontinued as soon as possible to avoid negative effects (e.g. ventilator/endotracheal tube–associated pneumonia); weaning from mechanical ventilation and adaptation of sedation and analgesia to individual needs should begin within the first 24 hours given hemodynamic, respiratory, and metabolic stability.

## Weaning from mechanical ventilation

There are no specific studies analyzing weaning from mechanical ventilation in patients with cardiogenic shock or patients with acute MI. Nevertheless, as in septic shock, it is prudent to wean from mechanical ventilation following an institutionalized weaning protocol; sedation of the patient should be monitored using a sedation scale (e.g. Sedation Agitation Scale (SAS) [106], Richmond Agitation Sedation scale (RASS) [107]) to avoid administration of excessive sedative drugs. In general the lowest amount of sedative drugs to obtain the desired sedation depth should be used. Furthermore, all patients should be evaluated daily for their readiness to wean. Patients can be considered to be ready for wean if they fulfill the following criteria: (1) clear evidence of reversal or stability of the cause of acute ventilatory failure; (2) adequate gas exchange indicated by a $PaO_2/FiO_2$ ratio above 150–200 at a PEEP of 5–8 cm $H_2O$; (3) pH above 7.25; (4) cardiovascular stability (no active myocardial ischemia or hypotension necessitating vasopressor drug therapy); and (5) ability to make an inspiratory effort [108].

The mental status of the patient must be adequate to allow for a full inspiratory effort on command. The required cardiovascular stability suggests that the patient should be weaned from the IABP before weaning from the ventilator. However, there are conflicting views and no trials on this subject. It has been argued that the IABP in place might help wean the patient off the ventilator. We recommend that, in general, patients be weaned from the IABP before the ventilator in light of the need for intensive physiotherapy after extubation to avoid alveolar atelectasis and promote removal of endotracheal secretion, which is hindered by an IABP in place. Continued inotropic therapy may facilitate successful weaning from the respirator in those with persistent severe LV dysfunction.

Once a patient is considered ready to wean, we recommend a spontaneous breathing trial as the above criteria alone do not predict successful weaning from the ventilator. This spontaneous breathing trial can be performed using a T-tube with CPAP or a T-tube with low levels of pressure support (5–8 cm $H_2O$) for 30 minutes. During this trial, the clinical condition of the patient (tachycardia, tachypnea >35/min, hypotension, hypertension, diaphoresis, signs of distress, hypoxemia $SaO_2$ <90%) and the shallow breathing index (the ratio between tidal volume and respiratory rate) should be closely monitored. If abnormalities in any of these parameters are observed (the shallow breathing index should be below 105 L/min), the patient is considered to have failed the spontaneous breathing trial. In this case, mechanical ventilatory support that allows nonfatiguing breathing should be reinstituted and readiness to wean and a spontaneous breathing trial should be reassessed daily.

If a spontaneous breathing trial is unsuccessful, correction of reversible causes of failure should be attempted. This includes fluid restriction, administration of bronchodilators if the patient exhibits signs of bronchospasm or has known obstructive pulmonary disease, physiotherapy/mobilization in order to prevent recurrent atelectasis, and optimization of nutritional status.

Successful completion of the spontaneous breathing trial is highly predictive of successful extubation. However, the reintubation rate varies with the underlying disease and has been reported to occur in 2–25% of patients despite a successful spontaneous breathing trial [109–112]. The success of extubation does not increase with a longer duration of spontaneous breathing trial [113] and does not depend on whether pressure support or CPAP only is applied when performing the trial [112]. The mortality of patients requiring reintubation is higher than that of patients with successful extubation and increases with the delay between extubation and reintubation [114]. At times it may be necessary to institute non-invasive ventilation by face mask immediately after extubation in order to prevent respiratory failure ("NIPPV as a method to wean").

## Summary for clinical practice (see also algorithm in Fig. 3.4)

In a patient with cardiogenic shock the most common indications for mechanical ventilation are respiratory failure and securing the airway to prevent aspiration in those who are unconscious. Low cardiac output with severe lactic acidosis may also warrant mechanical ventilation. In patients with hypoxemic respiratory failure, a trial of non-invasive mechanical ventilation is warranted as this might prevent the need for invasive mechanical ventilation with its associated complications. CPAP and NIPPV seem to be equivalent in this setting. However, if patients are hypercapnic as well as hypoxemic, NIPPV should probably be utilized. Close observation is required to immediately detect signs of respiratory fatigue in patients on a non-invasive ventilation trial. If non-invasive ventilation does not reverse hypoxemia, relieve respiratory distress (decrease work of breathing), provide adequate ventilation, and prevent respiratory muscle fatigue, the patient should be intubated and ventilated invasively. In patients with respiratory failure who are candidates for immediate revascularization, invasive mechanical ventilation should be instituted to avoid further delay of revascularization and facilitate the intervention.

In case of invasive mechanical ventilation, ventilation should start with a PEEP of 5 or above, a tidal volume of 6 mL/kg body weight, an $FiO_2$ of 100% with a respiratory rate of 12–15 per minute in order to guarantee adequate oxygenation, provided that peak airway pressures are kept below 30 cm $H_2O$ and $CO_2$ can be adequately eliminated to avoid the negative consequences of high airway pressures on one side and respiratory acidosis on the other side on hemodynamics. Thereafter the settings should be adapted to individual needs. The principles of a protective ventilation strategy should be applied (tidal volume of not more than 6 mL/kg body weight) whenever possible, taking care to avoid negative effects of hypercapnia and acidosis on hemodynamics. High levels of PEEP should also be avoided to avoid negative effects on hemodynamics unless it is required for progressive hypoxemic failure. Spontaneous ventilation should be allowed as soon as hemodynamic and respiratory stability are achieved. The readiness to be weaned from the ventilator should be assessed daily and follow institutionalized weaning protocols. A spontaneous breathing trial for 30 min should precede extubation, as successfully passing this test will improve the likelihood of a successful extubation. Failure to pass such a test should lead to reinstitution of mechanical ventilation and reassessment the next day.

## References

1. Sleeper L, Jacobs A, LeJemtel T, Webb J, Hochman J. A mortality model and severity scoring system for cardiogenic shock complicating acute myocardial infarction. *Circulation* 2000;102:11–795.

2. Alexander JH, Reynolds HR, Stebbins AL, et al. Effect of tilarginine acetate in patients with acute myocardial infarction and cardiogenic shock: the TRIUMPH randomized controlled trial. *JAMA* 2007;297:1657–66.

3. Sakr Y, Reinhart K, Vincent JL, et al. Does dopamine administration in shock influence outcome? Results of the Sepsis Occurrence in Acutely Ill Patients (SOAP) study. *Crit Care Med* 2006;34:589–97.

4. Antman EM, Anbe DT, Armstrong PW, et al. ACC/AHA guidelines for the management of patients with ST-elevation myocardial infarction: a report of the American College of Cardiology/American Heart Association Task Force on Practice Guidelines (Committee to Revise the 1999 Guidelines for the Management of Patients with Acute Myocardial Infarction). *Circulation* 2004;110:e82–292.

5. Nieminen MS, Bohm M, Cowie MR, et al. Executive summary of the guidelines on the diagnosis and treatment of acute heart failure: the Task Force on Acute Heart Failure of the European Society of Cardiology. *Eur Heart J* 2005;26:384–416.

6. Stamm C, Friehs I, Cowan DB, et al. Dopamine treatment of postischemic contractile dysfunction rapidly induces calcium-dependent pro-apoptotic signaling. *Circulation* 2002;106:I290–8.

7. Richard C, Ricome JL, Rimailho A, Bottineau G, Auzepy P. Combined hemodynamic effects of dopamine and dobutamine in cardiogenic shock. *Circulation* 1983;67:620–6.

8. Schulz R, Rose J, Martin C, Brodde OE, Heusch G. Development of short-term myocardial hibernation. Its limitation by the severity of ischemia and inotropic stimulation. *Circulation* 1993;88:684–95.

9. Leier CV, Binkley PF. Parenteral inotropic support for advanced congestive heart failure. *Prog Cardiovasc Dis* 1998;41:207–24.

10. Lowes BD, Tsvetkova T, Eichhorn EJ, Gilbert EM, Bristow MR. Milrinone versus dobutamine in heart failure subjects treated chronically with carvedilol. *Int J Cardiol* 2001;81:141–9.

11. Denton MD, Chertow GM, Brady HR. "Renal-dose" dopamine for the treatment of acute renal failure: scientific rationale, experimental studies and clinical trials. *Kidney Int* 1996;50:4–14.

12. Bellomo R, Chapman M, Finfer S, Hickling K, Myburgh J. Low-dose dopamine in patients with early renal dysfunction: a placebo-controlled randomised trial. Australian and New Zealand Intensive Care Society (ANZICS) Clinical Trials Group. *Lancet* 2000;356:2139–43.

13. Tune JD, Richmond KN, Gorman MW, Feigl EO. Control of coronary blood flow during exercise. *Exp Biol Med (Maywood)* 2002;227:238–50.

14. De Backer D, Creteur J, Silva E, Vincent JL. Effects of dopamine, norepinephrine, and epinephrine on the splanchnic circulation in septic shock: which is best? *Crit Care Med* 2003;31:1659–67.

15. Communal C, Singh K, Pimentel DR, Colucci WS. Norepinephrine stimulates apoptosis in adult rat ventricular myocytes by activation of the beta-adrenergic pathway. *Circulation* 1998;98:1329–34.

16. Jones CJ, DeFily DV, Patterson JL, Chilian WM. Endothelium-dependent relaxation competes with alpha 1- and alpha 2-adrenergic constriction in the canine epicardial coronary microcirculation. *Circulation* 1993;87:1264–74.

17. Singh K, Xiao L, Remondino A, Sawyer DB, Colucci WS. Adrenergic regulation of cardiac myocyte apoptosis. *J Cell Physiol* 2001;189:257–65.

18. Annane D, Vignon P, Renault A, et al. Norepinephrine plus dobutamine versus epinephrine alone for management of septic shock: a randomised trial. *Lancet* 2007;370:676–84.

19. Myburgh JA, Higgins A, Jovanovska A, Lipman J, Ramakrishnan N, Santamaria J, CAT Study investigators. A comparison of epinephrine and norepinephrine in critically ill patients. *Intensive Care Med* 2008;34:2226–34.

20. Cuffe MS, Califf RM, Adams KF Jr, et al. Short-term intravenous milrinone for acute exacerbation of chronic heart failure: a randomized controlled trial. *JAMA* 2002;287:1541–7.

21. Felker GM, Benza RL, Chandler AB, et al. Heart failure etiology and response to milrinone in decompensated heart failure: results from the OPTIME-CHF study. *J Am Coll Cardiol* 2003;41:997–1003.

22. Fuhrmann J. Levosimendan in advanced cardiogenic shock improved survival compared with enoximone. *Circulation* 2004;A:2253.

23. Fuhrmann JT, Schmeisser A, Schulze MR, et al. Levosimendan is superior to enoximone in refractory cardiogenic shock complicating acute myocardial infarction. *Crit Care Med* 2008;36:2257–66.

24. Toller WG, Stranz C. Levosimendan, a new inotropic and vasodilator agent. *Anesthesiology* 2006;104:556–69.

25. Hasenfuss G, Pieske B, Castell M, et al. Influence of the novel inotropic agent levosimendan on isometric tension and calcium cycling in failing human myocardium. *Circulation* 1998;98:2141–7.

26. Boknik P, Neumann J, Kaspareit G, et al. Mechanisms of the contractile effects of levosimendan in the mammalian heart. *J Pharmacol Exp Ther* 1997;280:277–83.

27. Gross GJ, Peart JN. KATP channels and myocardial preconditioning: an update. *Am J Physiol Heart Circ Physiol* 2003;285:H921–30.

28. Mebazaa A, Nieminen MS, Packer M, et al. Levosimendan vs dobutamine for patients with acute decompensated heart failure: the SURVIVE Randomized Trial. *JAMA* 2007;297:1883–91.

29. Moiseyev VS, Poder P, Andrejevs N, et al. Safety and efficacy of a novel calcium sensitizer, levosimendan, in patients with left ventricular failure due to an acute myocardial infarction. A randomized, placebo-controlled, double-blind study (RUSSLAN). *Eur Heart J* 2002;23:1422–32.

30. Follath F, Cleland JG, Just H, et al. Efficacy and safety of intravenous levosimendan compared with dobutamine in severe low-output heart failure (the LIDO study): a randomised double-blind trial. *Lancet* 2002;360:196–202.

31. Delle Karth G, Buberl A, Geppert A, et al. Hemodynamic effects of a continuous infusion of levosimendan in critically ill patients with cardiogenic shock requiring catecholamines. *Acta Anaesthesiol Scand* 2003;47:1251–6.

32. Rokyta R Jr, Pechman V. The effects of levosimendan on global haemodynamics in patients with cardiogenic shock. *Neuro Endocrinol Lett* 2006;27:121–7.

33. Garcia-Gonzalez MJ, Dominguez-Rodriguez A, Ferrer-Hita JJ. Utility of levosimendan, a new calcium sensitizing agent, in the treatment of cardiogenic shock due to myocardial stunning in patients with ST-elevation myocardial infarction: a series of cases. *J Clin Pharmacol* 2005;45:704–8.

34. Russ MA, Prondzinksy R, Christoph A, et al. Hemodynamic improvement following levosimendan treatment in patients with acute myocardial infarction and cardiogenic shock. *Crit Care Med* 2007;35:2732–9.

35. Garcia-Gonzalez MJ, Dominguez-Rodriguez A, Ferrer-Hita JJ, Abreu-Gonzalez P, Munoz MB. Cardiogenic shock after primary percutaneous coronary intervention: effects of levosimendan compared with dobutamine on haemodynamics. *Eur J Heart Fail* 2006;8:723–8.

36. Schwarte LA, Picker O, Bornstein SR, Fournell A, Scheeren TW. Levosimendan is superior to milrinone and dobutamine in selectively increasing microvascular gastric mucosal oxygenation in dogs. *Crit Care Med* 2005;33:135–42; discussion 246–7.

37. Coopersmith CM. Levosimendan and gut mucosal blood flow—not all inotropes are created equal. *Crit Care Med* 2005;33:246–7.

38. Cleland JG, Freemantle N, Coletta AP, Clark AL. Clinical trials update from the American Heart Association: REPAIR-AMI, ASTAMI, JELIS, MEGA, REVIVE-II, SURVIVE, and PROACTIVE. *Eur J Heart Fail* 2006;8:105–10.

39. Lindner KH, Dirks B, Strohmenger HU, et al. Randomised comparison of epinephrine and vasopressin in patients with out-of-hospital ventricular fibrillation. *Lancet* 1997;349:535–7.

40. Overgaard C, Dzavik V. Inotropes and vasopressors: review of physiology and clinical use in cardiovascular disease. *Circulation* 2008;118:1047–56.

41. Hupf H, Grimm D, Riegger GA, Schunkert H. Evidence for a vasopressin system in the rat heart. *Circ Res* 1999;84:365–70.

42. Guillon G, Grazzini E, Andrez M, et al. Vasopressin: a potent autocrine/paracrine regulator of mammal adrenal functions. *Endocr Res* 1998;24:703–10.

43. Tayama E, Ueda T, Shojima T, et al. Arginine vasopressin is an ideal drug after cardiac surgery for the management of low systemic vascular resistant hypotension concomitant with pulmonary hypertension. *Interact Cardiovasc Thorac Surg* 2007;6:715–19.

44. Huter L, Schwarzkopf K, Preussler NP, et al. Effects of arginine vasopressin on oxygenation and haemodynamics during one-lung ventilation in an animal model. *Anaesth Intensive Care* 2008;36:162–6.

45. Liard JF. Vasopressin-induced changes in cardiac vagal tone and oxygen consumption in dogs. *Am J Physiol* 1994;266:R838–49.

46. Salzman AL, Vromen A, Denenberg A, Szabo C. K(ATP)-channel inhibition improves hemodynamics and cellular energetics in hemorrhagic shock. *Am J Physiol* 1997;272:H688–94.

47. Kusano E, Tian S, Umino T, et al. Arginine vasopressin inhibits interleukin-1 beta-stimulated nitric oxide and cyclic guanosine monophosphate production via the V1 receptor in cultured rat vascular smooth muscle cells. *J Hypertens* 1997;15:627–32.

48. Hamu Y, Kanmura Y, Tsuneyoshi I, Yoshimura N. The effects of vasopressin on endotoxin-induced attenuation of contractile responses in human gastroepiploic arteries in vitro. *Anesth Analg* 1999;88:542–8.

49. Landry DW, Oliver JA. The pathogenesis of vasodilatory shock. *N Engl J Med* 2001;345:588–95.

50. Sharshar T, Carlier R, Blanchard A, et al. Depletion of neurohypophyseal content of vasopressin in septic shock. *Crit Care Med* 2002;30:497–500.

51. Landry DW, Levin HR, Gallant EM, et al. Vasopressin deficiency contributes to the vasodilation of septic shock. *Circulation* 1997;95:1122–5.
52. Day TA, Randle JC, Renaud LP. Opposing alpha- and beta-adrenergic mechanisms mediate dose-dependent actions of noradrenaline on supraoptic vasopressin neurones in vivo. *Brain Res* 1985;358:171–9.
53. Holmes CL, Walley KR, Chittock DR, Lehman T, Russell JA. The effects of vasopressin on hemodynamics and renal function in severe septic shock: a case series. *Intensive Care Med* 2001;27:1416–21.
54. Dunser MW, Mayr AJ, Ulmer H, et al. Arginine vasopressin in advanced vasodilatory shock: a prospective, randomized, controlled study. *Circulation* 2003;107:2313–19.
55. Okamura T, Ayajiki K, Fujioka H, Toda N. Mechanisms underlying arginine vasopressin-induced relaxation in monkey isolated coronary arteries. *J Hypertens* 1999;17:673–8.
56. Mayr V, Luckner G, Jochberger S, et al. Arginine vasopressin in advanced cardiovascular failure during the post-resuscitation phase after cardiac arrest. *Resuscitation* 2007;72:35–44.
57. Jolly S, Newton G, Horlick E, et al. Effect of vasopressin on hemodynamics in patients with refractory cardiogenic shock complicating acute myocardial infarction. *Am J Cardiol* 2005;96:1617–20.
58. Hochman JS. Cardiogenic shock complicating acute myocardial infarction: expanding the paradigm. *Circulation* 2003;107:2998–3002.
59. Schulz R, Wambolt R. Inhibition of nitric oxide synthesis protects the isolated working rabbit heart from ischaemia-reperfusion injury. *Cardiovasc Res* 1995;30:432–9.
60. Cotter G, Kaluski E, Blatt A, et al. L-NMMA (a nitric oxide synthase inhibitor) is effective in the treatment of cardiogenic shock. *Circulation* 2000;101:1358–61.
61. Cotter G, Kaluski E, Milo O, et al. LINCS: L-NAME (a NO synthase inhibitor) in the treatment of refractory cardiogenic shock: a prospective randomized study. *Eur Heart J* 2003;24:1287–95.
62. Dzavik V, Cotter G, Reynolds HR, et al. Effect of nitric oxide synthase inhibition on haemodynamics and outcome of patients with persistent cardiogenic shock complicating acute myocardial infarction: a phase II dose-ranging study. *Eur Heart J* 2007;28:1109–16.
63. Ho KM, Sheridan DJ. Meta-analysis of frusemide to prevent or treat acute renal failure. *BMJ* 2006;333:420.
64. Sahu A, Cooper HA, Panza JA. The initial anion gap is a predictor of mortality in acute myocardial infarction. *Coron Artery Dis* 2006;17:409–12.
65. Chiolero RL, Revelly JP, Leverve X, et al. Effects of cardiogenic shock on lactate and glucose metabolism after heart surgery. *Crit Care Med* 2000;28:3784–91.
66. Stacpoole PW, Wright EC, Baumgartner TG, et al. Natural history and course of acquired lactic acidosis in adults. DCA-Lactic Acidosis Study Group. *Am J Med* 1994;97:47–54.
67. Cooper DJ, Walley KR, Wiggs BR, Russell JA. Bicarbonate does not improve hemodynamics in critically ill patients who have lactic acidosis. A prospective, controlled clinical study. *Ann Intern Med* 1990;112:492–8.
68. Chaudhuri A, Janicke D, Wilson MF, et al. Anti-inflammatory and profibrinolytic effect of insulin in acute ST-segment-elevation myocardial infarction. *Circulation* 2004;109:849–54.

69. Malmberg K, Ryden L, Hamsten A, et al. Effects of insulin treatment on cause-specific one-year mortality and morbidity in diabetic patients with acute myocardial infarction. DIGAMI Study Group. Diabetes Insulin-Glucose in Acute Myocardial Infarction. *Eur Heart J* 1996;17:1337–44.

70. Diaz R, Paolasso EA, Piegas LS, et al. Metabolic modulation of acute myocardial infarction. The ECLA (Estudios Cardiologicos Latinoamerica) Collaborative Group. *Circulation* 1998;98:2227–34.

71. Ceremuzynski L, Budaj A, Czepiel A, et al. Low-dose glucose-insulin-potassium is ineffective in acute myocardial infarction: results of a randomized multicenter Pol-GIK trial. *Cardiovasc Drugs Ther* 1999;13:191–200.

72. Timmer JR, Svilaas T, Ottervanger JP, et al. Glucose-insulin-potassium infusion in patients with acute myocardial infarction without signs of heart failure: the Glucose-Insulin-Potassium Study (GIPS)-II. *J Am Coll Cardiol* 2006;47:1730–1.

73. van der Horst IC, Zijlstra F, van't Hof AW, et al. Glucose-insulin-potassium infusion inpatients treated with primary angioplasty for acute myocardial infarction: the glucose-insulin-potassium study: a randomized trial. *J Am Coll Cardiol* 2003;42:784–91.

74. Mehta SR, Yusuf S, Diaz R, et al. Effect of glucose-insulin-potassium infusion on mortality in patients with acute ST-segment elevation myocardial infarction: the CREATE-ECLA randomized controlled trial. *JAMA* 2005;293:437–46.

75. Hansen TK, Thiel S, Wouters PJ, Christiansen JS, Van den Berghe G. Intensive insulin therapy exerts antiinflammatory effects in critically ill patients and counteracts the adverse effect of low mannose-binding lectin levels. *J Clin Endocrinol Metab* 2003;88:1082–8.

76. Worthley MI, Holmes AS, Willoughby SR, et al. The deleterious effects of hyperglycemia on platelet function in diabetic patients with acute coronary syndromes mediation by superoxide production, resolution with intensive insulin administration. *J Am Coll Cardiol* 2007;49:304–10.

77. Langley J, Adams G. Insulin-based regimens decrease mortality rates in critically ill patients: a systematic review. *Diabetes Metab Res Rev* 2007;23:184–92.

78. Weston C, Walker L, Birkhead J. Early impact of insulin treatment on mortality for hyperglycaemic patients without known diabetes who present with an acute coronary syndrome. *Heart* 2007;93:1542–6.

79. van den Berghe G, Wouters P, Weekers F, et al. Intensive insulin therapy in the critically ill patients. *N Engl J Med* 2001;345:1359–67.

80. Van den Berghe G, Wilmer A, Hermans G, et al. Intensive insulin therapy in the medical ICU. *N Engl J Med* 2006;354:449–61.

81. Goldberg PA, Siegel MD, Sherwin RS, et al. Implementation of a safe and effective insulin infusion protocol in a medical intensive care unit. *Diabetes Care* 2004;27:461–7.

82. Brunkhorst FM, Engel C, Bloos F, et al. Intensive insulin therapy and pentastarch resuscitation in severe sepsis. *N Engl J Med* 2008;358:125–39.

83. Wagner RL, White PF, Kan PB, Rosenthal MH, Feldman D. Inhibition of adrenal steroidogenesis by the anesthetic etomidate. *N Engl J Med* 1984;310:1415–21.

84. Vinclair M, Broux C, Faure P, et al. Duration of adrenal inhibition following a single dose of etomidate in critically ill patients. *Intensive Care Med* 2008;34:714–9.

85. Riker RR, Shehabi Y, Bokesch PM, et al. For the SEDCOM (Safety and Efficacy of Dexmedetomidine Compared With Midazolam) Study Group. Dexmedetomidine vs. midazolam for sedation of critically ill patients. A randomized Trial. *JAMA* 2009;301:489–499.

86. Levine GN, Hochman JS. Thrombolysis in acute myocardial infarction complicated by cardiogenic shock. *J Thromb Thrombolysis* 1995;2:11–20.

87. Rozenfeld V, Cheng JW. The role of vasopressin in the treatment of vasodilation in shock states. *Ann Pharmacother* 2000;34:250–4.

88. Rawles JM, Kenmure AC. Controlled trial of oxygen in uncomplicated myocardial infarction. *Br Med J* 1976;1:1121–3.

89. Aubier M, Viires N, Syllie G, Mozes R, Roussos C. Respiratory muscle contribution to lactic acidosis in low cardiac output. *Am Rev Respir Dis* 1982;126:648–52.

90. Pang D, Keenan SP, Cook DJ, Sibbald WJ. The effect of positive pressure airway support on mortality and the need for intubation in cardiogenic pulmonary edema: a systematic review. *Chest* 1998;114:1185–92.

91. Bersten AD, Holt AW, Vedig AE, Skowronski GA, Baggoley CJ. Treatment of severe cardiogenic pulmonary edema with continuous positive airway pressure delivered by face mask. *N Engl J Med* 1991;325:1825–30.

92. Masip J, Betbese AJ, Paez J, et al. Non-invasive pressure support ventilation versus conventional oxygen therapy in acute cardiogenic pulmonary oedema: a randomised trial. *Lancet* 2000;356:2126–32.

93. Mehta S, Jay GD, Woolard RH, et al. Randomized, prospective trial of bilevel versus continuous positive airway pressure in acute pulmonary edema. *Crit Care Med* 1997;25:620–8.

94. Park M, Sangean MC, Volpe Mde S, et al. Randomized, prospective trial of oxygen, continuous positive airway pressure, and bilevel positive airway pressure by face mask in acute cardiogenic pulmonary edema. *Crit Care Med* 2004;32:2407–15.

95. Masip J, Roque M, Sanchez B, et al. Noninvasive ventilation in acute cardiogenic pulmonary edema: systematic review and meta-analysis. *JAMA* 2005;294:3124–30.

96. Gray A, Goodacre S, Newby DE, et al. Noninvasive ventilation in acute cardiogenic pulmonary edema. *N Engl J Med* 2008;359:142–51.

97. Peter JV, Moran JL, Phillips-Hughes J, Warn D. Noninvasive ventilation in acute respiratory failure—a meta-analysis update. *Crit Care Med* 2002;30:555–62.

98. Lesage A, Ramakers M, Daubin C, et al. Complicated acute myocardial infarction requiring mechanical ventilation in the intensive care unit: prognostic factors of clinical outcome in a series of 157 patients. *Crit Care Med* 2004;32:100–5.

99. Kontoyannis DA, Nanas JN, Kontoyannis SA, Stamatelopoulos SF, Moulopoulos SD. Mechanical ventilation in conjunction with the intra-aortic balloon pump improves the outcome of patients in profound cardiogenic shock. *Intensive Care Med* 1999;25:835–8.

100. Koreny M, Heinz G, Geppert A, et al. Mechanical ventilation and intra-aortic counterpulsation in cardiogenic shock. *Intensive Care Med* 2000;26:356–7.

101. Ventilation with lower tidal volumes as compared with traditional tidal volumes for acute lung injury and the acute respiratory distress syndrome. The Acute Respiratory Distress Syndrome Network. *N Engl J Med* 2000;342:1301–8.

102. Esteban A, Anzueto A, Frutos F, et al. Characteristics and outcomes in adult patients receiving mechanical ventilation: a 28-day international study. *JAMA* 2002;287:345–55.

103. Stewart TE, Meade MO, Cook DJ, et al. Evaluation of a ventilation strategy to prevent barotrauma in patients at high risk for acute respiratory distress syndrome. Pressure- and Volume-Limited Ventilation Strategy Group. *N Engl J Med* 1998;338:355–61.

104. Putensen C. Principles of mechanical ventilation. In Kuhlen R, Moreno R, Ranieri M, and Rhodes A (eds). *25 years of Progress and Innovation in Intensive Care Medicine.* 101–108.

105. Brower RG, Lanken PN, MacIntyre N, et al. Higher versus lower positive end-expiratory pressures in patients with the acute respiratory distress syndrome. *N Engl J Med* 2004;351:327–36.

106. Riker RR, Picard JT, Fraser GL. Prospective evaluation of the Sedation-Agitation Scale for adult critically ill patients. *Crit Care Med* 1999;27:1325–9

107. Sessler CN, Gosnell MS, Grap MJ, et al. The Richmond Agitation-Sedation Scale: validity and reliability in adult intensive care unit patients. *Am J Respir Crit Care Med* 2002;166:1338–44

108. MacIntyre NR, Cook DJ, Ely EW Jr, et al. Evidence-based guidelines for weaning and discontinuing ventilatory support: a collective task force facilitated by the American College of Chest Physicians; the American Association for Respiratory Care; and the American College of Critical Care Medicine. *Chest* 2001;120:375S–95S.

109. Demling RH, Read T, Lind LJ, Flanagan HL. Incidence and morbidity of extubation failure in surgical intensive care patients. *Crit Care Med* 1988;16:573–7.

110. Brochard L, Rauss A, Benito S, et al. Comparison of three methods of gradual withdrawal from ventilatory support during weaning from mechanical ventilation. *Am J Respir Crit Care Med* 1994;150:896–903.

111. Esteban A, Frutos F, Tobin MJ, et al. A comparison of four methods of weaning patients from mechanical ventilation. Spanish Lung Failure Collaborative Group. *N Engl J Med* 1995;332:345–50.

112. Esteban A, Alia I, Gordo F, et al. Extubation outcome after spontaneous breathing trials with T-tube or pressure support ventilation. The Spanish Lung Failure Collaborative Group. *Am J Respir Crit Care Med* 1997;156:459–65.

113. Esteban A, Alia I, Tobin MJ, et al. Effect of spontaneous breathing trial duration on outcome of attempts to discontinue mechanical ventilation. Spanish Lung Failure Collaborative Group. *Am J Respir Crit Care Med* 1999;159:512–18.

114. Epstein SK, Ciubotaru RL, Wong JB. Effect of failed extubation on the outcome of mechanical ventilation. *Chest* 1997;112:186–92.

# Chapter 4

# Left ventricular pump failure: general considerations for management

Arashk Motiei, David R. Holmes, Jr., and Christopher E. Buller

## Introduction

Cardiogenic shock is a clinical state characterized by tissue hypoperfusion resulting from cardiac dysfunction. It is most commonly caused by left ventricular (LV) failure consequent to acute myocardial ischemia or infarction. Cardiogenic shock can also be due to fulminant myocarditis, severe valvular heart disease, sustained bradyarrhythmias, decompensated chronic heart failure, mechanical complications of myocardial infarction, pericardial tamponade, hypertrophic cardiomyopathy, and the apical ballooning syndrome.

Shock resulting from acute ischemia or infarction develops in 5–9% of patients hospitalized with ST-segment elevation myocardial infarction (STEMI) [1–3]. It is also seen in patients with non–ST-segment elevation myocardial infarction (NSTEMI) or unstable angina with a frequency that is approximately half that seen with STEMI [4–6]. While previous publications indicate that the incidence of shock complicating acute myocardial infarction (MI) had not changed significantly over the course of the past few decades [7,8], more recent data suggest a decline in its incidence that may be attributable to improvements in the early mechanical and pharmacologic management of patients with acute coronary syndromes [9]. Whether due to LV pump failure or other mechanisms, cardiogenic shock remains one of the most serious consequences of acute myocardial ischemia or infarction with extraordinary inhospital mortality.

Although cardiogenic shock in the setting of myocardial infarction can be a manifestation of a mechanical complication [acute severe mitral regurgitation (MR), ventricular septal rupture, or ventricular free wall rupture with cardiac tamponade], right ventricular (RV) dysfunction, or sustained brady- or

*Cardiogenic Shock*. Edited by Judith S. Hochman and E. Magnus Ohman.
© 2009 American Heart Association, ISBN: 978-1-4051-7926-3

tachyarrhythmias, it is most commonly the result of extensive LV dysfunction (pump failure). In the multicenter SHOCK (SHould we emergently revascularize Occluded Coronary arteries for Cardiogenic shocK) registry, LV dysfunction was the predominant cause of shock in 78.5% of cases [10]. The focus of this chapter is largely on this common subgroup.

## Pathophysiology

The primary event in cardiogenic shock due to pump failure is an abrupt decline in LV systolic function resulting in reduced cardiac output with consequent critical reduction in regional tissue perfusion. Autopsy studies have shown that cardiogenic shock in the setting of myocardial infarction is usually associated with necrosis totaling more than 40% of the LV myocardium [10,11]. It is therefore more common with anterior myocardial infarctions, which tend to involve a larger mass of myocardium, than with inferior, posterior, or lateral wall infarctions. Cardiogenic shock due to LV failure resulting in part from stunned myocardium is also recognized.

According to the traditional conceptual model of this condition, a reduction in tissue perfusion leads to the activation of the sympathetic system through baroreceptors and the renin–angiotensin–aldosterone axis through renal hypoperfusion. These compensatory mechanisms serve to restore blood pressure through increased heart rate, increased contractility of noninfarcted myocardium, systemic vasoconstriction, and sodium–water retention. However, these acute responses also increase myocardial oxygen consumption, shorten the diastolic coronary perfusion period, and increase LV afterload. Especially in the presence of multivessel coronary artery disease, these adaptive responses may initiate a vicious cycle that results in further deterioration of LV systolic and diastolic function. In patients with LV failure, infarct expansion leads to early compensation with acute LV dilation, which in turn helps in the maintenance of stroke volume. However, this leads to an increase in wall stress, resulting in an increase in myocardial oxygen demand.

In nearly half of all patients with cardiogenic shock, LV size is small or normal [12]. In these cases, the transiently adaptive mechanism of acute dilation has failed. Since multiple pathophysiologic mechanisms are involved, the extent of LV dysfunction is not the sole determinant of the development of this syndrome. Indeed, many patients present with severe LV dysfunction in the setting of acute MI without the manifestations of cardiogenic shock. LV systolic function may be only moderately depressed in patients who develop cardiogenic shock; the mean ejection fraction (EF) in the SHOCK trial was 30%. The distribution of LVEF in patients with cardiogenic shock overlaps with that of post-MI patients with or without heart failure [13] (Fig. 4.1). LV systolic function has been observed to be similar in the acute phase of cardiogenic shock and 2 weeks later, by which time the overall clinical scenario is different [14]. A subgroup of

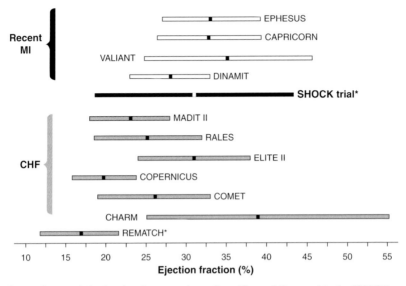

**Fig. 4.1** Range of ejection fractions seen in studies of heart failure and in the SHOCK trial [15]. This figure compares the range of left ventricular ejection fraction (mean ± SD) in the SHOCK trial with such ranges in studies of recent myocardial infarction (above SHOCK) and studies of heart failure (below SHOCK). Note that the range of LVEF in the SHOCK trial overlaps with these trials, although LVEF in SHOCK was obtained on support measures. REMATCH (Randomized Evaluation of Mechanical Assistance for the Treatment of Congestive Heart failure) studied LVAD use as destination therapy. *Note Measured on support. EPHESUS, Eplerenone Post–acute myocardial infarction Heart failure Efficacy and SUrvival Study; CAPRICORN, CArvedilol Post infaRct SurvIval CONtRol in LV dysfunctioN; VALIANT, VALsartan In Acute myocardial iNfarcTion; DINAMIT, Defibrillator IN Acute myocardial InfarcTion; MADIT II, Multicenter Automatic Defibrillator Implantation Trial II; RALES, Randomized ALdactone Evaluation Study; ELITE II, Evaluation of Losartan In The Elderly II; COPERNICUS, CarvedilOl ProspEctive RaNdomIzed CUmulative Survival study; COMET, Carvedilol Or Metoprolol European Trial; and CHARM, Candesartan in Heart failure: Assessment of moRtality and Morbidity. (Reprinted with permission from Reynolds HR, Hochman JS. *Circulation* 2008;117(5):686–97.)

patients present with cardiogenic shock in the setting of preserved LVEF in the absence of severe mitral regurgitation (MR) [16]. Although these observations suggest that the extent of LV dysfunction as measured by the LVEF correlates imperfectly with the clinical manifestations of low cardiac output and hypotension, EF retains significant prognostic impact [12].

Wide interpatient variability is observed not only in LVEF and size, but also in systemic vascular resistance (SVR) [12,17]. Moreover, the hemodynamic profile observed in many patients is characterized by inappropriately low systemic vascular resistance. These findings have led investigators to hypothesize that a systemic inflammatory response syndrome (SIRS) may develop in a subset of patients with cardiogenic shock, which has sparked interest in the role of inflammatory cytokines in the pathophysiology of cardiogenic shock. The activation of proinflammatory cytokines in SIRS from any cause leads to high levels of iNOS, NO, and NO-derived species such as peroxynitrite. NO is synthesized at low levels by endothelial and myocardial cell endothelial nitric oxide synthase (eNOS). Under normal physiologic circumstances, it has cardioprotective characteristics [18,19]. However, in the setting of exposure to inflammatory mediators or trauma, many cell types express iNOS at pathophysiologic levels [20]. This can lead to the accumulation of toxic levels of NO and other NO-derived species that form after NO reacts with superoxide. In experimental models, high iNOS and NO levels are seen after MI and subsequent reperfusion [21]. These agents may contribute to the pathogenesis of cardiogenic shock through a plethora of mechanisms, including systemic vasodilation, depression of myocardial contractility, suppression of myocardial respiration in nonischemic myocardium, reduced catecholamine sensitivity, and effects on glucose metabolism as well as effects on flow in the noninfarcted coronary vessels [17,22–24]. It therefore appears that the clinical picture of cardiogenic shock evolves under the influence of a complex interplay of factors including the compensatory mechanisms set in motion by tissue hypoperfusion and inflammation. This paradigm is illustrated in Fig. 4.1 [17]. These mechanisms offer intriguing targets for the future development of pharmaceutical agents for the medical management of cardiogenic shock. One such agent, an isoform-nonselective NOS inhibitor, L-$N$-monomethyl arginine (L-NMMA), was studied in the Tilarginine Acelate Injection in a Randomized International Study in Unstable MI Patients with Cardiogenic Shock (TRIUMPH) [25] trial in patients with MI and refractory cardiogenic shock in the presence of an open infarct artery. The enrollment for this trial was terminated at 398 patients on the basis of a prespecified futility analysis. There was no difference in 30-day all-cause mortality between patients who received L-NMMA (48%) versus placebo (42%) ($P = 0.24$) [25]. This may be a result of the fact that it is likely that multiple, redundant biochemical pathways are involved in the development of cardiogenic shock and that the inhibition of one mechanism alone may not be sufficient to either forestall or ameliorate the process.

## Clinical assessment

The classic clinical syndrome of cardiogenic shock due to LV failure is characterized by systemic hypotension (usually defined as a systolic blood pressure below 90 mm Hg, although patients requiring high-dose inotropic support to maintain a blood pressure of 90–100 mm Hg are also considered to be in shock) accompanied by symptoms or signs of tissue hypoperfusion and pulmonary congestion. The cardinal clinical signs of peripheral hypoperfusion include cool extremities and oliguria. Cerebral hypoperfusion may manifest as an altered sensorium, restlessness, or agitation.

Not all patients present with the entire constellation of clinical characteristics. While the combination of pulmonary congestion and peripheral hypoperfusion is the commonest presentation, nearly a quarter of patients with LV failure causing shock present with isolated tissue hypoperfusion in the absence of pulmonary congestion [26]. Occasional patients may demonstrate pulmonary congestion and hypotension in the absence of signs of tissue hypoperfusion [26]. Although classic teaching is that patients are tachycardic in the absence of chronotropic incompetence or medications that decrease heart rate, the average heart rate in the SHOCK registry and trial was 95 and 100 beats per minute, respectively [10,27]. Tachypnea and rales are usually present. Jugular venous distention may be seen. Cardiac examination most commonly demonstrates only faint heart sounds, though a third and/or fourth heart sound may be present. Murmurs indicative of concomitant mechanical complications such as mitral regurgitation and ventricular septal defect may be audible, although these findings are often subtle or obscured in a shock setting characterized by poor cardiac contractility and reduced gradients, rales or wheezes, and artifacts produced by intra-aortic balloon pumps (IABPs) and mechanical ventilation.

The majority of patients who eventually develop cardiogenic shock do not present in shock at the time of initial medical contact or hospitalization [1,3,4,28,29]. In the Global Use of Strategies to Open Occluded Coronary Arteries—I (GUSTO-I) trial, shock was present on admission in only 0.8% at hospitalization. An additional 5.3% developed shock after admission, either with sudden deterioration or following a gradual fall in cardiac output and blood pressure ("preshock"). Approximately 50% of patients who developed shock after admission did so within 24 hours of MI onset; most remaining cases occurred in the following 3 days, though isolated cases were delayed for up to 1 week [3]. Similarly, among patients with predominant LV dysfunction enrolled in the SHOCK trial, the median time from MI to shock onset was 5.5 hours, although 75% of patients developed shock within 24 hours [27]. In the SHOCK trial and registry, 26% of patients had cardiogenic shock on admission and 74% developed shock during hospitalization. Patients who presented with cardiogenic shock on admission had a shorter time from MI to cardiogenic shock (1.5 vs. 8.1 hours). While the majority of patients developed shock after admission, it is important to note that the patients who presented with shock had a worse initial hemodynamic profile. The use of aggressive treatment was less frequent in this group. Inhospital mortality was higher (75% vs. 56%; $P < 0.001$) with more rapid death (24-hour mortality 40% vs. 17%; $P < 0.001$) in cardiogenic shock on admission than in delayed cardiogenic shock patients. A similar reduction was seen in inhospital mortality with the use of emergency revascularization in both groups. After adjustment for clinical characteristics, cardiogenic shock on admission was an independent predictor of inhospital mortality but was no longer independent when variables derived from right heart catheterization were adjusted for [30].

Studies have been performed to predict the development of shock in patients with acute coronary syndromes. In one model, old age, systolic blood pressure, heart rate, and Killip class appeared to be strong predictors [31,32]. However, the positive predictive value of such models is limited and, as such, they are more helpful for identifying a low-risk group. In general, sustained relative hypotension, borderline tachycardia, and clinical or radiographic signs of pulmonary congestion are ominous signs that often precede the development of shock and frank tissue hypoperfusion. This constellation, often termed preshock, is typically accompanied by systolic blood pressure values above 90 mm Hg that are maintained through rising SVR coincident with falling cardiac output [33]. Clinically evident systemic hypoperfusion may not yet be present or appreciated. Nevertheless, prompt recognition of preshock by nurses and physicians caring for MI patients is pivotally important in order to initiate timely transfer, hemodynamic monitoring, cardiac catheterization, revascularization, and circulatory support.

A 12-lead electrocardiogram should be performed immediately on presentation to hospital. This may lead to the identification of MI and/or arrhythmias. A completely normal electrocardiogram suggests possibilities other than ischemic heart disease; a lack of extensive ST-segment elevations or depressions (severe) and/or Q-waves or other severe abnormality such as left bundle branch block (LBBB) suggests an etiology other than LV failure. Chest radiography may show cardiomegaly, pulmonary venous hypertension, or pulmonary edema. Blood counts may demonstrate a neutrophilic leukocytosis. Arterial blood gases may reveal hypoxemia and evidence of metabolic acidosis if tissue hypoperfusion has already developed. In the latter setting, an elevation in blood urea nitrogen, serum creatinine, and liver enzymes may also be seen.

Among MI patients with suspected shock, the likelihood of LV dysfunction as the primary etiology is especially high in patients with extensive ECG changes in the precordial leads. Most patients who have cardiogenic shock from LV pump failure show evidence of elevated filling pressures as manifested by rales or pulmonary congestion or pulmonary edema on chest radiography. In contrast, the clinical picture for shock due to RV infarction is a hypotensive patient with inferior myocardial infarction without evidence of pulmonary congestion by physical examination or chest radiography (see Chapter 5).

## Diagnostic evaluation

### Echocardiography

Once a diagnosis of cardiogenic shock due to LV failure is suspected on clinical grounds, echocardiography provides key confirmatory information. Transthoracic echocardiography can assess right- and left ventricular function. Other mechanical complications such as acute papillary muscle rupture with mitral regurgitation, ventricular septal defect, or ventricular free wall rupture with cardiac tamponade can also be readily diagnosed. These mechanical causes or contributors to shock may be easily missed during clinical examinations in patients with poor contractility and low output, and respiratory distress. Referral centers accepting patients with cardiogenic shock should ensure that echocardiography can be performed expeditiously at the patient bedside or in the cardiac catheterization laboratory in order to minimize delays in cardiac catheterization, circulatory support and revascularization. When an echocardiogram is not available before catheterization, right heart catheterization and left ventricular angiography can detect most contributory mechanical lesions.

In an analysis from the SHOCK trial, an echocardiogram and an angiogram before revascularization were available in 127 patients [34]. Although the median EF derived by echocardiography and LV angiography was identical (30%), the positive correlation was weak ($R^2 = 0.209$, $P = 0.019$). Patients with a larger number of diseased vessels had worse MR by echocardiography ($P = 0.005$). There was a significant but weak association between LV angiographic MR grade and echocardiographic MR severity ($R^2 = 0.162$, $P = 0.015$), but there was no association between culprit vessel and degree of MR [35]. Both short- and long-term mortality appear to be associated with initial LV systolic function and MR as assessed by echocardiography, and a benefit of early revascularization (ERV) is noted regardless of baseline EF or MR [12]. In the hypotensive patient, alternate diagnostic possibilities such as acute right heart failure from pulmonary embolism and other pathologies such as significant valvular disease can be diagnosed. In the patient with LV failure, the finding of RV enlargement and hypokinesis interestingly seems to identify a subgroup of patients with predominant inferior infarction and improved prognosis compared with patients with predominant LV failure alone [35]. Diastolic function abnormalities are often seen, and LV filling patterns are commonly observed to be restrictive [36].

In some circumstances, particularly in patients with chronic obstructive pulmonary disease or in supine, mechanically ventilated patients, it can be difficult to obtain adequate echocardiographic images. Here transesophageal echocardiography is a useful alternative. In general, this can be performed safely at the bedside. However, in patients who are not intubated but are exhibiting a tenuous respiratory status, the procedure does carry some risk, since use of sedation and esophageal intubation with the attendant risk of aspiration may precipitate acute respiratory failure that would usually mandate endotracheal intubation and mechanical ventilation.

Echocardiography is especially useful in undifferentiated patients with shock or hypotension, particularly when clinical findings are discordant or suggest multiple etiologies. A common scenario is the patient admitted to a medical intensive care unit with shock of unknown etiology and elevated biomarkers of cardiac injury, but with an unremarkable ECG. In such cases, documentation of normal or hyperdynamic LV function and normal RV size and function is a good way of excluding a significant cardiogenic component and will obviate the need for emergency cardiac catheterization and its attendant risks. Rapid echocardiography is also useful prior to catheterization for those with onset of shock late after MI onset. In contrast, patients presenting in shock with extensive anterior STEMI need not have intervention delayed by an echo.

## Hemodynamic assessment

Invasive hemodynamic assessment using pulmonary artery (PA) catheterization may be useful to confirm and characterize the initial shock state and for guiding therapy. The typical hemodynamic profile of a patient in cardiogenic shock is reduced cardiac index (less than 2.2 L/min/m$^2$), pulmonary artery wedge pressure of at least 15 mm Hg (usually considerably higher), and systemic blood pressure <90 mm Hg (Table 4.1). The presence of low filling

**Table 4.1** Hemodynamic characteristics of patients in the SHOCK trial ($n = 278$).

| | |
|---|---|
| SBP (mm Hg) | $90 \pm 21$ |
| DBP (mm Hg) | $56 \pm 15$ |
| MAP (mm Hg) | $67 \pm 16$ |
| RAP (mm Hg) | $15 \pm 8$ |
| PAWP (mm Hg) | $24 \pm 7$ |
| Cardiac index (L/min/m$^2$) | $1.80 \pm 0.61$ |
| CPI (W/m$^2$) | $0.27 \pm 0.12$ |
| SVR index (dyne $\cdot$ s $\cdot$ cm$^{-5}$ $\cdot$ m$^2$) | 2,468 (1,923–3,111) |
| SVI (mL/m$^2$) | $18.8 \pm 7.2$ |
| SWI (g/m/m$^2$) | 10.0 (6.5–14.3) |
| LV work index (kg/m/min/m$^2$) | $1.1 \pm 0.6$ |
| Coronary perfusion pressure (mm Hg) | $34 \pm 14$ |
| RV SBP (mm Hg) | $43 \pm 15$ |
| RV DBP (mm Hg) | $16 \pm 9$ |
| PA SBP (mm Hg) | $41 \pm 12$ |
| PA DBP (mm Hg) | $24 \pm 8$ |

*Note:* Values are given as the median (IQR) or mean ± SD, unless otherwise indicated. LV, left ventricular; SBP, systolic BP; DBP, diastolic BP; MAP, mean arterial pressure; RAP, mean right atrial pressure; CPO, cardiac power output; CPI, cardiac power index; SVR, systemic vascular resistance; RV, right ventricular; PA, pulmonary artery; PAWP, pulmonary artery wedge pressure; LVEF, left ventricular ejection fraction. All values recorded on support measures. (Reprinted with permission from Jeger RV, Lowe AM, Buller CE, et al. *Chest* 2007;132(6):1794–803.)

pressures from hypovolemia can be easily established and can lead to appropriate volume resuscitation. The presence of peripheral vasoconstriction or, in some patients, a distributive physiology characterized by low systemic vascular resistance can be determined. The degree of global perfusion impairment can be assessed by determining mixed venous oxygen saturations, which can then be tracked longitudinally to determine trends and responses to therapeutic interventions. Finally, pulmonary artery catheterization findings can suggest other causes of cardiogenic shock complicating acute MI, including ventricular septal rupture (oxygen saturation step-up across the right ventricle), acute severe MR (pulmonary artery wedge CV waves exceeding 10 mm Hg above mean wedge pressure), and RV shock [disproportionately high right-sided filling pressures accompanied by further elevation on spontaneous inspiration—Kussmauls' sign (Table 4.2)].

In using a flow-directed pulmonary artery (Swan-Ganz) catheter, it is important to be mindful of several issues. Accurate and reproducible hemodynamic measurements demand careful and frequent flushing and calibration, confirmation of appropriate waveforms (free of artifacts from catheter thrombosis, kinking, or migration). When uncertainty exists regarding differentiation of pulmonary artery and pulmonary wedge waveforms, it may be useful to confirm catheter tip position by obtaining a sample for oximetry. Over time, PA catheters tend to soften and thus migrate distally, leading to spontaneous wedging even when the balloon tip is not inflated. Beyond erroneous interpretation of values obtained from unintentionally wedged catheters, this phenomenon can lead to pulmonary infarction or if the balloon tip is unwittingly inflated in this position, PA rupture and massive hemoptysis. PA catheters traversing the tricuspid annulus and right ventricle can also be highly arryhthmogenic, leading to repeated episodes of ventricular tachycardia or fibrillation indistinguishable from spontaneous electrical storm. The development of repetitive ventricular arrhythmias in a shock patient with indwelling PA catheter should prompt consideration of the catheter, rather than the illness, as cause. Finally, patients with cardiogenic shock initially manifest high ventricular filling pressures not because of volume overload but because of poor cardiac performance. When interpreting the wedge pressure, one must remember that volume is only one of its many important determinants. LV compliance is another important factor. In the setting of acute MI, the reduced LV compliance leads to an elevated LV filling pressure at any given ventricular volume. Aggressive diuretic interventions intended to "normalize" the right- and left-sided filling pressures can exacerbate the low-output state and should be avoided.

Routine PA catheterization in intensive care units is controversial. Indeed, a frequently cited meta-analysis failed to show clear evidence of benefit but was based on studies in patients who were critically ill from a wide variety of causes [27]. No randomized studies have evaluated the utility of indwelling PA catheters for patients with cardiogenic shock. Nevertheless their use in MI

**Table 4.2** Hemodynamic patterns.

| | RA | RVS | RVD | PAS | PAD | PAW | CI | SVR |
|---|---|---|---|---|---|---|---|---|
| Normal values | <6 | <25 | 0–12 | <25 | 0–12 | <6–12 | ≥2.5 | (800–1600) |
| MI without pulmonary edema* | — | — | — | — | — | ~13 (5, 18) | ~2.7 (2.2–4.3) | — |
| Pulmonary edema | ↔↑ | ↔↑ | ↔↑ | ↑ | ↑ | ↑ | ↔↓ | ↑ |
| Cardiogenic shock | | | | | | | | |
| LV failure | ↔↑ | ↔↑ | ↔↑ | ↔↑ | ↑ | ↑ | → | ↔↑ |
| RV failure† | ↑ | ↓↔↑‡ | ↑ | ↓↔↑‡ | ↔↓↑‡ | ↓↔↑‡ | → | ↑ |

There is significant patient-to-patient variation. Pressures in RA, right atrium; RVS/D, right ventricular systolic/diastolic; PAS/D, pulmonary artery systolic/diastolic; PAW, pulmonary artery wedge are in mm Hg; CI, cardiac index (L/min/m$^2$); SVR, systemic vascular resistance (dynes/sec/cm$^5$); MI, myocardial infarction; and P/SBF, pulmonary/systemic blood flow.

*Forrester et al. classified nonreperfused MI patients into four hemodynamic subsets (*N Engl J Med* 1976;295:1356–62). PAWP and CI in clinically stable subset 1 patients are shown. Values in parenthesis represent range.

†"Isolated" or predominant RV failure.

‡PAW and PA pressures may rise in RV failure after volume loading due to RV dilation, right to left shift of the interventricular septum, resulting in impaired LV filling. When biventricular failure is present, the patterns are similar to those shown for LV failure.

Reprinted with permission from Hochman JS and Ingbar D, Cardiogenic Shock and Pulmonary Edema in Fauci AS, Braunwald E, Kasper DL et al., Harrison's Principles of Internal Medicine 17th Edition, McGraw-Hill Medical, 2008.

patients with shock is a class IIa recommendation in the ACC/AHA STEMI guidelines [38]. An observational analysis from 2401 GUSTO-I patients with cardiogenic shock found lower mortality among patients managed with PA catheters (45.2%) than among those not managed with PA catheters (63.4%) [39].

In a report from the GUSTO IIb and GUSTO III trials, PA catheterization was found to have been performed in 735 patients, with a median time to insertion of 24 hours [40]. Patients undergoing PA catheterization were older, more often diabetic, and more likely to present with ST-segment elevation or Killip class III or IV. U.S. patients were 3.8 times more likely than non–U.S. patients to undergo PA catheterization. Patients managed with PA catheterization also underwent more procedures, including percutaneous intervention (40.7% vs. 18.1%), coronary artery bypass graft (CABG) surgery (12.5% vs. 7.7%), and endotracheal intubation (29.3% vs. 2.2%). Raw and adjusted 30-day mortality was higher overall among patients managed with PA catheterization [OR 8.7 (CI 7.3–10.2) and 6.4 (CI 5.4–7.6), respectively] but not in the subgroup of patients with cardiogenic shock [OR 0.99 (CI 0.80–1.23)][40].

The Evaluation Study of Congestive Heart Failure and Pulmonary Artery Catheterization Effectiveness (ESCAPE) trial studied the effectiveness of PA catheterization in patients hospitalized with severe symptomatic and chronic recurrent heart failure. The addition of PA catheterization to careful clinical assessment was associated with a higher frequency of adverse events but did not affect overall mortality and hospitalization [41].

In the absence of more definitive data to guide practice, a clinician's decision to place a PA catheter in the setting of cardiogenic shock must be individualized. Experience suggests they are most useful in patients with sustained shock requiring titration of inotropes and vasoactive agents, when uncertainty regarding the cardiogenic nature of shock or pulmonary edema exists, when shock without pulmonary congestion develops, or when oxygenation is compromised despite high inspired fractional oxygen content ($FiO_2$). Conversely, patients in whom the diagnosis is clear and who are improving rapidly following revascularization are unlikely to benefit. The placement of an arterial line for real-time monitoring of blood pressure is also recommended, particularly when vasopressor or inotropic agents are administered.

## Coronary angiography

Emergency coronary angiography in the setting of cardiogenic shock complicating MI is indicated in order to determine the distribution and extent of coronary artery obstruction and guide emergency revascularization [42]. Revascularization is discussed in greater detail below and in Chapters 10 and 11. In patients presenting with cardiogenic shock complicating suspected but unconfirmed MI (usually a consequence of ambiguous ECG changes), early coronary angiography should be undertaken to establish the etiology. In the absence of obstructive coronary artery disease, right ventricular, left ventricular, valvular, and subvalvular function should be assessed. If normal, there should be a reevaluation of the cardiogenic nature of the shock state. Those with abnormal LV function may have other causes of cardiogenic shock, such as fulminant myocarditis (which can mimic STEMI with localized ST-segment elevation and regional wall motion abnormalities) or takotsubo cardiomyopathy (see Chapter 8).

Left ventriculography should be strongly considered if the patient has not undergone echocardiography since the development of shock. Digital angiographic techniques with only small volumes of contrast are preferable. Ventriculography will quantify LV dysfunction, reveal regional wall motion abnormalities, and identify clinically unsuspected mitral regurgitation and ventricular septal or free wall ruptures.

# Management

Once the diagnosis is established and the hemodynamic state is characterized, the management of the patient is based on general measures, circulatory support, and in the common scenario of cardiogenic shock resulting from acute MI and pump failure, emergency reperfusion and revascularization. In patients with cardiogenic shock from a nonischemic etiology, management largely centers on circulatory support until surgical correction of the valvular or mechanical cause, recovery from myocarditis, or LV assist devices (LVAD) implantation and/or cardiac transplantation can be undertaken in suitable candidates. The concepts of circulatory support outlined below can, in general, be applied to all patients with pump failure from a variety of causes, but the discussion on revascularization and antiplatelet therapy applies most specifically to patients with cardiogenic shock complicating predominantly LV pump failure due to an acute ischemic syndrome.

# General measures

All patients should be treated with aspirin. In the intubated patient, aspirin may be administered via a nasogastric tube or in the form of a rectal suppository. Intravenous heparin should be administered.

All patients should undergo coronary angiography to determine their coronary anatomy. If, following coronary angiography, percutaneous coronary intervention (PCI) is the chosen reperfusion strategy, glycoprotein IIb/IIIa inhibitors should be given immediately before the PCI procedure. Glycoprotein IIb/IIIa inhibitors should be individualized in patients undergoing rescue or adjunctive PCI after fibrinolysis, and are generally avoided within 4 hours of fibrinolytic administration or in those perceived to be at increased bleeding risk. If coronary angiography reveals extensive multivessel disease that requires urgent CABG surgery, and if both surgeon and operating room are available, glycoprotein IIb/IIIa inhibitors should be withheld.

Beta-blockers and angiotensin-converting enzyme (ACE) inhibitors should be avoided until the recovery period when the patient has a sustained period of stable blood pressure in the absence of mechanical or pharmacologic circulatory support. Beta-blockers should be initiated in preparation for discharge at a low dose with planned out-of-hospital gradual dose increases, with a regimen similar to those used for chronic heart failure patients. Indeed, early intravenous beta-blockade has been shown to be associated with a higher incidence of the development of cardiogenic shock in patients with acute MI who have evidence of rales or risk factors for shock and for this reason are to be avoided in these patients [43]. Calcium channel blockers should be avoided because of their negative inotropic effects. In the setting of arrhythmias, agents with negative inotropic and vasodilatory properties such as procainamide and quinidine should be avoided. If the need for an antiarrhythmic drug arises, amiodarone is generally a safe and well-tolerated agent that has less negative inotropic effects. However, rapid infusion of this agent can lower blood pressure, thereby contributing to compromise of systemic perfusion in shock patients (see Chapter 3).

Management of volume and preload in patients with both hypotension and pulmonary congestion is especially challenging. When a PA catheter is used, a preliminary goal should be to achieve and maintain a pulmonary artery wedge pressure of 18–25 mm Hg. Competing demands of cardiac output, arterial pressure, heart rate, and arterial oxygenation can generally be optimized within this range by stepwise titration of volume, inotropes, vasoactive agents, and circulatory support devices. However, the goal of achieving adequate systemic perfusion and oxygenation should be guided by clinical measures and should not be lost amid preoccupation with specific hemodynamic values. Patients with evidence of pulmonary congestion should be treated with diuretics, but overdiuresis should be avoided. Those with euvolemic status before the onset of shock have relative intravascular hypovolemia soon after the onset of pulmonary edema due to extravasation of fluid into the lungs. In the situation of acute respiratory failure from pulmonary edema, mechanical ventilation is typically required. The role of noninvasive positive pressure ventilation, endotracheal intubation, and mechanical ventilation is discussed in Chapter 3.

## Circulatory support

Circulatory support is one of the most important aspects of the management of cardiogenic shock. The goal of circulatory support is to reverse the state of tissue hypoperfusion induced by systemic hypotension. This is accomplished by pharmacologic and mechanical means.

# Pharmacologic circulatory support

Pharmacologic circulatory support generally implies the use of inotropic and vasopressor agents. To date, no large-scale controlled studies have compared various inotropes, alone or in combination, for the treatment of cardiogenic shock. All inotropic and vasoconstrictive pharmacologic agents increase myocardial oxygen consumption directly or indirectly. Moreover, those that contribute to tachycardia shorten the diastolic interval required for myocardial perfusion. Use of these agents should therefore be considered adjunctive or temporizing; the hemodynamic stability they provide in the short term is obtained at the expense of additional myocardial stress and ischemia.

Dopamine, commonly a first-line pharmacologic agent for cardiogenic shock, has direct inotropic effects mediated through beta-adrenergic stimulation. At higher doses it achieves vasopressor effects through peripheral alpha-adrenergic stimulation. Dobutamine has cardiac effects similar to dopamine, but when used alone it can worsen hypotension by causing peripheral vasodilation. Norepinephrine, an alpha-adrenergic stimulator with much less pronounced beta-adrenergic activity, is a useful second-line agent when dopamine or dopamine/dobutamine combination therapy is inadequate. All adrenergic agents with beta-adrenergic properties can contribute to excessive tachycardia and tachyarrhythmias. Phenylephrine (a highly selective alpha-adrenergic agonist) and vasopressin (a direct vasoconstrictor) may be useful adjuncts that can enable down-titration of beta-adrenergic catecholamines when necessary. As monotherapies, however, they reduce cardiac output by increasing afterload alone and there is a paucity of systematic data in cardiogenic shock.

Milrinone is a phosphodiesterase inhibitor that mediates its effects by causing an increase in intracellular cyclic adenosine monophosphate without employing adrenergic receptors. This agent has salutary effects on myocardial contractility. However, it also causes vasodilation and is therefore not recommended as a first-line agent in the hypotensive patient. If used, it may need to be combined with an agent such as dopamine.

# Mechanical circulatory support

In contrast to pharmacologic circulatory support, mechanical circulatory supports reduce cardiac work and myocardial oxygen consumption, and in complimentary fashion directly or indirectly improve myocardial perfusion. These technologies are discussed in detail in Chapter 9.

# Intra-aortic balloon pump

Intra-aortic balloon counterpulsation (IABP) provides systemic circulatory support by directly augmenting diastolic arterial pressure (balloon inflation phase) and by increasing LV stroke volume (by lowering LV afterload, balloon deflation phase). These same effects simultaneously improve coronary perfusion pressure in the critical diastolic phase of myocardial blood flow and reduce myocardial oxygen consumption by reducing LV volume and wall stress. Guidelines recommend the use of intra-aortic balloon counterpulsation in patients who fail to demonstrate immediate improvement in hemodynamic parameters with general supportive measures and simple pharmacologic therapy. Balloon pumps provide an important bridge to angiography and revascularization in the shock patient as well as critical circulatory support through the period of additional ischemic stress imposed by PCI or CABG procedures. However, based on a lack of randomized trial outcome data for IABP use in conjunction with PCI, new trials have been developed. IABP devices are unsuitable for patients with advanced atherosclerotic aortoiliac disease and for those with moderate or severe aortic valve insufficiency.

Intra-aortic balloon counterpulsation has been used in patients with acute MI and cardiogenic shock since the 1970s [44]. Several small retrospective studies conducted in the 1990s found a reduction in the inhospital mortality of patients treated with a combination of thrombolytic therapy and IABP [45–48]. In the GUSTO-I trial, there was a trend toward lower mortality in patients treated with IABP, although this was not a significant independent predictor of the outcome [49]. In the SHOCK trial registry of patients with predominant LV failure, patients treated with IABP in combination with thrombolytic therapy had the lowest inhospital mortality [50]. In the National Registry of Myocardial Infarction-2 (NRMI-2) database, the use of IABP in combination with thrombolysis was associated with a significant reduction in mortality from 67% to 49% [51]. To date, only one clinical trial has addressed the role of IABP in addition to thrombolytic therapy for acute MI. The Thrombolysis And Counterpulsation To Improve Cardiogenic Shock (TACTICS) trial randomized a total of 57 patients with STEMI and hypotension or heart failure to thrombolysis alone or to thrombolysis with IABP. In the group assigned to thrombolysis alone, 30% crossed over and received IABP. There was a trend toward a lower mortality at 6 months in the group treated with IABP and thrombolysis (34%) compared with the group treated with thrombolytics alone (43%) [52]. Although the independent effect of IABP use on mortality in conjunction with mechanical reperfusion has not been shown, its use facilitates the safe performance of percutaneous intervention.

## Percutaneous left ventricular assist devices

Percutaneous LVADs have recently emerged as an option for temporary circulatory support in the patient with LV failure. Currently, two devices are available for clinical use in North America. (A complete discussion of LVADs can be found in Chapter 9.) The TandemHeart (Cardiac Assist Inc, Pittsburgh, Pennsylvania,

USA) device has a 21F drainage cannula that is placed in the left atrium via a transseptal puncture. Oxygenated blood is aspirated from the left atrium and circulated back through the femoral artery by a centrifugal pump using a 15–17F cannula. The device can pump at a maximum of 7500 rpm, achieving flow rates of up to 3.5 L/min. The device produces a significant improvement in cardiac output and blood pressure and brings about a reduction in pulmonary artery wedge pressure [53]. There are anecdotal reports of the device being used successfully in patients with cardiogenic shock and worsening hemodynamics despite the use of vasopressors and balloon counterpulsation [54–56]. It has also been used for circulatory support in patients undergoing high-risk PCI [53,57–59].

The device has been compared with IABP in one small multicenter trial with 42 patients. Cardiogenic shock was due to MI in 70% of the patients and decompensated heart failure in most of the remaining patients. The mean duration of support was 2.5 days. Compared with IABP, the TandemHeart device achieved significantly greater increases in cardiac index and mean arterial blood pressure, and significantly greater decreases in pulmonary artery wedge pressure. Overall 30-day survival was not significantly different between the two groups. However, there was a trend toward a higher incidence of complications with the use of the TandemHeart device. The complications related to the large size of the cannulas need for transseptal puncture and included local vascular complications such as bleeding (42%) and distal limb ischemia (21%). Although not statistically significantly different, these complications occurred with a lower frequency in patients treated with IABP [60].

In a single-center study, patients in cardiogenic shock after acute MI with intended PCI of the infarct-related artery were randomized to either IABP ($n = 20$) or percutaneous VAD support ($n = 21$). The primary outcome measure, cardiac power index, as well as other hemodynamic and metabolic variables could be improved more effectively by VAD support. However, complications like severe bleeding (19 vs. 8, $P = 0.002$) or limb ischemia (7 vs. 0, $P = 0.009$) occurred more frequently after VAD support, whereas 30-day mortality was similar (IABP 45% vs. VAD 43%, log-rank, $P = 0.86$) [61]. Given the limited data that are presently available on this device, it appears that it is best suited for a scenario in which standard medical therapy with vasopressors and balloon counterpulsation has failed. This device should be used only by experienced teams because of the large bore of the catheters and the need for transseptal procedures.

Another device is the Impella Recover system (Impella Cardiosystems AG, Aachen, Germany) which has a caged blood flow inlet that is placed retrograde into the left ventricle to aspirate oxygenated blood, which is then injected into the ascending aorta by means of a microaxial pump [62]. Currently two types are available: the Impella Recover LP 2.5 and LP 5.0 models. The Impella Recover LP 2.5 is a 12F catheter well suited for percutaneous implantation, whereas the larger Impella Recover LP 5.0 catheter requires surgical cutdown of the femoral artery for insertion. The device has been used in patients with cardiogenic shock complicating acute MI, in those with postcardiotomy shock and fulminant myocarditis, and in those undergoing high-risk PCI [62–68]. Ongoing studies are comparing this device with IABP in patients with cardiogenic shock. Compared with TandemHeart, the Impella percutaneous device does not deliver as full circulatory support in terms of liters of flow per minute. In addition, hematologic abnormalities have been reported with it.

## Percutaneous cardiopulmonary bypass

Percutaneous cardiopulmonary bypass systems, often referred to as extracorporeal membrane oxygenators (ECMOs), have also been used to support patients with hemodynamic collapse or cardiogenic shock [69]. Such systems consist mainly of a blood pump and an oxygenator, 16–18F arterial cannulas in the descending aorta and an 18F venous cannula advanced into the right atrium. These are connected to an external pump and a membrane oxygenator. Blood is aspirated from the right atrium and pumped through a heat exchanger and membrane oxygenator, and then returned into the femoral artery. Continuous flow is provided with maintenance of a pulsatile arterial pressure unless the circulation is completely supported by the cardiopulmonary bypass device. The disadvantages include the large size of the cannulas with the risks of vascular hemorrhagic and ischemic complications. Trained perfusionists are required to operate these systems. The support time is usually limited to less than 6 hours. There are limited reports of the successful use of this approach in patients who have sustained hemodynamic collapse in the catheterization laboratory or who are in cardiogenic shock [70–76].

## Surgically implanted LVADs

There are limited data on the use of surgically implanted LVADs for circulatory support in patients in cardiogenic shock. The largest series comes from a multicenter trial that reported a 24% mortality rate with the use of LVADs in 17 patients with cardiogenic shock from acute MI [77]. Another report [78] documented an 85% rate of successful bridge to transplantation and a 29% mortality rate with the use of LVAD support in 7 patients with cardiogenic shock from acute MI. In the largest experience [79], 49 patients received LVAD support for cardiogenic shock in the setting of acute MI. The VAD support successfully bridged 38 (74%) patients to heart transplantation. Of the 38 patients who received transplants, 33 (87%) were eventually discharged from the hospital. The overall inhospital mortality rate for patients with cardiogenic shock was 33%.

One of the concerns that surgeons have when implanting an LVAD into a patient with an acute anterior wall myocardial infarction is the safety of apical cannulation in the presence of acutely infarcted apical myocardium, which is usually necrotic and friable. This can lead to ventricular disruption and bleeding from the cannulation site. These complications, when they occur, can have lethal consequences. LVADs have also been used in patients with myocarditis as a bridge to recovery or heart transplantation [80–82]. In general, where possible, the surgical placement of an LVAD should be considered for suitable candidates in the situation of cardiogenic shock refractory to conventional measures, as a bridge to recovery or transplantation.

## Reperfusion therapy

Emergency mechanical revascularization of occluded coronary arteries by PCI or CABG is a key intervention in cardiogenic shock due to LV failure complicating myocardial infarction (Fig. 4.2). While revascularization should be performed as early as possible, the time window for proven benefit is considerably longer than the 6- to 12-hour window established for primary PCI in uncomplicated STEMI, and extends to >24 hours after the onset of MI. This extended window of benefit is believed to exist because of the vicious cycle of hypotension and myocardial ischemia that characterizes shock due to LV ischemia and infarction. The importance of this approach was established in the SHOCK trial, which compared early revascularization to initial medical stabilization with delayed revascularization in patients in cardiogenic shock from STEMI [42]. The 30-day mortality rate was 46.7% in the early revascularization group and 56% in the initial medical stabilization group ($P = 0.11$). Survival curves continued to diverge such that the 6- and 12-month mortality rates were significantly lower for patients assigned to emergency revascularization (12-month mortality: 53.3% vs. 66.4%, $P < 0.03$), and this difference was maintained up to 11 (median 6) years [83–84]. Moreover, patients younger than 75 years had a significant reduction in mortality by 30 days.

The Swiss Multicenter Trial of Angioplasty for Shock [(S)MASH trial] randomized 55 patients with refractory shock to either PCI or conventional medical therapy. This trial was terminated prematurely due to slow enrollment, largely due to perceived benefits of ERV as demonstrated by retrospective studies. The mortality in the PCI group was lower at 69% compared with 78% for patients treated with conventional care, but this difference was not statistically significant [85]. Based on these data, the AHA/ACC guidelines specify emergency revascularization as a class 1A indication for patients <75 years with ST-segment elevation or LBBB who develop shock within 36 hours of MI and who are suitable for revascularization that can be performed within 18 hours of shock onset. The apparent lack of efficacy of emergency revascularization in patients >75 years enrolled in the SHOCK trial was likely related to chance imbalance of baseline characteristics in this small subgroup [86]. Multiple registry studies and the overall SHOCK trial results support a survival benefit with ERV in selected elderly patients without advanced comorbidities [87–89]. The

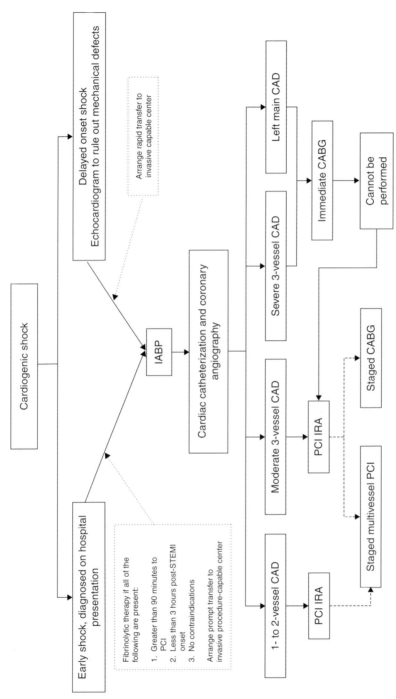

**Fig. 4.2** Recommendations for initial reperfusion strategy when cardiogenic shock complicates STEMI. (Reprinted with permission from Antman EM, Anbe DT, Armstrong PW, et al. *Circulation* 2004;110:e82–293.)

AHA/ACC guidelines give a class IIA recommendation for ERV in patients aged 75 or older, who are suitable candidates [38].

The choice of revascularization strategy (PCI vs. CABG) in SHOCK trial was left to physician discretion, though emergency surgery was encouraged in patients with severe 3-vessel or left main coronary artery disease. A comparison between PCI and CABG in 128 patients with predominant LV failure, who underwent ERV in the SHOCK trial, showed that the 47 patients selected for surgery had a higher frequency of diabetes and more extensive multivessel or left main disease. Despite these differences, the survival rates were 55.6% in the PCI group compared with 57.4% in the CABG group at 30 days ($P = 0.86$) and 51.9% compared with 46.8%, respectively, at 1 year ($P = 0.71$). This observation speaks to the important role of early CABG in shock patients, and may reflect more complete revascularization. Among patients with multivessel disease assigned early revascularization in SHOCK trial, complete revascularization was achieved in 87% who underwent CABG versus 23% of those who had PCI [91]. Nevertheless, long-term follow-up demonstrated similar survival for those who underwent CABG versus PCI [83]. Other potential benefits of early CABG include LV decompression, cardioplegia, and myocardial cooling as discussed in Chapter 11.

Based on SHOCK trial data, PCI appears to be appropriate in patients with 1- or 2-vessel disease amenable to PCI. For left main or severe 3-vessel disease, CABG may be the preferred strategy. CABG surgery is clearly indicated when concomitant mechanical complications warranting surgical repair coexist. If timely surgical revascularization is not available, left main or multivessel PCI is preferable to delaying surgery. Current guidelines discourage the treatment of nonculprit stenoses during primary PCI for uncomplicated MI. In the setting of cardiogenic shock, however, nonculprit stenoses, particularly if sufficiently severe to be contributing to ischemia, should be considered for intervention during the initial PCI procedure.

When mechanical reperfusion for STEMI patients with shock is not immediately available, fibrinolytic therapy is likely beneficial. No adequately powered prospective trial exists to definitively address this, although observational data provide insights that can inform clinical care. In GISSI-I (Gruppo Italiano per lo Studio della Streptochinasi nell'Infarto Miocardico), a small cohort of patients characterized at baseline as Killip class IV did not appear to derive benefit from streptokinase versus placebo [92]. In the Fibrinolytic Therapy Trialists (FTT) Collaborative group overview, the point estimate of benefit from fibrinolytic therapy over placebo was consistent with 7 lives saved per 100 patients treated, but this apparent, large, absolute benefit was not statistically significant [93].

An analysis of the SHOCK trial registry implied both a benefit attributable to fibrinolytic therapy alone and a plausible and potentially important positive interaction between fibrinolytic therapy and IABP [50]. Four categories of patients were compared: (1) fibrinolytic therapy plus IABP (19%; $n = 160$),

(2) IABP only (33%; $n = 279$); (3) fibrinolytic therapy only (15%; $n = 132$); neither fibrinolytic therapy nor IABP (33%; $n = 285$). A significant difference in unadjusted inhospital mortality between these groups was observed: 47%, 52%, 63%, and 77%, respectively, $P < 0.0001$. While these outcomes were confounded by intergroup differences in baseline characteristics and revascularization rates, favorable outcome associated with fibrinolytic treatment persisted after adjustment. The apparent interaction between fibrinolysis and IABP is supported by experimental results demonstrating reduced thrombus dissolution in a canine model of coronary thrombosis accompanied by hypotension. These experiments demonstrated recovery of thrombolytic efficacy when hypotension was reversed [94]. A post hoc analysis of the SHOCK trial found that patients assigned medical therapy had lower 12-month mortality if they had been treated with fibrinolytics than if they had not (60% vs. 78%) [94]. Finally, small retrospective series suggest that transfer of fibrinolytic-treated shock patients to tertiary centers for early revascularization is safe and associated with outcomes comparable to those achieved at centers with on-site early revascularization [45,47]. In total, the available data have led to a class I recommendation for the use of fibrinolytic therapy for STEMI patients with cardiogenic shock, who cannot undergo immediate emergency revascularization and do not have a contraindication to fibrinolysis [38].

It should be emphasized that nonrandomized studies have suggested a superiority of mechanical reperfusion to fibrinolytic therapy in patients with MI and in cardiogenic shock [3]. The SHOCK trial confirmed that ERV with either CABG or primary or rescue PCI for failed fibrinolysis was superior to fibrinolytic administration when possible, followed by late revascularization as clinically determined. The use of fibrinolysis as a reperfusion strategy should be reserved for circumstances where mechanical approaches are not readily available, including for patients who present early after MI onset but have long transport times to PCI- and CABG-capable facilities.

In STEMI complicated by cardiogenic shock, interhospital transfer of patients is difficult because of patients' hemodynamic instability. SHOCK trial and registry investigators reported the effect of ERV and the interaction with fibrinolytic therapy and intra-aortic balloon counterpulsation in transfer and direct-admit patients with cardiogenic shock [95]. Fibrinolytic therapy was administered in 49% of transfer patients at a median of 2.2 (interquartile range 1.1–4.5) hours after STEMI onset but 3.0 (interquartile range 0.2–12.7) hours before cardiogenic shock onset. In 81% of transfer patients treated with fibrinolysis, treatment was started before cardiogenic shock onset, and most transfer patients had cardiogenic shock before arriving at a hospital with revascularization capability. Compared with transfer patients without fibrinolysis, patients treated with fibrinolysis were younger and less likely to have diabetes, prior MI, or prior CABG and had better renal function. Transfer patients treated with fibrinolysis more often had ST-segment elevations but less often had LBBB on the initial electrocardiogram. More often the left anterior and right coronary artery and less often the left circumflex artery was the culprit artery compared with patients without fibrinolysis. Among transfer patients who underwent coronary angiography, those treated with fibrinolysis tended to have TIMI (thrombolysis in myocardial infarction) 0/1 flow less often (57% vs. 70%), but TIMI 2 flow (16% vs. 10%) and TIMI 3 flow more often (27% vs. 20%, overall $P = 0.051$). Inhospital mortality was lower in transfer patients treated with fibrinolysis than in patients without (43% vs. 55%, $P = 0.0071$). In transfer patients treated with fibrinolysis for STEMI (most often before cardiogenic shock), inhospital mortality was similar in both early revascularization and no/late revascularization groups (44% vs. 41%, $P = 0.69$), but was lower when patients who were not treated with fibrinolysis for STEMI subsequently received ERV for shock compared with no/late revascularization (40% vs. 63%, $P = 0.0016$). The interaction between early revascularization and fibrinolysis was significant (interaction $P = 0.011$) [95]. However, in the SHOCK trial, rescue PCI resulted in a treatment benefit that was similar to primary PCI when compared to initial medical stabilization. The transfer study suggests that mostly younger and healthier patients are selected for transfer and more aggressive therapy. Because transferred patients had similar mortality rates when adjusted for age, blood pressure, angiography, and ERV, the authors suggested that patients not transferred to tertiary care centers would also have had lower mortality rates if reperfusion strategies had been pursued as frequently as in transfer patients.

The AirPAMI trial [96] was the only randomized trial studying the interhospital transfer of patients with complicated STEMI. This study randomized 138 patients with risk factors including age >70, anterior STEMI, Killip class II or III, a heart rate >100 beat/min, or systolic blood pressure <100 mm Hg to on-site fibrinolysis in hospitals without revascularization capability versus transfer for primary PCI without fibrinolysis. The study showed a nonsignificant reduction in major adverse cardiac events in favor of the transfer group (8.4% vs. 13.6%, $P = 0.33$). On the other hand, the CAPTIM study [97,98] randomized patients with STEMI to fibrinolysis versus no fibrinolysis during transfer to hospitals with revascularization capability and found that the overall cardiogenic shock incidence during hospitalization was similar in patients who received fibrinolytic therapy and in patients without fibrinolysis (2.5% vs. 4.9%, $P = 0.09$). However, no cardiogenic shock occurred during transportation in patients receiving fibrinolysis compared with 2.1% incidence in patients without fibrinolysis ($P = 0.004$). Additionally, among patients randomized in the first 2 hours, cardiogenic shock occurred less frequently with fibrinolytic therapy than with PCI (1.3% vs. 5.3%, $P = 0.032$), whereas rates were similar in patients randomized later.

Data from a regional protocol for administration of half-dose fibrinolytic therapy for STEMI patients, including those with cardiogenic shock, in hospitals more than 60 miles away from a tertiary care center followed by transfer suggest outcomes that are comparable to direct-admission cardiogenic shock patients [99].

In most of these studies, it is difficult to assess the influence of fibrinolytic therapy and revascularization independently. Since most patients with STEMI who develop cardiogenic shock develop this problem after the initial presentation, the decision to use fibrinolysis versus PCI is likely to be driven by the circumstances of the original presentation with STEMI. In the case of patients who have cardiogenic shock at presentation, the current ACC/AHA guidelines advocate the use of prompt transfer to a facility with revascularization capability. Fibrinolytic therapy is supported if undue delays in transfer are expected, in particular if the elapsed time from MI onset is less than 3 hours. Furthermore, fibrinolysis should be administered in STEMI patients without contraindications who present in cardiogenic shock and are not candidates for invasive procedures. Additional evidence from randomized trials would be useful.

## Summary and conclusions

LV pump failure is the most common cause of cardiogenic shock and results from a number of underlying pathologies, with acute MI being the most frequent etiology. Early diagnosis and the aggressive institution of circulatory support should be followed by ERV when pump failure is due to acute myocardial infarction or unstable angina. Recent advances in our understanding of the pathophysiology of this condition, particularly the contribution of a systemic inflammatory response in some individuals, may yield novel therapeutic approaches. The advent of new and advanced circulatory support systems may also help in improving the outcomes of these patients in the future.

## References

1. Babaev A, Frederick PD, Pasta DJ, et al. Trends in management and outcomes of patients with acute myocardial infarction complicated by cardiogenic shock. *JAMA* 2005;294:448–54.
2. Hands ME, Rutherford JD, Muller JE, et al. The in-hospital development of cardiogenic shock after myocardial infarction: incidence, predictors of occurrence, outcome and prognostic factors. The MILIS Study Group. *J Am Coll Cardiol* 1989;14:40–6; discussion 47–8.
3. Holmes DR Jr, Bates ER, Kleiman NS, et al. Contemporary reperfusion therapy for cardiogenic shock: the GUSTO-I trial experience. The GUSTO-I Investigators. Global Utilization of Streptokinase and Tissue Plasminogen Activator for Occluded Coronary Arteries. *J Am Coll Cardiol* 1995;26:668–74.
4. Holmes DR Jr, Berger PB, Hochman JS, et al. Cardiogenic shock in patients with acute ischemic syndromes with and without ST-segment elevation. *Circulation* 1999;100:2067–73.
5. Jacobs AK, French JK, Col J, et al. Cardiogenic shock with non-ST-segment elevation myocardial infarction: a report from the SHOCK Trial Registry. SHould we emergently revascularize Occluded coronaries for Cardiogenic shocK? *J Am Coll Cardiol* 2000;36 (3 Suppl A):1091–6.

6. Lindholm MG, Køber L, Boesgaard S, et al. Cardiogenic shock complicating acute myocardial infarction; prognostic impact of early and late shock development. *Eur Heart J* 2003;24(3):258–65.
7. Goldberg RJ, Samad NA, Yarzebski J, et al. Temporal trends in cardiogenic shock complicating acute myocardial infarction. *N Engl J Med* 1999;340(15):1162–8.
8. Hasdai D, Holmes DR Jr, Topol EJ, et al. Frequency and clinical outcome of cardiogenic shock during acute myocardial infarction among patients receiving reteplase or alteplase. Results from GUSTO-III. Global Use of Strategies to Open Occluded Coronary Arteries. *Eur Heart J* 1999;20(2):128–35.
9. Fox KA, Steg PG, Eagle KA, et al. Decline in rates of death and heart failure in acute coronary syndromes, 1999–2006. *JAMA* 2007;297(17):1892–900.
10. Hochman JS, Buller CE, Sleeper LA, et al. Cardiogenic shock complicating acute myocardial infarction–etiologies, management and outcome: a report from the SHOCK Trial Registry. SHould we emergently revascularize Occluded Coronaries for cardiogenic shocK? *J Am Coll Cardiol* 2000;36(3 Suppl A):1063–70.
11. Hollenberg SM, Kavinsky CJ, Parrillo JE. Cardiogenic shock. *Ann Intern Med* 1999;131(1):47–59.
12. Picard MH, Davidoff R, Sleeper IA, et al. Echocardiographic predictors of survival and response to early revascularization in cardiogenic shock. *Circulation* 2003;107(2): 279–84.
13. Ramanathan K, Harkness SM, Nayar AC, et al. Cardiogenic shock in patients with preserved left ventricular systolic function: characteristics and insight into mechanisms. *J Am Coll Cardiol* 2004;43:241A.
14. Yehudai L, Reynolds HR, Schwarz SA, et al. Serial echocardiograms in patients with cardiogenic shock: analysis of the SHOCK Trial. *J Am Coll Cardiol* 2006;47 (Suppl A):111A.
15. Reynolds HR, Hochman JS. Cardiogenic shock: current concepts and improving outcomes. *Circulation* 2008;117(5):686–97.
16. Reynolds HR, Anand SK, Fox JM, et al. Restrictive physiology in cardiogenic shock: observations from echocardiography. *Am Heart J* 2006;151(890):e9–15.
17. Hochman JS. Cardiogenic shock complicating acute myocardial infarction: expanding the paradigm. *Circulation* 2003;107(24):2998–3002.
18. Rubbo H, Darley-Usmar V, Freeman BA. Nitric oxide regulation of tissue-free radical injury. *Chem Res Toxicol* 1996;9(9):809–20.
19. Wink DA, Hanbauer I, Krishna MC, et al. Nitric oxide protects against cellular damage and cytotoxicity from reactive oxygen species. *Proc Natl Acad Sci USA* 1993;90:9813–17.
20. Li H, Forstermann U. Nitric oxide in the pathogenesis of vascular disease. *J Pathol* 2000;190:244–54.
21. Wildhirt SM, Dudek RR, Suzuki H, et al. Involvement of inducible nitric oxide synthase in the inflammatory process of myocardial infarction. *Int J Cardiol* 1995(50): 253–61.
22. Depr'e C, Vanoverschelde JL, Goudemant JF, et al. Protection against ischemic injury by nonvasoactive concentrations of nitric oxide synthase inhibitors in the perfused rabbit heart. *Circulation* 1995;92(7):1911–18.
23. Schulz R, Wambolt R. Inhibition of nitric oxide synthesis protects the isolated working rabbit heart from ischaemia-reperfusion injury. *Cardiovasc Res* 1995;30(3):432–9.

24. Ziolo MT, Katoh H, Bers DM. Expression of inducible nitric oxide synthase depresses beta-adrenergic-stimulated calcium release from the sarcoplasmic reticulum in intact ventricular myocytes. *Circulation* 2001;104(24):2961–6.
25. TRIUMPH Investigators, Alexander JM, Raynolds HR, et al. Effect of Tilarginine acetate in patients with acute myocardial infarction and cardiogenic shock. *JAMA* 2007;297:1657–66.
26. Menon V, White H, LeJemtel T, et al. The clinical profile of patients with suspected cardiogenic shock due to predominant left ventricular failure: a report from the SHOCK Trial Registry. SHould we emergently revascularize Occluded Coronaries in cardiogenic shocK? *J Am Coll Cardiol* 2000;36(3 Suppl A):1071–6.
27. Hochman JS, Sleeper LA, Webb JG, et al. Early revascularization in acute myocardial infarction complicated by cardiogenic shock. SHOCK Investigators. Should We Emergently Revascularize Occluded Coronaries for Cardiogenic Shock. *N Engl J Med* 1999;341(9):625–34.
28. Webb JG, Sleeper LA, Buller CE, et al. Implications of the timing of onset of cardiogenic shock after acute myocardial infarction: a report from the SHOCK Trial Registry. SHould we emergently revascularize Occluded Coronaries for cardiogenic shocK? *J Am Coll Cardiol* 2000;36(3 Suppl A):1084–90.
29. Hasdai D, Harrington RA, Hochman JS, et al. Platelet glycoprotein IIb/IIIa blockade and outcome of cardiogenic shock complicating acute coronary syndromes without persistent ST-segment elevation. *J Am Coll Cardiol* 2000;36(3):685–92.
30. Jeger RV, Harkness SM, Ramanathan K, et al. Emergency revascularization in patients with cardiogenic shock on admission: a report from the SHOCK trial and registry. *Eur Heart J* 2006;27(6):664–70.
31. Hasdai D, Topol EJ, Califf RM, et al. Cardiogenic shock complicating acute coronary syndromes. *Lancet* 2000;356(9231):749–56.
32. Hasdai D, Califf RM, Thompson TD, et al. Predictors of cardiogenic shock after thrombolytic therapy for acute myocardial infarction. *J Am Coll Cardiol* 2000;35(1):136–43.
33. Menon V, Slater JN, White HD, et al, for the SHOCK Investigators. Acute myocardial infarction complicated by systemic hypoperfusion without hypotension: report of the SHOCK Trial Registry. *Am J Med* 2000;108:374–80 .
34. Berkowitz MJ, Picard MH, Harkness S, et al. Echocardiographic and angiographic correlations in patients with cardiogenic shock secondary to acute myocardial infarction. *Am J Cardiol* 2006;98(8):1004–8.
35. Mendes LA, Picard MH, Sleeper LA, et al. Cardiogenic shock: predictors of outcome based on right and left ventricular size and function at presentation. *Coron Artery Dis* 2005;16(4):209–15.
36. Reynolds HR, Anand SK, Fox JM, et al. Restrictive physiology in cardiogenic shock: observations from echocardiography. *Am Heart J* 2006;151(4):890, e9–15.
37. Jeger RV, Lowe AM, Buller CE, et al. Hemodynamic parameters are prognostically important in cardiogenic shock but similar following early revascularization or initial medical stabilization: a report from the SHOCK Trial. *Chest* 2007;132(6):1794–803.
38. Antman EM, Anbe DT, Armstrong PW, et al. ACC/AHA guidelines for the management of patients with ST-elevation myocardial infarction—executive summary: a report of the American College of Cardiology/American Heart Association Task Force on Practice Guidelines (Writing Committee to Revise the 1999 Guidelines for the

Management of Patients With Acute Myocardial Infarction). *Circulation* 2004;110(5): 588–636.

39. Hasdai D, Holmes DR Jr, Califf RM, et al. Cardiogenic shock complicating acute myocardial infarction: predictors of death. GUSTO Investigators. Global Utilization of Streptokinase and Tissue-Plasminogen Activator for Occluded Coronary Arteries. *Am Heart J* 1999;138(1 Pt 1):21–31.

40. Cohen MG, Kelly RV, Kong DF, et al. Pulmonary artery catheterization in acute coronary syndromes: Insights from the GUSTO IIb and GUSTO III trials. *Am J Med* 2005;118:482–8.

41. Binanay C, Califf RM, Hasselblad V, et al. Evaluation study of congestive heart failure and pulmonary artery catheterization effectiveness: the ESCAPE trial. *JAMA* 2005;294(13):1625–33.

42. Shah MR, Hasselblad V, Stevenson LW, et al. Impact of the pulmonary artery catheter in critically ill patients: meta-analysis of randomized clinical trials. *JAMA* 2005;294(13):1664–70.

43. Chen ZM, Pan HC, Chen YP, et al. Early intravenous then oral metoprolol in 45,852 patients with acute myocardial infarction: randomised placebo-controlled trial. *Lancet* 2005;366(9497):1622–32.

44. Scheidt S, Wilner G, Mueller H, et al. Intra-aortic balloon counterpulsation in cardiogenic shock. Report of a co-operative clinical trial. *N Engl J Med* 1973;288(19):979–84.

45. Kovack PJ, Rasak MA, Bates ER, et al. Thrombolysis plus aortic counterpulsation: improved survival in patients who present to community hospitals with cardiogenic shock. *J Am Coll Cardiol* 1997;29(7):1454–8.

46. Silverman AJ, Williams AM, Wetmore RW, Stomel RJ. Complications of intraaortic balloon counterpulsation insertion in patients receiving thrombolytic therapy for acute myocardial infarction. *J Interv Cardiol* 1991;4(1):49–52.

47. Stomel RJ, Rasak M, Bates ER. Treatment strategies for acute myocardial infarction complicated by cardiogenic shock in a community hospital. *Chest* 1994;105(4):997–1002.

48. Waksman R, Weiss AT, Gotsman MS, et al. Intra-aortic balloon counterpulsation improves survival in cardiogenic shock complicating acute myocardial infarction. *Eur Heart J* 1993;14(1):71–4.

49. Berger PB, Holmes DR Jr, Stebbins AL, et al. Impact of an aggressive invasive catheterization and revascularization strategy on mortality in patients with cardiogenic shock in the Global Utilization of Streptokinase and Tissue Plasminogen Activator for Occluded Coronary Arteries (GUSTO-I) trial. An observational study. *Circulation* 1997;96(1):122–7.

50. Sanborn TA, Sleeper LA, Bates ER, et al. Impact of thrombolysis, intra-aortic balloon pump counterpulsation, and their combination in cardiogenic shock complicating acute myocardial infarction: a report from the SHOCK Trial Registry. SHould we emergently revascularize Occluded Coronaries for cardiogenic shocK? *J Am Coll Cardiol* 2000;36(3 Suppl A):1123–9.

51. Barron HV, Every NR, Parsons LS, et al. The use of intra-aortic balloon counterpulsation in patients with cardiogenic shock complicating acute myocardial infarction: data from the National Registry of Myocardial Infarction 2. *Am Heart J* 2001;141(6):933–9.

52. Ohman EM, Nanas J, Stomel RJ, et al. Thrombolysis and counterpulsation to improve survival in myocardial infarction complicated by hypotension and suspected

cardiogenic shock or heart failure: results of the TACTICS Trial. *J Thromb Thrombolysis* 2005;19(1):33–9.

53. Vranckx P, Foley DP, de Feijter PJ, et al. Clinical introduction of the Tandemheart, a percutaneous left ventricular assist device, for circulatory support during high-risk percutaneous coronary intervention. *Int J Cardiovasc Intervent* 2003;5(1):35–9.

54. Chandra D, Kar B, Idelchik G, et al. Usefulness of percutaneous left ventricular assist device as a bridge to recovery from myocarditis. *Am J Cardiol* 2007;99(12):1755–6.

55. Idelchik GM, Loyalka P, Kar B. Percutaneous ventricular assist device placement during active cardiopulmonary resuscitation for severe refractory cardiogenic shock after acute myocardial infarction. *Tex Heart Inst J* 2007;34(2):204–8.

56. Khalife WI, Kar B. The TandemHeart pVAD in the treatment of acute fulminant myocarditis. *Tex Heart Inst J* 2007;34(2):209–13.

57. Kar B, Adkins LE, Civitello AB, et al. Clinical experience with the TandemHeart percutaneous ventricular assist device. *Tex Heart Inst J* 2006;33(2):111–5.

58. Aragon J, Lee MS, Kar S, et al. Percutaneous left ventricular assist device: "Tandem-Heart" for high-risk coronary intervention. *Catheter Cardiovasc Interv* 2005;65(3):346–52.

59. Kar B, Butkevich A, Civitello AB, et al. Hemodynamic support with a percutaneous left ventricular assist device during stenting of an unprotected left main coronary artery. *Tex Heart Inst J* 2004;31(1):84–6.

60. Burkhoff D, Cohen H, Brunckhorst C, et al. A randomized multicenter clinical study to evaluate the safety and efficacy of the TandemHeart percutaneous ventricular assist device versus conventional therapy with intraaortic balloon pumping for treatment of cardiogenic shock. *Am Heart J* 2006;152(3):469, e1–8.

61. Thiele H, Sick P, Boudriot E, et al. Randomized comparison of intra-aortic balloon support with a percutaneous left ventricular assist device in patients with revascularized acute myocardial infarction complicated by cardiogenic shock. *Eur Heart J* 2005;26:1276–83.

62. Henriques JP, Remmelink M, Baan J Jr, et al. Safety and feasibility of elective high-risk percutaneous coronary intervention procedures with left ventricular support of the Impella Recover LP 2.5. *Am J Cardiol* 2006;97(7):990–2.

63. Meyns B, Dens J, Sergeant P, et al. Initial experiences with the Impella device in patients with cardiogenic shock—Impella support for cardiogenic shock. *Thorac Cardiovasc Surg* 2003;51(6):312–17.

64. Siegenthaler MP, Brehm K, Strecker T, et al. The Impella Recover microaxial left ventricular assist device reduces mortality for postcardiotomy failure: a three-center experience. *J Thorac Cardiovasc Surg* 2004;127(3):812–22.

65. Garatti A, Colombo T, Russo C, et al. Impella recover 100 microaxial left ventricular assist device: the Niguarda experience. *Transplant Proc* 2004;36(3):623–6.

66. Jurmann MJ, Siniawski H, Erb M, et al. Initial experience with miniature axial flow ventricular assist devices for postcardiotomy heart failure. *Ann Thorac Surg* 2004;77(5):1642–7.

67. Valgimigli M, Steendijk P, Sianos G, et al. Left ventricular unloading and concomitant total cardiac output increase by the use of percutaneous Impella Recover LP 2.5 assist device during high-risk coronary intervention. *Catheter Cardiovasc Interv* 2005;65(2):263–7.

68. Minden HH, Lehmann H, Meyhöfer J, Butter C. Transradial unprotected left main coronary stenting supported by percutaneous Impella Recover LP 2.5 assist device. *Clin Res Cardiol* 2006;95(5):301–6.

69. Scholz KH. [Reperfusion therapy and mechanical circulatory support in patients in cardiogenic shock]. *Herz* 1999;24(6):448–64.

70. Shawl FA, Domanski MJ, Wish MH, et al. Emergency cardiopulmonary bypass support in patients with cardiac arrest in the catheterization laboratory. *Cathet Cardiovasc Diagn* 1990;19(1):8–12.

71. Reedy JE, Swartz MT, Raithel SC, et al. Mechanical cardiopulmonary support for refractory cardiogenic shock. *Heart Lung* 1990;19(5 Pt 1):514–23.

72. Reichman RT, Joyo CI, Dembitsky WP, et al. Improved patient survival after cardiac arrest using a cardiopulmonary support system. *Ann Thorac Surg* 1990;49(1):101–4; discussion 104–5.

73. Overlie PA, Walter PD, Hurd HP II, et al. Emergency cardiopulmonary support with circulatory support devices. *Cardiology* 1994;84(3):231–7.

74. Mooney MR, Arom KV, Joyce LD, et al. Emergency cardiopulmonary bypass support in patients with cardiac arrest. *J Thorac Cardiovasc Surg* 1991;101(3):450–4.

75. Hartz R, LoCicero J III, Sanders JH Jr, et al. Clinical experience with portable cardiopulmonary bypass in cardiac arrest patients. *Ann Thorac Surg* 1990;50(3):437–41.

76. Shawl FA, Domanski MJ, Hernandez TJ, Punja S. Emergency percutaneous cardiopulmonary bypass support in cardiogenic shock from acute myocardial infarction. *Am J Cardiol* 1989;64(16):967–70.

77. Farrar DJ, Lawson JH, Litwak P, Cederwall G. Thoratec VAD system as a bridge to heart transplantation. *J Heart Transplant* 1990;9(4):415–22; discussion 422–3.

78. Park SJ, Nguyen DQ, Bank AJ, et al. Left ventricular assist device bridge therapy for acute myocardial infarction. *Ann Thorac Surg* 2000;69(4):1146–51.

79. Leshnower BG, Gleason TG, O'Hara ML, et al. Safety and efficacy of left ventricular assist device support in postmyocardial infarction cardiogenic shock. *Ann Thorac Surg* 2006;81(4):1365–70; discussion 1370–1.

80. Vitali E, Lanfranconi M, Bruschi G, et al. Mechanical circulatory support in severe heart failure: single-center experience. *Transplant Proc* 2004;36(3):620–2.

81. Ueno T, Bergin P, Richardson M, Esmore DS. Bridge to recovery with a left ventricular assist device for fulminant acute myocarditis. *Ann Thorac Surg* 2000;69(1):284–6.

82. Weitkemper HH, El-Banayosy A, Arusoglu L, et al. Mechanical circulatory support: reality and dreams experience of a single center. *J Extra Corpor Technol* 2004;36(2):169–73.

83. Hochman JS, Sleeper LA, Webb JG, et al. Early revascularization and long-term survival in cardiogenic shock complicating acute myocardial infarction. *JAMA* 2006;295(21):2511–5.

84. Hochman JS, Sleeper LA, White HD, et al. One-year survival following early revascularization for cardiogenic shock. SHOCK Investigators. Should We Emergently Revascularize Occluded Coronaries for Cardiogenic Shock. *JAMA* 2001;285(2):190–2.

85. Urban P, Stauffer JC, Bleed D, et al. A randomized evaluation of early revascularization to treat shock complicating acute myocardial infarction. The (Swiss) Multicenter Trial of Angioplasty for Shock-(S)MASH. *Eur Heart J* 1999;20(14):1030–8

86. Dzavik V, Sleeper LA, Picard MH, et al. Outcome of patients aged ≥75 years in the SHould we emergently revascularize Occluded Coronaries in cardiogenic shocK (SHOCK) trial: do elderly patients with acute myocardial infarction complicated by cardiogenic shock respond differently to emergent revascularization? *Am Heart J* 2005;149(6):1128–34.

87. Dzavik V, Sleeper LA, Cocke TP, et al. Early revascularization is associated with improved survival in elderly patients with acute myocardial infarction complicated by cardiogenic shock: a report from the SHOCK Trial Registry. *Eur Heart J* 2003;24(9): 828–37.

88. Dauerman HL, Goldberg RJ, Malinski M, et al. Outcomes and early revascularization for patients ≥65 years of age with cardiogenic shock. *Am J Cardiol* 2001;87(7): 844–8.

89. Dauerman HL, Ryan TJ Jr, Piper WD, et al. Outcomes of percutaneous coronary intervention among elderly patients in cardiogenic shock: a multicenter, decade-long experience. *J Invasive Cardiol* 2003;15(7):380–4.

90. Antman EM, Anbe DT, Armstrong PW, et al. ACC/AHA guidelines for the management of patients with ST-elevation myocardial infarction. *Circulation* 2004;110:e82–293.

91. White HD, Assmann SF, Sanborn TA, et al. Comparison of percutaneous coronary intervention and coronary artery bypass grafting after acute myocardial infarction complicated by cardiogenic shock: results from the Should We Emergently Revascularize Occluded Coronaries for Cardiogenic Shock (SHOCK) trial. *Circulation* 2005;112(13):1992–2001.

92. Gruppo Italiano per lo Studio della Streptochinasi nell'Infarto Miocardico (GISSI). Effectiveness of intravenous thrombolytic treatment in acute myocardial infarction. *Lancet* 1986;1(8478):397–402.

93. Fibrinolytic Therapy Trialists' (FTT) Collaborative Group. Indications for fibrinolytic therapy in suspected acute myocardial infarction: collaborative overview of early mortality and major morbidity results from all randomised trials of more than 1000 patients. *Lancet* 1994;343(8893):311–22.

94. Prewitt RM. Thrombolytic therapy in patients where hypotension or cardiogenic shock complicate acute myocardial infarction. *Can J Cardiol* 1993;9:155–7.

95. Jeger RV, Tseng CH, Hochman JS, Bates ER. Interhospital transfer for early revascularization in patients with ST-elevation myocardial infarction complicated by cardiogenic shock—a report from the SHould we revascularize Occluded Coronaries for cardiogenic shocK? (SHOCK) trial and registry. *Am Heart J* 2006;152(4):686–92.

96. Grines CL, Westerhausen DR Jr, Grines LL, et al. A randomized trial of transfer for primary angioplasty versus on-site thrombolysis in patients with high-risk myocardial infarction: the Air Primary Angioplasty in Myocardial Infarction study. *J Am Coll Cardiol* 2002;39(11):1713–19.

97. Bonnefoy E, Lapostolle F, Leizorovicz A, et al. Primary angioplasty versus prehospital fibrinolysis in acute myocardial infarction: a randomised study. *Lancet* 2002;360(9336):825–9.

98. Steg PG, Bonnefoy E, Chabaud S, et al. Impact of time to treatment on mortality after prehospital fibrinolysis or primary angioplasty: data from the CAPTIM randomized clinical trial. *Circulation* 2003;108(23):2851–6.

99. Henry TD, Sharkey SW, Burke MN, et al. A regional system to provide timely access to percutaneous coronary intervention for ST-elevation myocardial infarction. *Circulation* 2007;116(7):721–8.

# Chapter 5

# Pathophysiology and management of shock due to right heart ischemia

James A. Goldstein

Based on early experiments of right ventricular (RV) performance, RV contraction was for many years considered unimportant in the circulation. The profound hemodynamic effects of RV systolic dysfunction were recognized when severe RV infarction (RVI) was first described [1–7]. Significant RVI occurs in association with acute transmural inferior–posterior left ventricular (LV) myocardial infarction (MI); the right coronary artery (RCA) is always the culprit vessel [3,5–9]. At necropsy, RVI inscribes a "tripartite" signature consisting of necrosis of the LV inferior–posterior wall, septum, and posterior RV free wall contiguous with the septum [3].

Nearly 50% of patients with acute inferior MI manifest echocardiographic evidence of RV ischemic dysfunction, characterized by RV free wall motion abnormalities and RV dilatation [5,6]. RVI may be silent, with hemodynamic compromise developing in less than 25% of cases, presenting in its most dramatic form as frank shock, with severe right heart failure, clear lungs, and low output despite intact global LV systolic function [2,4–7].

## Clinical presentations and evaluation

Patients with severe RVI but preserved global LV function may be hemodynamically compensated, manifested by elevated jugular venous pressure (JVP) but clear lungs, normal systemic arterial pressure, and intact perfusion [5–7]. When RVI leads to more severe hemodynamic compromise, cardiogenic shock (i.e. systemic hypotension and hypoperfusion despite adequate RV filling pressures) results. "Isolated" RV failure accounts for 2.8% of cases of cardiogenic shock complicating acute MI [10,11]. Patients with inferior MI may initially

*Cardiogenic Shock.* Edited by Judith S. Hochman and E. Magnus Ohman.
© 2009 American Heart Association, ISBN: 978-1-4051-7926-3

present without evidence of hemodynamic compromise, but subsequently develop hypotension precipitated by preload reduction attributable to nitroglycerin or associated with bradyarrhythmias [7]. When RVI develops in the setting of global LV dysfunction, the picture may be dominated by low output and pulmonary congestion with right heart failure.

## Noninvasive and hemodynamic evaluation

Although ST-segment elevation and loss of R wave in the right-sided electrocardiogram (ECG) leads ($V_{3R}$ and $V_{4R}$) are sensitive indicators of RVI when obtained early after infarct onset [5,7], they are not predictive of the magnitude of RV dysfunction nor its hemodynamic impact. Echocardiography (echo) is the most effective tool for delineation of the presence and severity of RV dilatation and depression of global RV performance [7]. Echo also delineates the extent of reversed septal curvature, which confirms the presence of significant adverse diastolic interactions, the degree of paradoxical septal motion indicative of compensatory systolic interactions, and the presence of severe right atrial (RA) enlargement which may indicate concomitant ischemic RA dysfunction and/or tricuspid regurgitation.

Although the magnitude of hemodynamic derangements is related to the extent of RV free wall contraction abnormalities [5–9], some patients tolerate severe RV systolic dysfunction without hemodynamic compromise, whereas others develop life-threatening low output, emphasizing that additional factors modulate the clinical expression of RVI. Although acute ischemic RV dysfunction may result in hemodynamic compromise associated with higher in-hospital morbidity and mortality [8–12], most patients manifest spontaneous early hemodynamic improvement and later recovery of RV function, even in the absence of reperfusion of the infarct-related artery [5,8,13,14]. In fact, chronic right heart failure attributable to RVI is rare [7]. The term RV "infarction" is, to an extent, a misnomer, for in most cases acute RV ischemic dysfunction appears to represent viable myocardium. These responses are in marked contrast to the effects of ischemia on the left ventricle [15].

## Differential diagnosis of right ventricular ischemia

Important clinical entities to consider in patients who present with low-output hypotension, clear lungs, and disproportionate right heart failure include cardiac tamponade, constrictive pericarditis or restrictive cardiomyopathy, acute severe tricuspid regurgitation, severe pulmonary hypertension, acute pulmonary embolism, and right heart mass obstruction. The hemodynamic differentiation of these are shown in Table 5.1. The general clinical presentation of chest pain with acute inferior MI, together with echocardiographic documentation of RV dilatation and dysfunction, effectively exclude tamponade,

**Table 5.1** Hemodynamic patterns.

|  | RA | RVS | RVD | PAS | PAD | PAW | CI | SVR |
|---|---|---|---|---|---|---|---|---|
| Normal values | <6 | <25 | 0–12 | <25 | 0–12 | <6–12 | ≥2.5 | (800–1600) |
| Pulmonary edema | ↔↑ | ↔↑ | ↔↑ | ↑ | ↑ | ↑ | ↔↓ | ↑ |
| Cardiogenic shock |  |  |  |  |  |  |  |  |
| LV failure | ↔↑ | ↔↑ | ↔↑ | ↔↑ | ↑ | ↑ | ↓ | ↔↑ |
| RV failure† | ↑ | ↓↔↑* | ↑ | ↓↔↑* | ↔↓↑* | ↓↔↑* | ↓ | ↑ |
| Cardiac tamponade | ↑ | ↔↑ | ↑ | ↔↑ | ↔↑ | ↔↑ | ↓ | ↑ |

There is significant patient-to-patient variation. Abbreviations: RA, right atrium; RVS/D, right ventricular systolic/diastolic; PAS/D, pulmonary artery systolic/diastolic; PAW, pulmonary artery wedge (mm Hg). CI, cardiac index (L/min/m²); SVR, systemic vascular resistance (dynes/sec/cm⁵).

*PAW and PA pressures may rise in RV failure after volume loading due to RV dilation, right-to-left shift of the interventricular septum, resulting in impaired LV filling. When biventricular failure is present, the patterns are similar to those shown for LV failure. Values in parentheses represent range. Reprinted with permission from Hochman JS and Ingbar D. Cardiogenic Shock and Pulmonary Edema in Fauci AS, Braunwald E, Kasper DL et al., Harrison's Principles of Internal Medicine 17th Edition, McGraw-Hill Medical, 2008.

†"Isolated" or predominant RV failure.

constriction, and restriction. Echocardiography confirms primary tricuspid regurgitation. Severe pulmonary hypertension with RV decompensation may mimic severe RVI, but delineation of markedly elevated pulmonary artery systolic pressures by Doppler or invasive hemodynamic monitoring excludes RVI, in which RV pressure generation is depressed. Acute massive pulmonary embolism may also mimic severe RVI and, since the unprepared right ventricle cannot acutely generate elevated RV systolic pressures (>50–55 mm Hg), severe pulmonary hypertension may be absent. In such cases, absence of inferior LV MI by ECG and echo point to embolism, easily confirmed by CT or invasive angiography.

## Right ventricular mechanics and oxygen supply–demand

The right and left ventricles face dramatically different loading conditions and therefore differ markedly in their anatomy, mechanics, and metabolism. In contrast to the LV, a thick-walled pressure pump, the pyramidal-shaped right ventricle with its thin crescentic free wall is designed as a volume pump, ejecting into the lower resistance pulmonary circulation. RV systolic pressure and flow are generated by RV free wall shortening and contraction toward the septum from apex to outflow tract [7,16]. The septum is an integral architectural and mechanical component of the RV chamber and, even under physiologic conditions, LV-septal contraction contributes to RV performance. The right ventricle has a more favorable oxygen supply–demand profile than the left ventricle. RV oxygen demand is lower owing to lesser myocardial mass, preload, and afterload [17,18]. RV perfusion also is more favorable, due to a dual anatomic supply system from left coronary branches. The RV free wall is thinner, develops lower systolic intramyocardial pressure, and faces less diastolic intracavitary pressure, and lower coronary resistance favors acute collateral development to the RCA [19–21].

## Patterns of coronary compromise resulting in right ventricular ischemia

The RCA is the culprit vessel in RV ischemic dysfunction, typically proximal occlusion compromising flow to the major RV branches (Figs. 5.1 and 5.2) [6,8,9]. In contrast, distal RCA lesions or circumflex culprits that spare RV branch perfusion rarely compromise RV performance [9]. There are exceptions in which proximal occlusions do not result in RV ischemic dysfunction, attributable in most cases to restoration of RV free wall perfusion through prominent collaterals or spontaneous antegrade reperfusion. Occasionally, isolated RVI may develop from occlusion of a nondominant RCA or compromise of RV branches during percutaneous interventions.

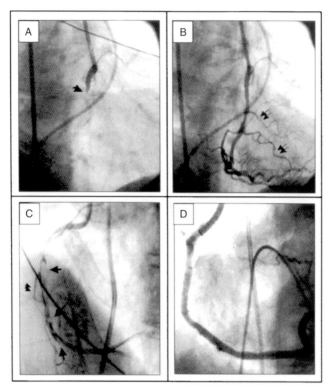

**Fig. 5.1** Angiograms showing successful and unsuccessful reperfusion in patients with RV infarction who underwent primary angioplasty. Panel A shows total occlusion of the right coronary artery proximal to RV branches (arrow) in a patient before angioplasty, and Panel B after angioplasty shows complete reperfusion in the right main coronary artery including the major RV branches (arrowheads). Panel C in another patient shows complete failure of RCA reperfusion (arrowhead), attributable to refractory dissection and thrombus (arrows). Panel D shows partial reperfusion in a third patient, with absence of flow in the RV branches, despite successful reperfusion of the right main coronary artery and its LV branches. (Reprinted with permission from Bowers TR, O'Neill WW, Grines C, et al. *N Engl J Med* 1998;338:933–40.)

## Effects of right ventricular systolic and diastolic dysfunction

Proximal RCA occlusion that compromises RV free wall perfusion results in RV free wall dyskinesis and depressed global RV performance reflected by a sluggish, depressed RV systolic waveform (Figs. 5.2–5.4) [6–8,19,20,22–26]. RV systolic dysfunction diminishes transpulmonary delivery of LV preload, leading to decreased cardiac output despite intact LV contractility.

Biventricular diastolic dysfunction contributes to hemodynamic compromise [6,7,19,20,22–27]. The ischemic RV is noncompliant, which impedes inflow

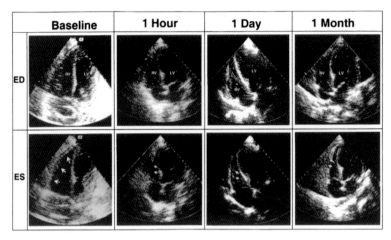

**Fig. 5.2** Echocardiographic images from a patient with acute inferior MI and RV ischemia undergoing successful angioplasty. End diastolic and end systolic images obtained at base line show severe RV dilatation with reduced LV diastolic size. At end systole, there was RV free wall dyskinesis (arrows), intact LV function, and compensatory paradoxical septal motion. One hour after angioplasty, there was striking recovery of RV free wall contraction (arrows), resulting in marked improvement in global RV performance and markedly reduced RV size and increased LV preload. At day 1, there was further improvement in RV function (arrows), which at 1 month was normal. Abbreviations: RV, right ventricle; LV, left ventricle. (Reprinted with permission from Bowers TR, O'Neill WW, Grines C, et al. *N Engl J Med* 1998;338:933–40.)

leading to rapid elevation of diastolic pressure. Acute RV dilatation and elevated diastolic pressure shift the interventricular septum toward the volume-deprived left ventricle, further impairing LV compliance and filling. Abrupt RV dilatation within the noncompliant pericardium elevates intrapericardial pressure, further impairing RV and LV compliance and filling. These effects contribute to the pattern of equalized diastolic pressures and the RV "dip-and-plateau" characteristic of RVI [4,6,22–26].

## Determinants of right ventricular performance in severe right ventricular ischemia: importance of systolic ventricular interactions

Despite the absence of RV free wall motion, an active albeit depressed RV systolic waveform is generated by systolic interactions mediated by primary septal contraction and mechanical displacement of the septum into the RV cavity associated with paradoxical septal motion (Fig. 5.2) [6,7,19,20,22–26]. In the LV, acute ischemia results in regional dyskinesis; such dysynergic segments are stretched in early isovolumic systole by neighboring contracting segments through regional intraventricular interactions that dissipate the functional work

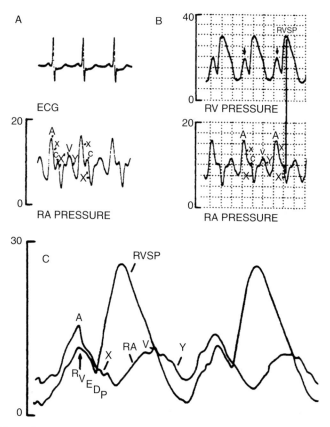

**Fig. 5.3** Hemodynamic recordings from a patient with RA pressure W pattern, timed to ECG (A) and RV pressures (B, C). Peaks of W are formed by prominent A waves with associated sharp X systolic descent, followed by a comparatively blunted Y descent. Peak RVSP is depressed, RV relaxation is prolonged, and there is a dip and rapid rise in RV diastolic pressure. (Reprinted with permission from Goldstein JA, Barzilai B, Rosamond TL, et al. *Circulation* 1990;82:359–68.)

of these neighboring regions [28]. The ischemic dyskinetic RV free wall behaves similarly and must be stretched to the maximal extent of its systolic lengthening through interventricular interactions before providing a stable buttress upon which actively contracting segments can generate effective stroke work, thereby imposing a mechanical disadvantage that reduces contributions to cardiac performance [19,20,25,27]. The compensatory contributions of LV-septal contraction are emphasized by the deleterious effects of LV-septal dysfunction which exacerbates the hemodynamic compromise associated with RVI [26]. In contrast, inotropic stimulation enhances LV-septal contraction and thereby augments RV performance through augmented compensatory systolic interactions.

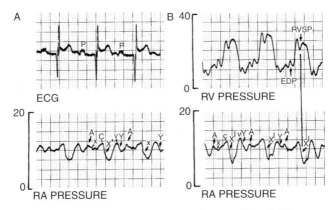

**Fig. 5.4** RA M pressure pattern timed to electrocardiogram (A) and RV pressure (B). M pattern comprises a depressed A wave, X descent before a small C wave, a prominent X descent, a small V wave, and a blunted Y descent. Peak RV systolic pressure (RVSP) is depressed and bifid (arrow) with delayed relaxation and an elevated end-diastolic pressure (EDP). (All pressures are measured in mm Hg). (Reprinted with permission from Goldstein JA, Barzilai B, Rosamond TL, et al. *Circulation* 1990;82:359–68.)

## Compensatory role of augmented right atrial contraction

The hemodynamic benefits of augmented atrial contraction to performance of the ischemic LV are well documented [29]. Similarly, augmented RA booster pump transport is an important compensatory mechanism that optimizes RV performance and cardiac output [24,26]. When RVI develops from occlusions compromising RV but sparing RA branches, RV diastolic dysfunction imposes increased preload and afterload on the right atrium, resulting in enhanced RA contractility that augments RV filling and performance. This is reflected in the RA waveform as a "W" pattern characterized by a rapid upstroke and increased peak A wave amplitude, sharp X descent reflecting enhanced atrial relaxation, and blunted Y descent owing to pandiastolic RV dysfunction (Fig. 5.3). Conversely, more proximal RCA occlusions compromising atrial as well as RV branches result in ischemic depression of atrial function, which compromises RV performance and cardiac output [6,24,26]. RA ischemia manifests hemodynamically as more severely elevated mean RA pressure and inscribes an "M" pattern in the RA waveform characterized by depressed A wave and X descent, as well as blunted Y descent (Fig. 5.4).

Ischemic atrial involvement is not rare, with autopsy studies documenting atrial infarction in up to 20% of cases of ventricular infarction, with RA involvement five times more common than left [6,7,30,31]. Under conditions of acute RV dysfunction, loss of augmented RA transport due to ischemic depression of atrial contractility or AV dyssynchrony precipitates more severe hemodynamic compromise [24,32]. RA dysfunction decreases RV filling, which impairs global RV systolic performance, thereby resulting in further decrements in LV preload and cardiac output [19,20,25,26]. Impaired RA contraction diminishes atrial relaxation; thus, RA ischemia impedes venous return and right heart filling owing to loss of atrial suction associated with atrial relaxation during the X descent [7,24–26,33].

## Rhythm disorders and reflexes associated with right ventricular ischemia

High-grade atrioventricular (AV) block and bradycardia-hypotension without AV block commonly complicate inferior MI and have been attributed predominantly to the effects of AV nodal ischemia and cardioinhibitory (Bezold-Jarisch) reflexes arising from stimulation of vagal afferents in the ischemic LV inferoposterior wall [34–38]. Patients with acute RVI are at increased risk for both high-grade AV block and bradycardia-hypotension without AV block [8,12,38–40]. Recent findings have documented that, during acute coronary occlusion, bradycardia-hypotension and AV block are far more common in patients with proximal RCA lesions (Fig. 5.5), inducing RV and LV inferior–posterior ischemia, compared with more distal occlusions compromising LV perfusion but sparing the RV branches [39]. These observations suggest that the ischemic right heart may elicit cardioinhibitory-vasodilator reflexes. In patients with inferior MI, similar bradycardic-hypotensive reflexes may be elicited during reperfusion (Fig. 5.6), and they also appear to be more common with proximal versus distal RCA lesions [39]. Following successful thrombolysis or primary angioplasty of the acutely occluded RCA, transient but profound bradycardia-hypotension may develop paradoxically in a patient whose rhythm and blood pressure were stable during occlusion [39,40].

Patients with RVI are prone to in-hospital ventricular tachyarrhythmias [8,12,41], which should not be unexpected given that the ischemic RV is often massively dilated. Autonomic denervation in the peri-infarct area may also play a role [41]. Supraventricular tachycardias including atrial fibrillation also may develop, attributable to atrial ischemia/infarction, distension, and elevated atrial pressures.

## Natural history of right ventricular ischemic dysfunction

In marked contrast to the effects of coronary occlusion on segmental and global LV function, the natural history of RV performance following RVI is quite favorable. Although RVI may result in profound acute hemodynamic effects, arrhythmias, and higher in-hospital mortality, many patients improve spontaneously within 3 to 10 days regardless of the patency status of the infarct-related artery [5,13]. Within 3 to 12 months, global RV performance typically recovers [13,14]. Chronic unilateral right heart failure secondary to RVI is rare [14].

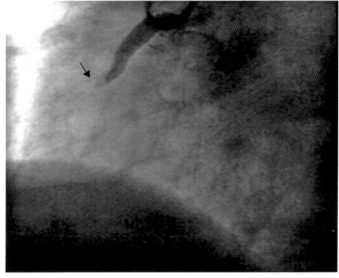

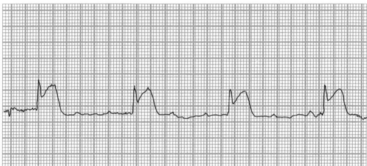

**Fig. 5.5** Patient with proximal RCA occlusion (arrow) complicated by third-degree AV block. (Reprinted with permission from Goldstein JA, Lee DT, Pica MC, et al. *Coron Artery Dis* 2005;16:265–74.)

Observations from experimental animal studies confirm spontaneous recovery of RV function despite chronic RCA occlusion attributable to the more favorable oxygen supply–demand characteristics of the RV in general and the beneficial effects of collaterals in particular [19,20]. Similarly, in patients with chronic proximal RCA occlusion, RV function is typically maintained at rest and augments appropriately during stress [14]. This dramatic spontaneous recovery of RV function and trivial infarction contrast sharply with the response of the left ventricle to equivalent ischemic insults [42,43]. The relative resistance of the RV free wall to infarction is undoubtedly attributable to more favorable oxygen supply–demand characteristics [7]. Pre-infarction angina appears to reduce the risk of developing RVI, possibly due to preconditioning [43].

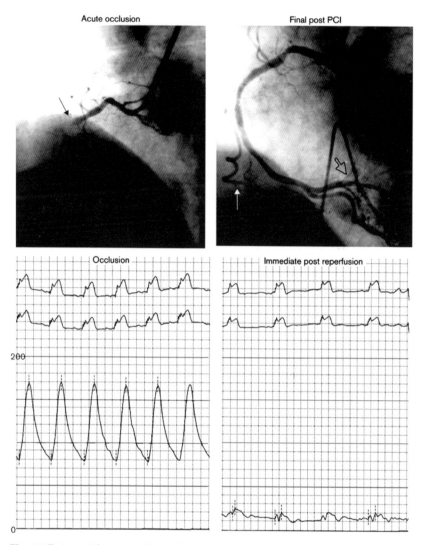

**Fig. 5.6** Patient with proximal RCA (left panel, arrow) compromising the RV branches (right panel, solid arrow) as well as the LV and AV nodal branches (right panel, open arrow), who developed profound reperfusion-induced bradycardia–hypotension. During occlusion, there was sinus rhythm with normal blood pressure (left panel, second and third rows, respectively). Reperfusion by primary percutaneous transluminal coronary angioplasty resulted in abrupt but transient sinus bradycardia with profound hypotension (right panel, second and third rows, respectively). Abbreviation: PCI, percutaneous coronary intervention. (Reprinted with permission from Goldstein JA, Lee DT, Pica MC, et al. *Coron Artery Dis* 2005;16:265–74.)

## Mechanical complications associated with right ventricular ischemia

Patients with acute RVI may suffer additional mechanical complications that may compound hemodynamic compromise and confound the clinical-hemodynamic picture. Ventricular septal rupture is a particularly disastrous complication, adding substantial overload stress to the ischemically dysfunctional right ventricle, precipitating pulmonary edema, elevating pulmonary pressures and resistance, and exacerbating low output [44]. Surgical repair is imperative but may be technically difficult owing to extensive necrosis involving the LV inferior–posterior free wall, septum, and apex. RV dysfunction increases the surgical mortality rate.

Severe right heart dilatation and diastolic pressure elevation associated with RVI may stretch open a patent foramen ovale, precipitating acute right-to-left shunting manifest as systemic hypoxemia or paradoxic emboli. Although most resolve as right heart pressures diminish with recovery of RV performance, some may require closure [45]. Severe tricuspid regurgitation may also complicate RVI, developing as a result of primary papillary muscle ischemic dysfunction or rupture as well as secondary functional regurgitation attributable to severe RV and tricuspid valve annular dilatation [46].

## Therapy

Therapeutic options for management of right heart ischemia (Table 5.2) follow directly from the pathophysiology. Treatment modalities include: (1) restoration of physiologic rhythm; (2) optimization of ventricular preload; (3) optimization of oxygen supply and demand; (4) parenteral inotropic support for persistent hemodynamic compromise; (5) reperfusion; and (6) mechanical support with intra-aortic balloon counterpulsation and RV assist devices.

## Optimization of rhythm

Patients with RVI are particularly prone to the adverse effects of bradyarrhythmias. The depressed ischemic right ventricle has a relatively fixed stroke volume, as does the preload-deprived left ventricle [7,19,20,39]. Therefore, biventricular output is exquisitely heart rate-dependent, and bradycardia even in the absence of AV dyssynchrony may be deleterious to patients with RVI. For similar reasons, chronotropic competence is critical. However, not only are such patients notoriously prone to reflex-mediated frank bradycardia, but they often manifest a relative inability to increase sinus rate in response to low output, owing to excess vagal tone, ischemia, or pharmacologic agents. Given that the ischemic right ventricle is dependent on atrial transport, the loss of RA contraction due to AV dyssynchrony further exacerbates difficulties with RV filling and contributes to hemodynamic compromise [7,24,32]. Although atropine may restore physiologic rhythm in some patients, temporary pacing is often required. Ventricular

**Table 5.2** RV infarction: ACC/AHA guidelines for the management of patients with ST-elevation MI, executive summary.

**Class I**

1. Patients with inferior STEMI and hemodynamic compromise should be assessed with a precordial V4R lead to detect ST-segment elevation and an echocardiogram to screen for RV infarction (Level of evidence B).

2. The following principles of apply to therapy of patients with STEMI and RV infarction and ischemic dysfunction:
   a. Early reperfusion should be achieved if possible (Level of evidence C).
   b. AV synchrony should be achieved, and bradycardia should be corrected (Level of evidence C).
   c. RV preload should be optimized, which usually requires initial volume challenge in patients with hemodynamic instability provided the jugular venous pressure is normal or low (Level of evidence C).
   d. RV afterload should be optimized, which usually requires therapy for concomitant LV dysfunction (Level of evidence C).
   e. Inotropic therapy should be used for hemodynamic instability not responsive to volume challenge (Level of evidence C).

**Class IIa**

1. After infarction that leads to clinically significant RV dysfunction, it is reasonable to delay CABG surgery for 4 weeks to allow recovery of contractile performance (Level of evidence C).

Reprinted with permission from Antman EM, Anbe DT, Armstrong PW, et al. *J Am Coll Cardiol* 2004;44:671–719.

pacing alone may suffice, especially if the bradyarrhythmias are intermittent, but some patients require temporary AV sequential pacing.

## Optimization of ventricular preload

In patients with RVI, the dilated, noncompliant right ventricle is exquisitely preload-dependent, as is the left ventricle, which is stiff but preload-deprived. Therefore, any factor that reduces ventricular preload tends to be detrimental. Accordingly, vasodilators and diuretics are contraindicated. Although experimental animal studies of RVI demonstrate hemodynamic benefit from volume loading [21], clinical studies have reported variable responses to volume challenge [2,5,6,47–49]. These conflicting results may reflect a spectrum of initial volume status in patients with acute RVI, with those patients who are relatively volume-depleted benefiting, and those who are more replete manifesting a flat or negative response of cardiac output to fluid administration. Nevertheless, an initial volume challenge is appropriate for patients manifesting low output without pulmonary congestion if the estimated central venous pressure is less than 15 mm Hg. For those unresponsive to an initial trial of fluids, determination of filling pressures and subsequent hemodynamically monitored volume challenge may be appropriate, combined with inotropic therapy for those with adequate filling pressures. The optimal filling pressure is typically 10–15 mm Hg, but varies among patients and should be empirically determined. Caution should be exercised to avoid excessive volume administration beyond that documented to augment output, since cardiac output may fall with RV overdistention. The mechanisms include: impaired LV filling, which results from excessive RV dilatation and ventricular interdependence, and/or reduced contractility based on the right ventricle operating on the "descending limb" of the Starling curve. Perhaps reflecting the adverse effect of volume overloading, the mean RA pressure was 25 mm Hg in patients with "isolated" RV shock in the SHOCK registry [11]. Abnormalities of volume retention and impaired diuresis may be related in part to impaired responses of atrial natriuretic factor [50].

## Anti-ischemic therapy

Treatment of RVI should focus on optimizing oxygen supply and demand to optimize recovery of both RV function and LV function. However, most anti-ischemic agents exert hemodynamic effects that may be deleterious in patients with RVI. Beta blockers and some calcium-channel blockers may reduce heart rate and depress conduction, thereby increasing the risk of bradyarrhythmias and heart block in these chronotropically dependent patients. The vasodilator properties of nitrates and calcium-channel blockers may precipitate hypotension. In general, these drugs should be avoided in patients with RVI.

## Reperfusion therapy

### Effects of reperfusion on ischemic right ventricular dysfunction

Although RV function may recover despite persistent RCA occlusion, acute RV ischemia contributes to early morbidity and mortality [6,12]. Furthermore, spontaneous recovery of RV contractile function and hemodynamics may be slow. The beneficial effects of successful reperfusion in patients with predominant LV infarction are well documented [51,52]. Observations in experimental animals [20] and in humans [8,53] demonstrate the beneficial effects of reperfusion on recovery of RV performance. In patients, successful mechanical reperfusion of the RCA, including the major RV branches, leads to immediate improvement in and later complete recovery of RV free wall function and global RV performance (Figs. 5.1, 5.2, and 5.7). Such reperfusion-mediated recovery of RV performance is associated with excellent clinical outcomes. In contrast, failure to restore flow to the major RV branches is associated with a lack of recovery of RV performance and refractory hemodynamic compromise leading to high in-hospital mortality, even if flow was restored in the main RCA (Fig. 5.1). Successful mechanical

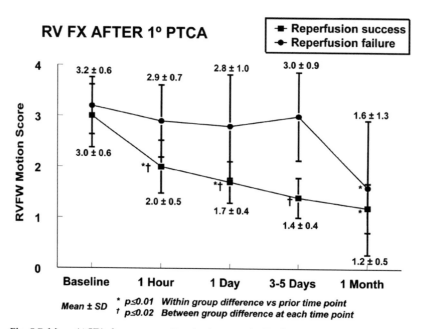

**Fig. 5.7** Mean (±SD) changes over time in the score for RV free wall motion in patients with successful reperfusion and those with unsuccessful reperfusion. An asterisk denotes $P \le 0.01$ for the comparison with the most recent score in the same group. A dagger denotes $P \le 0.02$ for the comparison between groups at one point in time. (Reprinted with permission from Bowers TR, O'Neill WW, Grines C, et al. *N Engl J Med* 1998;338:933–40.)

reperfusion has also led to superior late survival of patients with shock due to predominant RVI versus those with LV shock [10,54].

Although evidence suggests that patients with inferior MI benefit from timely thrombolytic reperfusion, the specific short- and long-term responses of those with RVI have not been adequately evaluated. Some thrombolytic studies suggested that RV function improves only in patients in whom RCA patency is achieved [55–58], whereas others report little benefit [59,60]. Recent prospective reports demonstrate that successful thrombolysis imparts survival benefit in those with RV involvement and that failure to restore infarct-related artery patency is associated with persistent RV dysfunction and increased mortality [60]. Unfortunately, patients with RVI appear to be particularly resistant to fibrinolytic recanalization, owing to extensive clot burden in the proximal RCA together with impaired coronary delivery of fibrinolytic agents attributable to hypotension. There also appears to be a higher incidence of reocclusion following thrombolysis of the RCA.

It is important to consider RVI in the elderly separately. Early reports suggested elderly patients with RVI suffer 50% in-hospital mortality and that hemodynamic compromise in such cases is irreversible. However, recent studies have documented survival of the majority of elderly RVI patients undergoing successful mechanical reperfusion, including those with hemodynamic compromise [53].

## Inotropic stimulation

Parenteral inotropic support is usually effective in stabilizing hemodynamically compromised patients not fully responsive to volume resuscitation and restoration of physiologic rhythm [7]. The mechanisms by which inotropic stimulation improves low output and hypotension in patients with acute RVI have not been well studied. However, experimental animal investigations suggest that inotropic stimulation enhances RV performance by increasing LV-septal contraction, which augments septal-mediated systolic ventricular interactions [24,26]. Although an inotropic agent such as dobutamine that has the least deleterious effects on afterload, oxygen consumption, and arrhythmias is the preferred initial drug of choice, patients with severe hypotension may require agents with pressor effects (such as dopamine) for prompt restoration of adequate coronary perfusion pressure. The "inodilator" agents such as milrinone have not been studied in patients with RVI, but their vasodilator properties could exacerbate hypotension.

## Mechanical assist devices

Intra-aortic balloon pumping may be beneficial in patients with RVI and refractory low output and hypotension. Although there is little research to shed light on the mechanisms by which it exerts salutary effects, balloon assist likely does not directly improve RV performance, but rather stabilizes blood pressure and thereby improves perfusion pressure throughout the coronary tree in severely hypotensive patients. Since RV myocardial blood flow is dependent on perfusion pressure, balloon pumping may also improve RV perfusion and thereby benefit RV function, particularly if the RCA has been recanalized or if there is collateral supply to an occluded vessel. Intra-aortic balloon pumping may also potentially improve LV performance in patients with hypotension and depressed LV function. Since performance of the dysfunctional RV is largely dependent on LV septal contraction, RV performance may also benefit. Additionally, reduction of elevated pulmonary artery wedge pressure reduces RV afterload, which may be accomplished by inhaled nitrous oxide [61]. Recent reports suggest percutaneous RV assist devices can improve hemodynamics in patients with refractory life-threatening low output, providing the reperfused RV with a bridge to recovery [62]. Successful treatment of RV failure by atrial septostomy to augment left heart filling [63] should be considered only as a desperation intervention when all other measures have failed (see Table 5.2).

# Summary

Although right ventricular infarction has been misclassified as benign, when it is associated with cardiogenic shock it has a very poor prognosis and requires special attention to the therapies that can improve survival. Rapid clinical detection with expedited reperfusion with primary PCI is the cornerstone of this approach. While right heart catheterization has lately been neglected in the diagnostic approach for patients with cardiogenic shock, it is essential for the patient with right ventricular involvement. In addition, it allows the clinician to follow the very complex hemodynamic picture as it evolves in the patients with right ventricular failure. However, caution should be applied during invasive hemodynamic evaluation as catheter manipulation within the ischemic RV may provoke malignant ventricular arrhythmias. The use of this comprehensive approach, that also includes echocardiographic evaluation, can ensure better outcomes for the patients with cardiogenic shock with right ventricular involvement.

# References

1. Starr I, Jeffers WA, Meade RH Jr. The absence of conspicuous increments of venous pressure after severe damage to the right ventricle of the dog, with a discussion of the relation between clinical congestive failure and heart disease. *Am Heart J* 1943;26:291–301.
2. Cohn JN, Guiha NH, Broder MI, et al. Right ventricular infarction. Clinical and hemodynamic features. *Am J Cardiol* 1974;33:209–14.
3. Andersen HR, Falk E, Nielsen D. Right ventricular infarction: frequency, size and topography in coronary heart disease: a prospective study compromising 107 consecutive autopsies from a coronary care unit. *J Am Coll Cardiol* 1987;10:1223–32.
4. Lorell B, Leinbach RC, Pohost GM, et al. Right ventricular infarction: clinical diagnosis and differentiation from cardiac tamponade and pericardial constriction. *Am J Cardiol* 1979;43:465–71.
5. Dell'Italia LJ, Starling MR, Crawford MH, et al. Right ventricular infarction: identification by hemodynamic measurements before and after volume loading and correlation with noninvasive techniques. *J Am Coll Cardiol* 1984;4:931–9.
6. Goldstein JA, Barzilai B, Rosamond TL, et al. Determinants of hemodynamic compromise with severe right ventricular infarction. *Circulation* 1990;82:359–68.
7. Goldstein JA. State of the art review: pathophysiology and management of right heart ischemia. *J Am Coll Cardiol* 2002;40:841–53.
8. Bowers TR, O'Neill WW, Grines C, et al. Effect of reperfusion on biventricular function and survival after right ventricular infarction. *N Engl J Med* 1998;338:933–40.
9. Bowers TR, O'Neill WW, Pica M, et al. Patterns of coronary compromise resulting in acute right ventricular ischemic dysfunction. *Circulation* 2002;106(9):1104–9.
10. Hochman JS, Buller CE, Sleeper LA, et al. Cardiogenic shock complicating acute myocardial infarction- etiologies, management and outcome: overall findings of the SHOCK Trial registry. *J Am Coll Cardiol* 2000;36:1063–70.

11. Jacobs AK, Leopold JA, Bates E, et al. Cardiogenic shock caused by right ventricular infarction. A report from the SHOCK registry. *J Am Coll Cardiol* 2003;41:1273–9.

12. Zehender M, Kasper W, Kauder E, et al. Right ventricular infarction as an independent predictor of prognosis after acute inferior myocardial infarction. *N Engl J Med* 1993;328:981–8.

13. Dell'Italia LJ, Lembo NJ, Starling MR, et al. Hemodynamically important right ventricular infarction: follow-up evaluation of right ventricular systolic function at rest and during exercise with radionuclide ventriculography and respiratory gas exchange. *Circulation* 1987;75:996–1003.

14. Lim ST, Marcovitz P, Pica M, et al. Right ventricular performance at rest and during stress with chronic proximal occlusion of the right coronary artery. *Am J Cardiol* 2003;92:1203–6.

15. Bates ER, Califf RM, Stack RS, et al. Thrombolysis and angioplasty in myocardial infarction (TAMI–1) trial: influence of infarct location on arterial patency, left ventricular function and mortality. *J Am Coll Cardiol* 1989;1:12–18.

16. Santamore WP, Lynch PR, Heckman JL, et al. Left ventricular effects on right ventricular developed pressure. *J Appl Physiol* 1976;41:925–30.

17. Kusachi S, Nishiyama O, Yasuhara K, et al. Right and left ventricular oxygen metabolism in open-chest dogs. *Am J Physiol* 1982;243:H761–6.

18. Ohzono K, Koyanagi S, Urabe Y, et al. Transmural distribution of myocardial infarction: difference between the right and left ventricles in a canine model. *Circ Res* 1986;59:63–73.

19. Laster SB, Shelton TJ, Barzilai B, et al. Determinants of the recovery of right ventricular performance following experimental chronic right coronary artery occlusion. *Circulation* 1993;88:696–708.

20. Laster SB, Ohnishi Y, Saffitz JE, et al. Effects of reperfusion on ischemic right ventricular dysfunction: disparate mechanisms of benefit related to duration of ischemia. *Circulation* 1994;90:1398–1409.

21. Raffenbeul W, Urhaler F, Lichtlen P, et al. Quantitative difference in "critical" stenosis between right and left coronary artery in man. *Circulation* 1980;62:1188–96.

22. Goldstein JA, Vlahakes GJ, Verrier ED, et al. The role of right ventricular systolic dysfunction and elevated intrapericardial pressure in the genesis of low output in experimental right ventricular infarction. *Circulation* 1982;65:513–22.

23. Goldstein JA, Vlahakes GJ, Verrier ED, et al. Volume loading improves low cardiac output in experimental right ventricular infarction. *J Am Coll Cardiol* 1983;2:270–8.

24. Goldstein JA, Harada A, Yagi Y, et al. Hemodynamic importance of systolic ventricular interaction, augmented right atrial contractility and atrioventricular synchrony in acute right ventricular dysfunction. *J Am Coll Cardiol* 1990;16:181–9.

25. Goldstein JA, Tweddell JS, Barzilai B, et al. Right atrial ischemia exacerbates hemodynamic compromise associated with experimental right ventricular dysfunction. *J Am Coll Cardiol* 1991;18:1564–72.

26. Goldstein JA, Tweddell JS, Barzilai B, et al. Importance of left ventricular function and systolic interaction to right ventricular performance during acute right heart ischemia. *J Am Coll Cardiol* 1992;19:704–11.

27. Coma-Canella I, Lopez-Sendon J. Ventricular compliance in ischemic right ventricular dysfunction. *Am J Cardiol* 1980;45:555–61.

28. Akaishi M, Weintraum WS, Schneider RM, et al. Analysis of systolic bulging: mechanical characteristics of acutely ischemic myocardium in the conscious dog. *Circ Res* 1986;8:209–17.

29. Rahimtoola SH, Ehsani A, Sinno MZ, et al. Left atrial transport function in myocardial infarction. *Am J Med* 1975;9:686–94.

30. Cushing EH, Feil HS, Stanton EJ, et al. Infarction of the cardiac auricles (atria): clinical, pathological, and experimental studies. *Br Heart* 1942;4:17–34.

31. Lasar EJ, Goldberger JH, Peled H, et al. Atrial infarction: diagnosis and management. *Am Heart J* 1988;6:1058–63.

32. Topol EJ, Goldschlager N, Ports TA, et al. Hemodynamic benefit of atrial pacing in right ventricular myocardial infarction. *Ann Intern Med* 1982;6:594–7.

33. Kalmanson D, Veyrat C, Chiche P. Atrial versus ventricular contribution in determining systemic venous return. *Cardiovasc Res* 1971;5:293–302.

34. Adgey AAJ, Geddes JS, Mulholland C, et al. Incidence, significance, and management of early bradyarrhythmia complicating acute myocardial infarction. *Lancet* 1968;2(7578):1097–101.

35. Tans A, Lie K, Durrer D. Clinical setting and prognostic significance of high degree atrioventricular block in acute inferior myocardial infarction: a study of 144 patients. *Am Heart J* 1980;99:4–8.

36. Mark A. The Bezold-Jarisch reflex revisited: clinical implications of inhibitory reflexes originating in the heart. *J Am Coll Cardiol* 1983;1:90–102.

37. Wei JY, Markis JE, Malagold M, et al. Cardiovascular reflexes stimulated by reperfusion of ischemic myocardium in acute myocardial infarction. *Circulation* 1983;67:796–801.

38. Mavric Z, Zaputovic L, Matana A, et al. Prognostic significance of complete atrioventricular block in patients with acute inferior myocardial infarction with and without right ventricular involvement. *Am Heart J* 1990;19:823–8.

39. Goldstein JA, Lee DT, Pica MC, et al. Patterns of coronary compromise leading to bradyarrhythmias and hypotension in inferior myocardial infarction. *Coron Artery Dis* 2005;16:265–74.

40. Gacioch GM, Topol EJ. Sudden paradoxic clinical deterioration during angioplasty of the occluded right coronary artery in acute myocardial infarction. *J Am Coll Cardiol* 1989;14:1202–9.

41. Elvan A, Zipes D. Right ventricular infarction causes heterogeneous autonomic denervation of the viable peri-infarct area. *Circulation* 1998;97:484–92.

42. Bush, LR, Buja LM, Samowitz W, et al. Recovery of left ventricular segmental function after long-term reperfusion following temporary coronary occlusion in conscious dogs. *Circ Res* 1983;3:248–63.

43. Shiraki H, Yoshikawa U, Anzai T, et al. Association between preinfarction angina and a lower risk of right ventricular infarction. *N Engl J Med* 1998;338:941–7.

44. Moore CA, Nygaard TW, Kaiser DL, et al. Postinfarction ventricular septal rupture: the importance of location of infarction and right ventricular function in determining survival. *Circulation* 1986;74:45–55.

45. Gudipati CV, Nagelhout DA, Serota H, et al. Transesophageal echocardiographic guidance for balloon catheter occlusion of patent foramen ovale complicating right ventricular infarction. *Am Heart J* 1991;121(3 Pt 1):919–22.

46. Korr KS, Levinson H, Bough E, et al. Tricuspid valve replacement for cardiogenic shock after acute right ventricular infarction. *JAMA* 1980;244:1958–60.

47. Dell'Italia LJ, Starling MR, Blumhardt R, et al. Comparative effects of volume loading, dobutamine, and nitroprusside in patients with predominant right ventricular infarction. *Circulation* 1985;72,6:1327–35.

48. Siniorakis EE, Nikolaou NI, Sarantopoulos CD, et al. Volume loading in predominant right ventricular infarction: bedside hemodynamics using rapid response thermistors. *Eur Heart J* 1994;15:1340–7.

49. Ferrario M, Poli A, Previtali M, et al. Hemodynamics of volume loading compared with Dobutamine in severe right ventricular infarction. *Am J Cardiol* 1994;74: 329–33.

50. Robalino BD, Petrella RW, Jubran FY, et al. Atrial Natriuretic factor in patients with right ventricular infarction. *J Am Coll Cardiol* 1990;15:546–53.

51. O'Neill WW, Timmis GC, Bourdillon PD, et al. A prospective randomized clinical trial of intracoronary streptokinase versus coronary angioplasty for acute myocardial infarction. *N Engl J Med* 1986;314:812–18.

52. Berger PB, Ruocco NA, Ryan TJ, et al. Frequency and significance of right ventricular myocardial infarction treated with thrombolytic therapy (results from the thrombolysis in myocardial infarction (TIMI II Trial). *Am J Cardiol* 1993;71:1148–52.

53. Hanzel G, Merhi WM, O'Neill WW, et al. Impact of mechanical reperfusion on clinical outcome in elderly patients with right ventricular infarction. *Coron Artery Dis* 2006;17:517–21.

54. Brodie BR, Stuckey TD, Hansen C, et al. Comparison of late survival in patients with cardiogenic shock due to right ventricular infarction versus left ventricular pump failure following primary percutaneous coronary intervention for ST-elevation acute myocardial infarction. *Am J Cardiol* 2007;99:431–5.

55. Schuler G, Hofmann M, Schwarz F, et al. Effect of successful thrombolytic therapy on right ventricular function in acute inferior wall myocardial infarction. *Am J Cardiol* 1984;54:951–7.

56. Braat SH, Ramentol M, Halders S, et al. Reperfusion with streptokinase of an occluded right coronary artery: effects on early and late right ventricular ejection fraction. *Am Heart J* 1987;113:257–60.

57. Kinn JW, Ajluni SC, Samyn JG, et al. Rapid hemodynamic improvement after reperfusion during right ventricular infarction. *J Am Coll Cardiol* 1995;26:1230–4.

58. Roth A, Miller HI, Kaluski E, et al. Early thrombolytic therapy does not enhance the recovery of the right ventricle in patients with acute inferior myocardial infarction and predominant right ventricular involvement. *Cardiology* 1990;77:40–9.

59. Giannitsis E, Potratz J, Wiegand U, et al. Impact of early accelerated dose tissue plasminogen activator on in-hospital patency of the infarcted vessel in patients with acute right ventricular infarction. *Heart* 1997;77:512–16.

60. Zeymer U, Neuhaus KL, Wegscheider K, et al. Effects of thrombolytic therapy in acute inferior myocardial infarction with or without right ventricular involvement. *J Am Coll Cardiol* 1998;32:876–81.

61. Inglesis I, Shin JT, Lepore JJ, et al. Hemodynamic effects of inhaled nitric oxide in right ventricular myocardial infarction and cardiogenic shock. *J Am Coll of Cardiol* 2004;44:793–8.

62. Atiemo AD, Conte JV, Heldman AW. Resuscitation and recovery from acute right ventricular failure using a percutaneous right ventricular assist device. *Catheter Cardiovasc Interv* 2006;66:78–82.

63. Kernis SJ, Goldstein JA, Yerkey M, et al. Percutaneous atrial septostomy for urgent palliative treatment of severe refractory cardiogenic shock due to right ventricular infarction. *Catheterization and Cardiovascular Interventions* 2003;59:44–48.

64. Antman EM, Anbe DT, Armstrong PW, et al. ACC/AHA Guidelines for the management of patients with ST-elevation myocardial infarction-Executive summary. A report of the American College of Cardiology/American Heart Association Task Force on Practical Guidelines (Writing Committee to Revise the 1999 Guidelines for the management of patients with acute myocardial infarction. *J Am Coll Cardiol* 2004;44:671–719.

# Chapter 6

# Ventricular septal rupture and tamponade

Kellan E. Ashley and Venu Menon

## Introduction

Cardiogenic shock is the most common cause of in-hospital death following an acute myocardial infarction (MI). The etiology of shock in this setting is multifactorial; mechanical complications constitute a unique subset. Early recognition of the underlying pathology and prompt referral for surgical correction are crucial to achieving optimal patient outcome. Due to the complexity of management and the need for rapid surgical intervention, these patients should be transferred as expeditiously as possible to a surgical center that is well versed in their care. This chapter reviews the clinical profile, management, and outcome of cardiac rupture, which involves either the interventricular septum or the left ventricular (LV) free wall. Other mechanical complications, such as chordae rupture or ischemic mitral regurgitation (MR), are covered in Chapter 7.

## Common themes

### Pathogenesis

The pathogenesis, timing, and impact of reperfusion therapy on the incidence of ventricular septal and free wall rupture are similar. The classification of free wall rupture (Fig. 6.1) by Becker and van Mantgem [1] appears applicable to patients with and without reperfusion therapy. Type I rupture generally occurs within 24 hours of an acute infarction and is characterized by a slitlike tear through the full-thickness infarcted muscle with abrupt onset of symptoms. A ventricular septal rupture (VSR) is classically seen in the area bordering an akinetic, infarcted segment and an adjacent hyperdynamic, noninfarcted zone

*Cardiogenic Shock.* Edited by Judith S. Hochman and E. Magnus Ohman.
© 2009 American Heart Association, ISBN: 978-1-4051-7926-3

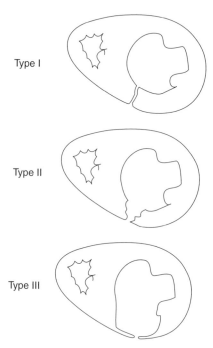

Type I

Type II

Type III

**Fig. 6.1** Morphological classification of myocardial rupture. (Reprinted with permission from Becker AE, van Mantgem JP. *Eur J Cardiol* 1975;3:349–58.)

(Fig. 6.2). Type II rupture progresses more slowly and is due to erosion of the infarct zone before rupture occurs. Consequently, there is some time delay between the infarction and the onset of rupture. Type III rupture is correlated with even older infarcts and is characterized by severe expansion of the infarct zone with marked wall thinning. When rupture occurs, it involves the center of the previously aneurysmally dilated segment.

## Incidence

The quality and nature of reperfusion of the infarct-related artery appears closely related to the incidence of rupture. The reported incidence of free wall rupture and ventricular septal rupture in the pre-reperfusion era were 6% and 1–3%, respectively [2,3]. The impact of reperfusion therapy on rupture incidence is highlighted in Fig. 6.3. In the GUSTO-I (Global Utilization of Streptokinase and TPA for Occluded Coronary Arteries) trial, the rate of VSR was found to be much lower (0.2%) [5]. The superior TIMI-3 (Thrombolysis In Myocardial Infarction—3) flow noted with t-PA over streptokinase led to a proposed etiology of the decreased rate of rupture [6]. In addition, the higher TIMI-3 flow rates achieved with angioplasty over t-PA in the PAMI (Primary Angioplasty in Myocardial Infarction) registry resulted in a further decline in the incidence

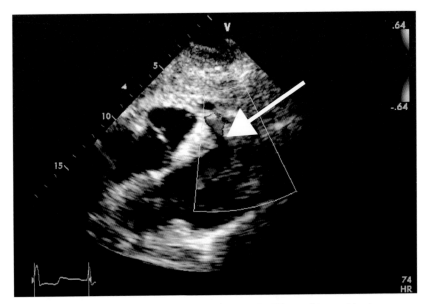

**Fig. 6.2** Full-thickness inferior myocardial infarct with VSR noted (arrow) in the area between an akinetic basal septum supplied by the RCA and a hyperkinetic midseptum supplied by the LAD. VSR, ventricular septal rupture; RCA, right coronary artery; LAD, left anterior descending.

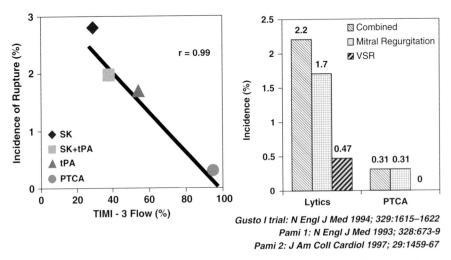

Gusto I trial: N Engl J Med 1994; 329:1615–1622
Pami 1: N Engl J Med 1993; 328:673-9
Pami 2: J Am Coll Cardiol 1997; 29:1459-67

**Fig. 6.3** Inverse relation between effectiveness of reperfusion strategy and incidence of observed rupture. (Reprinted with permission from Kinn JW, O'Neill WW, Benzuly KH, et al. *Cathet Cardiovasc Diagn* 1997;42(2):151–7.)

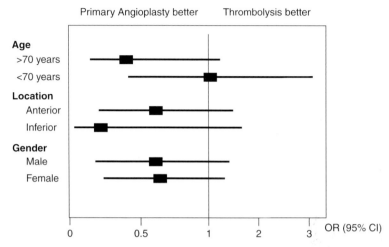

**Fig. 6.4** Effect of primary angioplasty compared with thrombolysis on the risk of free wall rupture according to age, gender, and infarct location. CI, confidence interval; OR, odds ratio. (Reprinted with permission from Moreno R, Lopez-Sendon J, Garcia E, et al. *J Am Coll Cardiol* 2002;39(4):598–603.)

of this complication [4]. As a result, the incidence of rupture can be expected to decline with the adoption of a primary angioplasty strategy. Moreno and colleagues evaluated 1375 patients admitted to the coronary care unit within 12 hours of an ST-segment elevation MI; 762 (55%) were treated with primary angioplasty and 613 (45%) with fibrinolytic therapy [7]. Although patients undergoing primary angioplasty were older, had worse Killip classification, experienced longer time from the onset of symptoms, and were more often female with hypertension, diabetes, and anterior location of the MI, the observed rate of free wall rupture was 3.3% with fibrinolysis compared to 1.8% with angioplasty (OR 0.46, 95% CI 0.22–0.96; $p = 0.037$) (Fig. 6.4).

## Timing of rupture

VSR is often mistakenly referred to as a late first-week complication following MI. Although mean times were noted to be 5–7 days after MI, rupture usually occurs in a bimodal distribution based on the type of rupture [1], with peaks on the first day and later that week. There is a shift in the timing from late to early rupture in fibrinolytic-treated patients [1,8]. Among fibrinolytic-treated patients in the GUSTO-I trial [5], the median time to diagnosis of VSR was 1 day. Similarly, in the SHOCK (SHould we emergently revascularize Occluded Coronaries in cardiogenic shocK?) trial [9], the median time to VSR was even shorter, occurring at 16 hours in the setting of suspected cardiogenic shock. A number of other factors appear to have contributed to this observation. Original surgical series may have been prone to survival bias. Consequently, only patients surviving the early phase and selected for surgery were accounted for in the analysis. With the advent of pulmonary artery catheterization in the 1970s and color Doppler echocardiography in the 1980s, early clinical diagnosis of VSR was enhanced. Of utmost importance, the myocardial hemorrhage and edema that accompany fibrinolytic reperfusion appear to have accelerated the onset of rupture in a vulnerable subset of patients. As a result, a new, distinct, early risk period for VSR has become apparent. The lack of mortality benefit (early hazard) noted at 24 hours for fibrinolytic therapy over placebo-treated patients is largely attributed to rupture.

## Vulnerable population

A number of clinical series have identified patient subsets at increased risk for mechanical complications post–MI. The elderly, hypertensive female appears most vulnerable to this complication. Rupture is commonly noted in the setting of a first transmural MI with a persistently occluded infarct-related artery or in the setting of late fibrinolytic reperfusion. A majority of patients with VSR have been shown to have either single- or double-vessel coronary artery disease, with total occlusion of the infarct-related artery [5,9]. A lack of collateral flow on angiography is a common feature, and the performance of primary percutaneous coronary intervention (PCI) is noted to reduce the risk of rupture. The multivariable predictors of VSR following fibrinolytic therapy are illustrated in Fig. 6.5, with age, anterior infarct location, female gender, and smoking status being the most significant variables [5].

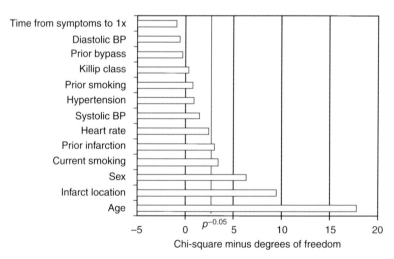

**Fig. 6.5** Relative importance of multivariable enrollment predictors of VSR in GUSTO-I. All factors from age to prior infarction have corresponding $P < 0.05$. BP, blood pressure; tx, treatment, VSR, ventricular septal rupture; GUSTO-I, Global Utilization of Streptokinase and TPA for Occluded Coronary Arteries. (Reprinted with permission from Crenshaw BS, Granger CB, Birnbaum Y, et al. *Circulation* 2000;101(1):27–32.)

# Ventricular septal rupture

## Classification

### Morphology

Based on morphologic characteristics, VSR can be classified as simple or complex. With a simple rupture, there is a through-and-through defect, with the perforation occurring at the same level on the left and right ventricular (RV) sides. In contrast, complex ruptures can have multiple irregular tracts in various directions through the ventricular septum, formed as a result of the extensive necrosis and hemorrhage of the myocardium [2]. These tracts can cover extensive areas and reach sites distant to the infarcted myocardium. Consequently, complex ruptures are more likely to involve surrounding structures, such as papillary muscles or the right ventricle [10]. Complex ruptures are seen more often with inferior infarcts; they more often result in the need for difficult surgical repair with worsened surgical outcome.

### Location

VSR occurs with both anterior and inferior MI. Anterior VSR is more common and occurs in the setting of infarction in the left anterior descending (LAD) coronary artery territory. The location of the VSR is usually the apical septum, with communication between the two ventricular chambers. Inferior VSRs are usually complex and involve the basal inferoposterior septum; RV involvement is common [2]. The culprit vessel is usually the right coronary artery (RCA), but a dominant circumflex involvement has also been seen.

### Hemodynamic stability

It is important to differentiate patients with VSR and cardiogenic shock from patients with stable hemodynamics. Although expeditious surgical correction is advocated for all patients, clinical outcomes among patients with cardiogenic shock remain dismal, even in experienced surgical centers. In contrast, relatively favorable results can be obtained in the hemodynamically stable patient.

### Hemodynamics (Table 6.1)

VSR results in an acute left-to-right shunt. The severity of the shunt depends on the size of the defect as well as the relative pulmonary and systemic vascular resistances. The size of the rupture may range from small (a few millimeters) to large (several centimeters). As a result, pulmonary blood flow is increased by the amount of the shunted blood, which eventually leads to secondary volume overload of the left atrium and left ventricle [2]. Shunting of blood from left to right decreases the effective cardiac output and may result in systemic hypotension and hypoperfusion. Ensuing systemic vasoconstriction results in an increase in the amount of shunted blood through the septum, and a vicious spiral ensues. This process may ultimately progress to LV failure and refractory

**Table 6.1** Hemodynamic patterns.

| | RA | RVS | RVD | PAS | PAD | PAW | CI | SVR |
|---|---|---|---|---|---|---|---|---|
| Normal values | <6 | <25 | 0–12 | <25 | 0–12 | <6–12 | ≥2.5 | (800–1600) |
| Cardiac tamponade | ↑ | ↔↑ | ↑ | ↔↑ | ↔↑ | ↔↑ | ↓ | ↑ |
| Cardiogenic shock | | | | | | | | |
|   LV failure | ↔↑ | ↔↑ | ↔↑ | ↔↑ | ↑ | ↑ | ↓ | ↔↑ |
|   RV failure* | ↑ | ↓↔↑† | ↑ | ↓↔↑† | ↔↓↑† | ↓↔↑† | ↓ | ↑ |
| Acute mitral regurgitation | ↔↑ | ↑ | ↔↑ | ↑ | ↑ | ↑ | ↔↓ | ↔↑ |
| Ventricular septal rupture | ↑ | ↔↑ | ↑ | ↔↑ | ↔↑ | ↔↑ | ↑PBF ↓SBF | ↔↑ |

There is significant patient-to-patient variation. Pressures in RA, right atrium; RVS/D, right ventricular systolic/diastolic; PAS/D, pulmonary artery systolic/diastolic; PAW, pulmonary artery wedge are in mm Hg. CI, cardiac index (L/min/m²) and SVR, systemic vascular resistance (dynes/sec/cm⁵). MI, myocardial infarction and P/SBF, pulmonary/systemic blood flow.

*"Isolated" or predominant RV failure.

†PAW and PA pressures may rise in RV failure after volume loading due to RV dilation, right to left shift of the interventricular septum, resulting in impaired LV filling. When biventricular failure is present, the patterns are similar to those shown for LV failure.

‡Forrester et al. classified nonreperfused MI patients into four hemodynamic subsets (*N Engl J Med* 1976;295:1356–62). PAWP and CI in clinically stable subset I patients are shown. Values in parentheses represent range. Reprinted with permission from Hochman JS and Ingbar D, Cardiogenic Shock and Pulmonary Edema in Fauci AS, Braunwald E, Kasper DL et al., Harrison's Principles of Internal Medicine 17th Edition, McGraw-Hill Medical, 2008.

hypotension, leading to shock [2]. Not all patients who suffer VSR post–MI experience shock, as small defects may be well compensated, at least temporarily. Expansion and extension of the septal perforation, with accompanying hemodynamic collapse, is often sudden and unpredictable. As a result, a strategy of watchful medical stabilization and deferred surgery cannot be advocated. In the SHOCK trial registry [8], VSR was the primary cause of cardiogenic shock in 3.9% of patients, third in incidence behind predominant LV dysfunction and severe MR.

## Diagnosis of ventricular septal rupture

### Overall approach

The diagnosis of VSR, and mechanical complications in general, is dependent on strong clinical suspicion. It is crucial for the clinician to determine the etiology of hemodynamic instability in each individual case. Hemodynamic collapse disproportionate to the degree of myocardium at risk should warrant immediate reevaluation. A detailed clinical examination and review of laboratory and therapeutic data is warranted. A comprehensive emergency echocardiogram greatly aids in this approach. An echo gives the clinician immediate insight into the status of overall LV function, contractility in the remote myocardium, involvement of the right ventricle, and valvular competence. The presence of significant eccentric mitral regurgitation (MR) or aortic insufficiency (AI) should prompt a transesophageal echocardiogram (TEE) to rule out a flail leaflet or a dissection flap in the aortic root when suspected. The presence of a VSR, free wall rupture, or tamponade can be easily excluded by this approach.

### Presentation and physical examination

Patients who suffer VSR may present with symptoms of chest pain and shortness of breath due to acute pulmonary edema and cardiogenic shock. Other symptoms related to end-organ hypoperfusion may also be present [2]. On examination, there is characteristically a new holosystolic murmur that is harsh and loud, located at the left sternal border, with radiation to the base and right parasternal area. There is an associated thrill in 50% of patients [10]. In the setting of a large defect, with acute elevation in pulmonary pressures or with low cardiac output and shock, there may be no thrill and the murmur may be difficult to auscultate. Mechanical ventilation and intra-aortic balloon pump (IABP) support may further hinder auscultation. Other physical examination findings can include an S3 gallop, an accentuated pulmonic component of S2, and the murmur of tricuspid regurgitation. It can be difficult to differentiate the murmur of VSR from the murmur of severe MR due to papillary muscle rupture. Generally, the murmur of VSR is louder and more often associated with a palpable thrill. Also, VSR is more likely to be accompanied by signs of RV failure and less likely to be associated with pulmonary edema than papillary muscle rupture [2]. Physical examination is not sufficient to confirm the diagnosis of VSR.

## EKG, chest x-ray, pulmonary artery catheterization

Electrocardiograms (ECG) are nonspecific and may show evidence of anterior or inferior MI. Chest x-ray is equally nonspecific, potentially showing evidence of cardiomegaly, pulmonary vascular congestion, or pleural effusions [11]. Although the use of pulmonary arterial catheterization in the cardiac care unit has dramatically decreased over time [12], it is helpful in the diagnosis and acute management of patients with VSR. The catheter can be used to obtain blood for oximetry from the right atrium, right ventricle, and pulmonary artery. In VSR, the characteristic step-up in oxygen saturation between the right atrium and right ventricle is diagnostic [10]. Pulmonary artery catheters also allow quantification of the shunt by comparison of the ratio of pulmonary to systemic blood flow, estimated from oxygen saturations obtained from the right atrium (mixed venous saturation), pulmonary artery, and any other peripheral artery (aortic saturation) [11]. The equation for calculation of the ratio of pulmonary to systemic flow, or shunt fraction ($Q_p / Q_s$), is shown:

$$Q_p/Q_s = [O_2 \, sat_{art} - O_2 \, sat_{mv}]/[O_2 \, sat_{pv} - O_2 \, sat_{pa}]$$

where $Q_p$ is pulmonary blood flow, $Q_s$ is systemic blood flow, $O_2 \, sat_{art}$ is peripheral arterial oxygen saturation, $O_2 \, sat_{mv}$ is mixed venous oxygen saturation, $O_2 \, sat_{pv}$ is pulmonary vein oxygen saturation, and $O_2 \, sat_{pa}$ is pulmonary arterial oxygen saturation. If the pulmonary vein oxygen saturation is not measured, it can be assumed to be 95%.

### Echocardiography

Two-dimensional echocardiography is the initial diagnostic method of choice and will confirm the presence of VSR in the majority of cases. Echocardiography allows direct visualization and definition of the site and size of the defect. The defect entry site on the LV aspect usually appears as an abrupt break in the septum, surrounded by a large area of akinesis. Color Doppler confirms the left-to-right shunt, and the defect size correlates closely with findings noted at surgery/autopsy. Unconventional views superimposed with color flow Doppler are usually required to identify the RV exit site. Echo also provides an estimation of LV and RV function, estimation of RV systolic pressure, and quantification of the left-to-right shunt [2]. If there are poor acoustic windows with transthoracic echocardiography, TEE can be employed to improve diagnostic accuracy. With three-dimensional echocardiography, the location, shape, and size of the septal defect can be delineated enface from both the LV and RV aspects.

### Left ventriculography

An unsuspected VSR may be diagnosed in the setting of ventriculography performed during routine angiography or following percutaneous intervention. Caution should be used before employing this modality in the

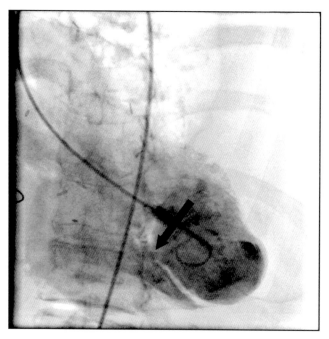

**Fig. 6.6** Left anterior oblique ventriculogram with slight cranial angulation in a 79-year-old woman with history of postbypass myocardial infarction (MI) complicated by ventricular septal rupture. The arrow highlights the large defect in the interventricular septum.

hemodynamically unstable patient, as it can acutely precipitate respiratory distress, pulmonary edema, and a need for mechanical ventilation [10]. If the ventriculogram is performed, ideally it should be filmed in the 60-degree left anterior oblique (LAO) projection with 15–20 degrees of cranial angulation, in order to better visualize the length of the interventricular septum and location of the defect (see Fig. 6.6) [13]. The patient should also inspire deeply prior to the cine run, as this minimizes diaphragmatic interference. However, in most situations, the standard 30-degree right anterior oblique (RAO) ventriculogram is done following coronary angiography. The LAO ventriculogram is generally not performed (unless the catheterization laboratory has biplane capabilities) in order to minimize contrast exposure, unless there is suspicion for VSR or need to visualize the septum and lateral walls. VSR can be diagnosed from the RAO ventriculogram, but it is somewhat more challenging. Figure 6.7 shows the slightly increased difficulty of visualizing the VSR from the RAO projection of the same patient as is shown in Fig. 6.6. Fortunately, in this example, the defect is large and easily visualized in the RAO projection. However, with smaller defects, it can be somewhat more difficult. Particular attention should be given

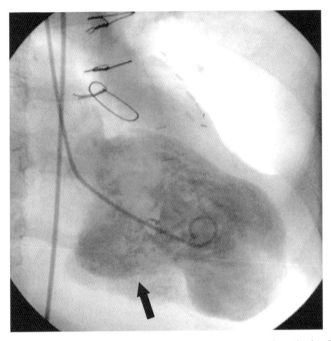

**Fig. 6.7** Right anterior oblique ventriculogram in the same patient described in Fig. 6.6. In this projection, the ventricular septal rupture can be harder to visualize. The defect in this example is large and indicated by the arrow. Faint filling of the right ventricle with contrast is noted.

to the inferomedial aspect of the RAO projection to look for faint filling of the right ventricle when performing ventriculography.

### Other imaging modalities

Both cardiac magnetic resonance imaging (MRI) and multidetector computed tomography (MDCT) are useful in making or confirming the diagnosis of VSR. However, these imaging modalities are generally limited to the hemodynamically stable patient. Therefore, these modalities are not helpful in the evaluation of the unstable patient in cardiogenic shock.

### Treatment

The key to successful therapy is rapid diagnosis, aggressive medical stabilization, and early surgical intervention.

### Medical therapy

Medical therapy consists of interventions to reverse the acute hemodynamic instability. Adequate oxygenation and ventilation should be ensured with face mask oxygen, noninvasive positive pressure ventilation, or intubation with mechanical ventilation [2] (see Chapter 3). Invasive monitoring with an arterial pressure line and a pulmonary artery catheter is useful in the acute management, as it allows continuous hemodynamic assessment. In the absence of significant hypotension and ready availability of an IABP, vasodilator therapy may be initiated in order to reduce systemic vascular resistance and, thus, the degree of the shunt. This is effectively achieved with a sodium nitroprusside infusion, which can be easily titrated intravenously [14]. In addition to reducing the degree of the shunt, nitroprusside improves effective cardiac output, enabling adequate blood flow to prevent vital end-organ dysfunction. Although vasopressors will increase the amount of left-to-right shunt, therapy should be initiated in the setting of refractory hypotension.

IABP placement should be strongly considered in all patients with VSR and is recommended by the current ACC/AHA guidelines [15]. The IABP improves hemodynamics by decreasing LV afterload. This increases systemic output and decreases the left-to-right shunt across the ventricular septum. This is medically stabilizing and should not delay definitive surgical therapy. Thiele and colleagues report on the impact of IABP in 23 patients with acute VSR. The use of IABP increased cardiac index, decreased left-to-right shunt, improved metabolic acidosis, and reduced lactate levels [16]. Patients should be transferred to an experienced surgical center promptly following diagnosis.

If the VSR is small, the patient may be relatively asymptomatic. Even in this scenario, medical therapy is only supportive, as most patients tend to deteriorate suddenly. The mortality rate in patients treated medically is 24% in the first 24 hours, 46% at 7 days, and 67–82% at 2 months [2]. In the absence of significant comorbidities, all patients should be offered definitive therapy with surgical intervention. In a single-center experience, long-term follow-up was reported on seven medically treated subjects who refused to undergo surgery for post–MI VSR. Most of these patients (six out of seven) had small anterior VSR (9.8 $\pm$ 2.8 mm) with $Q_p/Q_s$ 1.98 $\pm$ 0.55, and a mean pulmonary artery pressure of 28 $\pm$ 10.6 mm Hg in the setting of single-vessel disease [17]. Two patients were lost to follow-up after 6 months; both of them were in New York Heart Association (NYHA) class II heart failure at their last visit. One patient had sudden cardiac death after 4 years of follow-up, and prior to that point he had been in NYHA class II heart failure. The remaining four patients had been stable in NYHA class II heart failure managed medically over a mean follow-up of 3.75 years. The fact that several of these patients could be managed medically is quite uncommon. Likely contributors to the relative stability of these patients were the small defects, normal LV and RV function, and single-vessel coronary artery disease. Additionally, these patients were evaluated initially at a mean of 2.2 months post–MI, giving this very small case series a selection bias.

## Surgical therapy

Surgical therapy should be considered for all patients with VSR. The first surgical repair was performed by Cooley on April 5, 1956, in a patient with intractable heart failure and inferior VSR weeks after initial admission [18]. Unfortunately, the patient died 6 weeks later due to VSR recurrence, renal failure, and infectious complications. Despite significant advances since then, the surgical repair of VSR remains a major challenge. There was a long-held belief in the early experience with surgical correction of VSR that a waiting period was necessary to prepare the myocardium for surgical repair [2]. In the first few days to weeks post–MI, the myocardial infarct zone was thought to be too friable for repair. A waiting policy would let the margins of the rupture become fibrotic, making them more amenable to suturing. The risk of this approach was quickly recognized, and several case series confirmed that early surgical repair was the key to improving survival [19–21]. The outcomes of VSR once cardiogenic shock has developed remain dismal, as reflected by the 81% mortality rate in the SHOCK trial registry [9].

The ACC/AHA guidelines advocate urgent surgical repair of VSR with concomitant coronary artery bypass grafting (CABG) [15]. The data on CABG at the time of VSR repair have been conflicting, with some case series showing benefit [22–24], while others not [25–27]. In the absence of harm, revascularization with CABG at the time of surgical VSR repair appears reasonable in most patients. Table 6.2 summarizes the outcome of VSR in large published series since 2000, with an overall early mortality rate of 30–40%. Most of these series report only on the outcome of patients selected for surgical repair. Variable numbers in each series were considered to be in cardiogenic shock. As a result, the true mortality rate for patients with VSR, especially those in cardiogenic shock, is significantly underestimated, as noted by the 94% mortality for medically treated patients in the GUSTO-I trial [5]. Despite the increased vulnerability of women to develop rupture, they appear underrepresented in most surgical series.

Long-term follow-up has been reported. In one report [31], the 8-year survival rate was about 59%, and in the large Southampton experience, 5- and 10-year survival rates were 60% and 31%, respectively [32]. Similar to the findings in patients with LV failure in the randomized SHOCK trial [33], most survivors were noted to be in NYHA class I/II heart failure on follow-up.

Surgical outcomes appear closely related to clinical experience. In the Swedish Heart Surgery Registry, the mortality rate in large centers (>30 patients during study period) was 36%, compared to 54% mortality observed in small centers ($\leq$15 patients, $p = 0.06$) [29]. A number of reports have evaluated the predictors of poor surgical outcome in this patient population. Old age, the presence of cardiogenic shock, and RV involvement appear to be the dominant variables. RV dysfunction in the setting of a VSR is multifactorial and may be due to RV infarction, LV failure, and RV volume overload. While the volume overload

**Table 6.2** Large published case series of outcomes with post-myocardial infarction VSR from 2005 to 2007.

| Year published | First author | Number (undergoing repair) | Age | Male gender (%) | Anterior location (%) | Median days to diagnosis | Cardiogenic shock (%) | Surgical mortality (%) | Medical mortality (%) | Remarks |
|---|---|---|---|---|---|---|---|---|---|---|
| 2000 | Crenshaw [5] | 84 (34) | 72 | 43 | 70 | 1 day | 67 | 47 | 94 | All patients received fibrinolytic treatment for ST-segment elevation MI |
| 2000 | Menon [9] | 55 (31) | 72 | 42 | 48 | <1 day | 100 | 81 | 96 | All patients were in cardiogenic shock at diagnosis |
| 2000 | Deja [26] | 117 (117) | 66 | 64 | 69 | 6 days | 30 | 38 | — | Consecutive patients over 12 years from 1986 to 1998 |
| 2002 | Labrousse [25] | 85 (85) | 69 | 60 | 59 | 3 days | 19 | 42 | — | Consecutive series from 1971 to 2001 with preoperative IABP use in 95% |
| 2003 | Cerin [28] | 58 (58) | 73 | — | — | — | 41 | 52 | — | |
| 2003 | Barker [22] | 65 (65) | 64 | 61 | 48 | 5 days | 52.4% in those who had CABG (n = 42); 56.5% in those without CABG (n = 23) | 32 | — | Consecutive series from 1997 to 2002; superior outcome for patients undergoing CABG |
| 2005 | Jeppsson [29] | 189 (189) | 70 | 63 | 49 | 4 days | — | 41 | — | Consecutive series from 1992 to 1998 |
| 2006 | Mantovani [30] | 50 (50) | 66 | 52 | 60 | — | — | 36 | — | Consecutive series from 1983 from 2002 |

MI, myocardial infarction; IABP, intra-aortic balloon pump; CABG, coronary artery bypass grafting.

improves with surgery, involvement of the RV in the infarct is an ominous sign. In up to 28% of patients, there will be a residual septal defect after surgical repair [2]. These residual defects carry a high mortality rate and should be repaired if there is heart failure or if the calculated shunt ratio is greater than 2 [2]. Regardless of the surgical technique employed, the most common cause of death in the postoperative setting is LV failure [34].

The general approach to surgical repair is summarized below. Intraoperative TEE is a useful adjunct. The patient is placed on cardiopulmonary bypass with bicaval venous access as well as ascending aorta cannulation. If coronary bypass is pursued, it is undertaken first, before the ventricular septum is repaired, in order to improve myocardial protection [34]. The usual approach to the VSR is via incision through the infarcted area of the left ventricle. Debridement is usually required to remove necrotic tissue in order to prevent postoperative bleeding or a residual septal defect [2]. If the defect is small and apical, the apex of the heart, including the defect, can be amputated and the ventricle repaired with horizontal mattress sutures that are reinforced by Teflon strips [11]. If the defect is elsewhere, the technique employed is determined by its location. It is usually possible to patch the defect with prosthetic material (Dacron prosthetic patch, glutaraldehyde-fixed bovine pericardial patch). The perimeter of the defect is first covered with pledget, interrupted mattress sutures, and then the prosthetic patch is sewn into place [34].

An alternative technique may be employed in an attempt to maintain the native geometry of the left ventricle and thereby improve postoperative LV function. With this technique, the patch is placed in the LV cavity and excludes the septal defect as well as the infarcted myocardium from the remainder of the LV cavity. With this approach there is no myocardial resection, and no sutures are placed in friable, infarcted myocardium [34]. Other techniques such as a right atrial incision to repair posterior VSR may also be used in selected patients [35]. The mitral valve and papillary muscles should be inspected, regardless of surgical approach, in order to determine if repair or replacement of the mitral valve should be pursued [2].

**Percutaneous therapy**

Percutaneous closure with a catheter-based device is the best option for therapy in a select group of patients deemed unsuitable for surgical repair. The exact role of this procedure as a therapeutic option is currently not defined. These devices have been used in various settings—as primary therapy for post–MI VSR, as an adjunct for residual defect postsurgical repair, and as a bridge to surgical repair in the acutely unstable patient [36]. The procedure is not without risk, as there is a chance of enlarging the defect with device passage through the septum while it is still necrotic and friable [2]. Also, the location of the defect may not be amenable to percutaneous repair. There is risk of damaging surrounding structures, especially if the defect is basal and close to the mitral or tricuspid valves [2].

Most of the experience with percutaneous closure of VSR is limited to case reports. The devices used in these cases include the Rashkind double umbrella, the Clamshell double umbrella, the CardioSEAL device, and different Amplatzer devices [37]. In one of the larger series [37] of 18 patients, a device was successfully deployed in 16. The 30-day mortality rate was 28%, with a longer term mortality rate of 41%. The long-term follow-up in this study was less than 1 year. In another case series ($n = 18$) [38], with follow-up extended to a median of 54 months, similar mortality rates were reported. The limited transcatheter closure experience is subject to selection bias, with most of these procedures performed more than 2 weeks after the initial MI. Further prospective study is required to delineate the exact timing and patient profile that is optimal for this approach.

# Left ventricular free wall rupture and tamponade

LV free wall rupture is a relatively uncommon occurrence, but it accounts for approximately 15% of the inhospital mortality from MI [3]. Due to its acute presentation and propensity for rapid deterioration, free wall rupture was thought to result in virtually certain death from cardiac tamponade. However, if recognized early in its course and aggressively stabilized, free wall rupture may be amenable to surgical repair. This usually occurs in the setting of partial containment, when the pericardium seals the defect, with the formation of a pseudoaneurysm (false aneurysm) [10]. In contrast to a true LV aneurysm, whose walls consist of infarcted myocardium or scar, the walls of the pseudoaneurysm consist entirely of pericardium.

## Hemodynamics

After rupture of the free wall of the LV, there is rapid accumulation of blood in the pericardial space. Unless the defect is sealed by pericardium, electromechanical dissociation, cardiovascular collapse, and death rapidly ensue. In the setting of containment, the patient may present subacutely with local or generalized cardiac tamponade.

## Presentation

Patients with free wall rupture can present with chest pain that is either anginal or pleuritic, as well as nausea, emesis, and restlessness [2]. Instead of the more common presentation, which involves hypotension, electromechanical dissociation, and rapid deterioration, it is possible to have rupture with a brief period of symptoms followed by stabilization. This is usually due to subacute tamponade, likely because of latent sealing of the defect by the pericardium. This subacute presentation has been estimated to occur in up to one-third of patients with free wall rupture [10]. On rare occasions, patients remain asymptomatic and pseudoaneurysms may be incidentally discovered on routine echocardiographic follow-up.

## Diagnosis

Making the diagnosis requires a high index of suspicion, as some of the signs and symptoms can be very nonspecific. Engorged neck veins and the presence of a pulsus paradoxus may heighten clinical suspicion. The ECG is variable and can show signs of pericarditis, persistent ST-segment elevations, T-wave changes, or complete heart block [10]. Transthoracic two-dimensional echocardiography with color flow Doppler imaging is the diagnostic modality of choice. The echocardiogram may reveal a pericardial effusion with or without signs of tamponade (RA and RV diastolic collapse, respirophasic changes in mitral and tricuspid valve inflows), and evidence of a defect by color flow Doppler across the free wall of the left ventricle is confirmatory. The lack of a defect visualized by echocardiogram does not rule out the diagnosis of free wall rupture, however. Only 39% of patients in the SHOCK trial registry had evidence of a defect on transthoracic echocardiogram [3]. The use of contrast echocardiography can heighten diagnostic sensitivity. A pulmonary artery catheter may show evidence of tamponade with equalization of the diastolic pressures. Left ventriculography is not routinely useful for diagnosis of free wall rupture, as patients are generally too unstable to undergo angiography. However, subacute ruptures or pseudoaneurysms may be identified in the standard 30-degree RAO projection of the LV, which allows visualization of the anterior, apical, and inferior walls. The 60-degree LAO projection may also be used, which allows visualization of the septal, lateral, and posterior walls [13]. The role that newer imaging modalities may play in the diagnosis of free wall rupture is still undefined. Thus far, all information on cardiac MRI and MDCT is in the form of case reports. In general, most patients with free wall rupture are too hemodynamically unstable to undergo either cardiac MRI or MDCT. However, these modalities are becoming increasingly more useful in the evaluation of subacute rupture and pseudoaneurysms.

## Treatment

Rapid diagnosis, aggressive medical stabilization, and emergency surgical repair are the keys to a favorable outcome.

### Medical therapy

Aggressive supportive care is warranted using intravenous fluids or vasopressors to increase systemic blood pressure. Oxygenation and ventilation should be maintained with supplemental oxygen, noninvasive positive airway pressure ventilation, or intubation with mechanical ventilation (see Chapter 3). Occasionally, intra-aortic balloon counterpulsation is used, but it is not as effective in this setting as it is for VSR. Pericardiocentesis may be needed in the emergency stabilization of the patient to relieve tamponade [10]. Only the amount of fluid needed to stabilize the hemodynamics of the patient should be removed with pericardiocentesis. The goal is to get the patient to emergency open surgical repair. A pericardial drain may be left in place and clamped for future drainage if tamponade recurs before the patient can get to the operating room.

### Surgical therapy

Oftentimes in acute LV free wall rupture, the decision to go for open surgical repair has to be made based on a high index of suspicion, as the diagnostic testing is often equivocal or unable to localize the site of rupture [10]. As for VSR, the goal with surgical repair is to control the hemorrhage, perform a patch repair with the edges anchored into healthy myocardium, and attempt to maintain normal LV geometry [39]. The technique used depends on the site and nature of the rupture.

## Outcomes

Data from the SHOCK trial registry [3] showed the inhospital mortality rate in patients with free wall rupture and cardiogenic shock due to tamponade to be over 60%, which was similar to the mortality rate in the cohort of patients without free wall rupture. If patients survived to surgical repair (75%), there was a 62% mortality rate, which was worse in women. Overall, the mortality rate in the SHOCK trial registry was similar to the mortality rate observed in earlier trials. In the large Spanish series reported by Lopez Sendon and colleagues [40], 1247 patients were prospectively followed after acute MI, with 2.6% ($n = 33$) having free wall rupture. All 33 patients went for surgical repair, with 76% ($n = 25$) surviving the procedure. However, long-term survival was similar to that observed in the SHOCK trial registry, with only 48.5% of patients surviving long term.

## Conclusion

Mechanical complications in the setting of an acute MI continue to be associated with increased inhospital morbidity and mortality. Heightened clinical suspicion, prompt medical stabilization, and emergency surgical referral remain the keys to improving the outcome in this unique subset of patients. Advances in percutaneous therapies may permit definitive treatment for a broader group of patients. Adoption of a primary PCI strategy with early and effective reperfusion of the infarct-related artery will protect against this disastrous complication.

## References

1. Becker AE, van Mantgem JP. Cardiac tamponade. A study of 50 hearts. *Eur J Cardiol* 1975;3:349–58.
2. Birnbaum Y, Fishbein MC, Blanche C, Siegel RJ. Ventricular septal rupture after acute myocardial infarction. *New Engl Journal Med* 2002;347(18):1426–32.

3. Slater J, Brown RJ, Antonelli TA, et al. Cardiogenic shock due to cardiac free-wall rupture or tamponade after acute myocardial infarction: a report from the SHOCK Trial Registry. Should we emergently revascularize occluded coronaries for cardiogenic shock? *J Am Coll Cardiol* 2000;36(3 Suppl A):1117–22.

4. Kinn JW, O'Neill WW, Benzuly KH, Jones DE, Grines CL. Primary angioplasty reduces risk of myocardial rupture compared to thrombolysis for acute myocardial infarction. *Cathet Cardiovasc Diagn* 1997;42(2):151–7.

5. Crenshaw BS, Granger CB, Birnbaum Y, et al. Risk factors, angiographic patterns, and outcomes in patients with ventricular septal defect complicating acute myocardial infarction. GUSTO-I (Global Utilization of Streptokinase and TPA for Occluded Coronary Arteries) Trial Investigators. *Circulation* 2000;101(1):27–32.

6. The effects of tissue plasminogen activator, streptokinase, or both on coronary-artery patency, ventricular function, and survival after acute myocardial infarction. The GUSTO Angiographic Investigators. *N Engl J Med* 1993;329(22):1615–22.

7. Moreno R, Lopez-Sendon J, Garcia E, et al. Primary angioplasty reduces the risk of left ventricular free wall rupture compared with thrombolysis in patients with acute myocardial infarction. *J Am Coll Cardiol* 2002;39(4):598–603.

8. Hochman JS, Buller CE, Sleeper LA, et al. Cardiogenic shock complicating acute myocardial infarction—etiologies, management and outcome: a report from the SHOCK Trial Registry. Should we emergently revascularize occluded coronaries for cardiogenic shock? *J Am Coll Cardiol* 2000;36(3 Suppl A):1063–70.

9. Menon V, Webb JG, Hillis LD, et al. Outcome and profile of ventricular septal rupture with cardiogenic shock after myocardial infarction: a report from the SHOCK Trial Registry. should we emergently revascularize occluded coronaries in cardiogenic shock? *J Am Coll Cardiol* 2000;36(3 Suppl A):1110–6.

10. Topol EJ, Califf RM. *Textbook of Cardiovascular Medicine* (3rd edition). Philadelphia: Lippincott Williams & Wilkins, 2007.

11. Murday A. Optimal management of acute ventricular septal rupture. *Heart* 2003;89(12):1462–6.

12. Menon V, Hochman JS, Stebbins A, et al. Lack of progress in cardiogenic shock: lessons from the GUSTO trials. *Eur Heart J* 2000;21(23):1928–36.

13. Baim DS, Grossman W. *Grossman's Cardiac Catheterization, Angiography, and Intervention* (7th edition). Philadelphia: Lippincott, Williams & Wilkins, 2006.

14. Zipes DP, Braunwald E. *Braunwald's Heart Disease: A Textbook of Cardiovascular Medicine* (7th edition). Philadelphia: Elsevier Saunders, 2005.

15. Antman EM, Anbe DT, Armstrong PW, et al. ACC/AHA guidelines for the management of patients with ST-elevation myocardial infarction; A report of the American College of Cardiology/American Heart Association Task Force on Practice Guidelines (Committee to Revise the 1999 Guidelines for the Management of patients with acute myocardial infarction). *J Am Coll Cardiol* 2004;44(3):E1–211.

16. Thiele H, Lauer B, Hambrecht R, et al. Short- and long-term hemodynamic effects of intra-aortic balloon support in ventricular septal defect complicating acute myocardial infarction. *Am J Cardiology* 2003;92(4):450–4.

17. Sivadasan Pillai H, Tharakan J, Titus T, et al. Ventricular septal rupture following myocardial infarction. Long-term survival of patients who did not undergo surgery. Single-centre experience. *Acta Cardiol* 2005;60(4):403–7.

18. Cooley DA, Belmonte BA, Zeis LB, Schnur S. Surgical repair of ruptured interventricular septum following acute myocardial infarction. *Surgery* 1957;41(6):930–7.
19. Lemery R, Smith HC, Giuliani ER, Gersh BJ. Prognosis in rupture of the ventricular septum after acute myocardial infarction and role of early surgical intervention. *Am J Cardiol* 1992;70(2):147–51.
20. Daggett WM, Guyton RA, Mundth ED, et al. Surgery for post-myocardial infarct ventricular septal defect. *Ann Surg* 1977;186(3):260–71.
21. Scanlon PJ, Montoya A, Johnson SA, et al. Urgent surgery for ventricular septal rupture complicating acute myocardial infarction. *Circulation* 1985;72(3 Pt 2):II185–90.
22. Barker TA, Ramnarine IR, Woo EB, et al. Repair of post-infarct ventricular septal defect with or without coronary artery bypass grafting in the northwest of England: a 5-year multi-institutional experience. *Eur J Cardiothorac Surg* 2003;24(6):940–6.
23. Muehrcke DD, Daggett WM Jr, Buckley MJ, et al. Postinfarct ventricular septal defect repair: effect of coronary artery bypass grafting. *Ann Thorac Surg* 1992;54(5):876–82; discussion 82–3.
24. Pretre R, Ye Q, Grunenfelder J, Zund G, Turina MI. Role of myocardial revascularization in postinfarction ventricular septal rupture. *Ann Thorac Surg* 2000;69(1):51–5.
25. Labrousse L, Choukroun E, Chevalier JM, et al. Surgery for post infarction ventricular septal defect (VSD): risk factors for hospital death and long term results. *Eur J Cardiothorac Surg* 2002;21(4):725–31; discussion 31–2.
26. Deja MA, Szostek J, Widenka K, et al. Post infarction ventricular septal defect—can we do better? *Eur J Cardiothorac Surg* 2000;18(2):194–201.
27. Dalrymple-Hay MJ, Langley SM, Sami SA, et al. Should coronary artery bypass grafting be performed at the same time as repair of a post-infarct ventricular septal defect? *Eur J Cardiothorac Surg* 1998;13(3):286–92.
28. Cerin G, Di Donato M, Dimulescu D, et al. Surgical treatment of ventricular septal defect complicating acute myocardial infarction. Experience of a north Italian referral hospital. *Cardiovasc Surg* 2003;11(2):149–54.
29. Jeppsson A, Liden H, Johnsson P, Hartford M, Radegran K. Surgical repair of post infarction ventricular septal defects: a national experience. *Eur J Cardiothorac Surg* 2005;27(2):216–21.
30. Mantovani V, Mariscalco G, Leva C, Blanzola C, Sala A. Surgical repair of post-infarction ventricular septal defect: 19 years of experience. *Int J Cardiol* 2006; 108(2):202–6.
31. David TE, Armstrong S. Surgical repair of postinfarction ventricular septal defect by infarct exclusion. *Semin Thorac Cardiovasc Surg* 1998;10(2):105–10.
32. Dalrymple-Hay MJ, Monro JL, Livesey SA, Lamb RK. Postinfarction ventricular septal rupture: the Wessex experience. *Semin Thorac Cardiovasc Surg* 1998;10(2):111–16.
33. Sleeper LA, Ramanathan K, Picard MH, et al. Functional status and quality of life after emergency revascularization for cardiogenic shock complicating acute myocardial infarction. *J Am Coll Cardiol* 2005;46(2):266–73.
34. Sellke FW, Del Nido PJ, Swanson SJ, Sabiston DC, Spencer FC. *Sabiston & Spencer Surgery of the Chest* (7th edition). Philadelphia: Elsevier Saunders, 2005.
35. Massetti M, Babatasi G, Le Page O, et al. Postinfarction ventricular septal rupture: early repair through the right atrial approach. *J Thorac Cardiovasc Surg* 2000;119 (4 Pt 1):784–9.

36. Martinez MW, Mookadam F, Sun Y, Hagler DJ. Transcatheter closure of ischemic and post-traumatic ventricular septal ruptures. *Catheter Cardiovasc Interv* 2007;69(3):403–7.

37. Holzer R, Balzer D, Amin Z, et al. Transcatheter closure of postinfarction ventricular septal defects using the new Amplatzer muscular VSD occluder: results of a U.S. Registry. *Catheter Cardiovasc Interv* 2004;61(2):196–201.

38. Landzberg MJ, Lock JE. Transcatheter management of ventricular septal rupture after myocardial infarction. *Sem Thorac Cardiovasc Surg* 1998;10(2):128–32.

39. Park WM, Connery CP, Hochman JS, Tilson MD, Anagnostopoulos CE. Successful repair of myocardial free wall rupture after thrombolytic therapy for acute infarction. *Ann Thorac Surg* 2000;70(4):1345–9.

40. Lopez-Sendon J, Gonzalez A, Lopez de Sa E, et al. Diagnosis of subacute ventricular wall rupture after acute myocardial infarction: sensitivity and specificity of clinical, hemodynamic and echocardiographic criteria. *J Am Coll Cardiol* 1992;19(6):1145–53.

# Chapter 7

# Valvular heart disease in cardiogenic shock

Jason N. Katz, John G. Webb, and Michael H. Sketch, Jr.

Improvements in pharmacotherapeutics, interventional techniques, and health care delivery practices have allowed contemporary cardiologists to successfully alter the natural history of diseases that were once considered universally fatal. As a result, over the past several decades there has been a steady decline in the morbidity and mortality related to most cardiovascular maladies [1]. One major exception to these epidemiologic trends, however, has been in the care of patients with cardiogenic shock. Despite gaining substantial insight into the pathophysiology of acute coronary syndromes, nearly three quarters of patients who develop cardiogenic shock in the setting of myocardial infarction (MI) do not survive to hospital discharge [2]. Consequently, cardiogenic shock remains the most common mode of death for those hospitalized with acute MI.

What we do know about cardiogenic shock comes largely from reports of the SHOCK (SHould we emergently revascularize Occluded Coronaries for cardiogenic shocK) trial [3,4] and registry [5]. As a result of their influential findings, much of the interest in cardiogenic shock has focused predominantly on the acutely ischemic patient and the benefits of emergent restoration of coronary blood flow. An often overlooked finding from the SHOCK registry, however, was the suggestion that a substantial proportion (>8%) of patients with cardiogenic shock present with concomitant valvular heart disease [5,6]. This valvular pathology is not merely a consequence of infarction and shock, but rather is felt to contribute directly to the hemodynamic instability of afflicted patients.

Few studies to date have helped to elucidate the role of valvular heart disease in the pathogenesis of cardiogenic shock, although the available literature would suggest that not only is valvular disease a relatively common contributor

*Cardiogenic Shock.* Edited by Judith S. Hochman and E. Magnus Ohman.
© 2009 American Heart Association, ISBN: 978-1-4051-7926-3

to shock but, if not promptly identified and expeditiously managed, can be associated with catastrophic outcomes [7–12]. This chapter focuses on cardiogenic shock as a complication of valvular heart disease. The etiology of valvular dysfunction, whether a direct consequence of ischemic injury or thrombosis of a structurally normal valve or due to exacerbation of chronic valvular disease, will be described, and its influence on patient morbidity and mortality clarified. Additionally, management strategies for affected individuals will be explored in detail.

# Mitral valve disease

## Acute mitral regurgitation

Acute, severe mitral regurgitation (MR) results in a sudden overload of left atrial and left ventricular (LV) volume. In the absence of compensatory LV dilation and eccentric hypertrophy, which often accommodates the increased preload seen in chronic valvular insufficiency, stroke volume and cardiac output may be dramatically reduced. At the same time, the suddenly overloaded left heart is unable to handle the regurgitant volume, leading to pulmonary vascular congestion, overt pulmonary edema, and even cardiogenic shock.

Hemodynamically significant acute MR can result from a variety of disorders, including infective endocarditis, iatrogenic injury, and trauma. Additionally, acute ischemic injury during MI can cause the sudden onset of mitral insufficiency and concomitant cardiogenic shock. The management of patients with acute ischemic MR will be the focus of the remainder of this section.

Epidemiologic studies have suggested that the prevalence of papillary muscle dysfunction and severe, acute MR in patients with MI ranges from 17% to 55% [13,14]. Of the 1,160 patients with cardiogenic shock enrolled in the SHOCK registry, 7 to 8% presented with acute MR [5,6]. In general, results of small case series and autopsy studies indicate that patients presenting with acute MR were more commonly female, had predominant involvement of posterior and inferior myocardium, tended to have single-vessel obstructive coronary disease (most often the right coronary artery followed by the left circumflex artery), and often had no prior history of angina or MI [15–20].

SHOCK investigators more rigorously evaluated this population of patients with acute, severe MR and compared these individuals with a similar cohort of patients having predominant LV failure without associated mechanical sequelae [6]. Like previous studies, these investigators found that the population of patients with acute ischemic MR tended to have greater female representation and greater involvement of inferior and posterior myocardial territories with their infarct. It should be noted, however, that still nearly one-third of MR patients had evidence of anterior injury by electrocardiography. Additionally, patients with MR developed later shock (although most were within the first 24 hours of MI) than those in the comparative LV failure cohort and had significantly longer delays to potentially life-saving invasive therapies, including left

**Table 7.1** Acute MI associated cardiogenic shock due to predominant LV failure compared to acute severe mitral regurgitation

| | Severe MR | LV Failure | p-Value |
|---|---|---|---|
| *Baseline Features:* | | | |
| Female | 52% | 37% | 0.004 |
| Admit by Transfer | 65% | 42% | <0.004 |
| *Clinical Findings:* | | | |
| Anterior MI | 34% | 59% | <0.001 |
| Inferior MI | 55% | 44% | 0.039 |
| Posterior MI | 32% | 17% | 0.002 |
| ST-elevation at Shock | 41% | 63% | <0.001 |
| Time from MI to Shock (hrs)* | 12.8 (2.4,36.3) | 6.2 (1.7,20.1) | <0.001 |
| Pulmonary Edema on X-ray | 81% | 58% | <0.001 |
| LV Ejection Fraction (%)* | 36.5 (25,48) | 30.0 (20,40) | <0.001 |
| *Treatments:* | | | |
| Mechanical Ventilation | 93% | 75% | <0.001 |
| Inotropes | 88% | 71% | 0.002 |
| Right Heart Catheterization | 85% | 64% | <0.001 |
| Intraaortic Balloon Pump | 68% | 52% | 0.003 |
| Coronary Angiography | 76% | 61% | 0.006 |
| Angioplasty Attempted | 16% | 33% | 0.001 |
| Bypass Surgery | 43% | 15% | <0.001 |
| Transfusion | 64% | 39% | <0.001 |
| In-Hospital Mortality | 55% | 61% | 0.277 |

Marked differences in presentation, clinical characteristics, and treatment characterize those patients whose cardiogenic shock is associated with mitral regurgitation compared with those whose shock is associated primarily with left ventricular dysfunction. *Median (Q1,Q3).
Reprinted with permission from Thompson CR, Buller CE, Sleeper LA, et al. *J Am Coll Cardiol* 2000;36:1104–9.

heart catheterization and intra-aortic balloon counterpulsation, perhaps underscoring the clinical uncertainty surrounding the management of these complex patients (Table 7.1).

## Pathophysiology of acute ischemic mitral regurgitation in cardiogenic shock

Before embarking on further discussion of the relation between acute MR and cardiogenic shock, careful review of pathophysiology is warranted. Acute ischemic MR can occur as a consequence of either one of two unique clinical events: direct mechanical injury from infarction that results in papillary muscle rupture or chordal tear (structural MR) or dysfunction of the papillary muscle, and indirect disruption of the normal integrity of the mitral apparatus from pathologic ventricular remodeling (functional MR). Consideration of these two events may have significant implications in the diagnostic and therapeutic management strategies for affected patients. Furthermore, one must be mindful of the potential impact of pre-existing mitral insufficiency on the development of hemodynamically significant valvular regurgitation following ischemic insult.

*Structural mitral regurgitation*
Papillary muscle rupture inevitably leads to cardiogenic shock; mortality rates range from 70% to 90% without operative intervention. There is a bi-modal distribution in the timing of rupture; most occur within the first 24 hours and there is a second peak 2–7 days after the index MI [6,21]. Most of what is known about papillary muscle rupture complicating acute MI comes from autopsy series. In a study by Wei and colleagues [15], posterior LV involvement was a universal finding in fatal cases of papillary muscle rupture, and no individuals had evidence of anterior wall injury. For most patients, this was their first documented infarct, most had acute occlusions of the right coronary artery, and most had isolated involvement of the posterior papillary muscle. These findings have been corroborated in other necropsy series [22,23].

In comparing angiographic and clinical characteristics of patients with structural MR with those of patients with papillary muscle dysfunction but intact muscular integrity, Calvo and colleagues found results that closely mirrored previous autopsy findings [20]. Once again, patients with papillary muscle rupture had lower rates of prior angina or infarction, more commonly had inferior wall injury, had greater rates of single-vessel coronary disease, and had high mortality rates. These investigators also found that patients with papillary muscle rupture were older, more often required mechanical ventilation for associated respiratory failure, and had greater frequencies of infectious complications during hospitalization.

*Functional mitral regurgitation*
Unlike structural MR, functional MR is not due to direct ischemic injury to the mitral apparatus. Rather, functional MR is thought to result either from tethering forces that restrict the ability of the mitral leaflets to close or from a reduction in the mitral "closing force" due to LV systolic dysfunction [24]. A growing body of evidence supports a role for geometric distortion of the mitral apparatus resulting from progressive ventricular remodeling as the primary pathophysiologic mechanism [25]. Additionally, disagreement exists regarding the extent of ischemic injury required to invoke significant MR and shock. Some investigators argue that extensive MI and global remodeling is necessary [19,26]; Llaneras et al., for instance, demonstrated that in an animal model of ischemic MR, only large (involving 35 to 40% of the myocardial mass) posterior wall

infarctions could produce significant ischemic MR. Smaller territory infarction required either concomitant posterior papillary muscle rupture or significant LV dilatation to cause pathologic MR [19]. Others, however, in data largely derived from small necropsy series, have suggested that sufficient MR may develop due to dysfunction of only small areas of vital tissue [15,17,18]. It is noteworthy that the EF was depressed for those with severe MR in the SHOCK registry (median 37%) suggesting substantial LV damage, but 25% had an EF of 48% or higher suggesting more limited ischemic papillary muscle damage.

Evidence also indicates that mortality rates for functional MR are lower than for those patients with acute papillary muscle rupture, though individuals with functional MR still tend to have higher short-term and long-term mortality than comparable patients with MI but functionally normal valves [27].

## Diagnosis of acute ischemic mitral regurgitation

For structural MR, prompt diagnosis and immediate operative repair are essential for survival. Although there is controversy about the appropriate management of those with functional MR, evidence still supports early risk stratification and diagnostic evaluation, given the significant prognostic influence of this disease process.

While some patients may demonstrate classical findings of acute MR at the bedside, including a soft, low-pitched systolic murmur or prominent jugular venous v-waves (due to concomitant tricuspid insufficiency resulting from an elevated right ventricular pressure), the physical examination has been shown to be an insensitive tool for identifying those with ischemic MR [27,28].

In other instances, acute changes in waveforms derived from invasive hemodynamic monitoring may herald the development of severe mitral regurgitation. The Swan-Ganz catheter may reveal large v-waves, in addition to the other typical features of cardiogenic shock, including an elevated pulmonary artery wedge pressure, elevated right-sided pressures, and low mixed venous oxygen saturation (Table 7.2). However, for the majority of patients, more definitive diagnostic modalities are often required to identify acute MR.

Echocardiography is often the diagnostic study of choice to evaluate patients with acute MR and is considered an appropriate initial test for patients with suspected mechanical injury in the setting of MI [29]. Initially, echocardiography should focus on the presence of significant structural injury to the mitral valve, including flail leaflet or ruptured papillary muscle (Fig. 7.1). If absent, further echocardiographic evaluation of the mitral valve should include the application of commonly applied Doppler principles such as color flow (Fig. 7.2) and quantitative assessments of the effective regurgitant orifice, the regurgitant fraction, and the regurgitant volume, all of which have been shown to be predictive of mortality in small case series [30,31]. Additionally, the presence of systolic flow reversal in the pulmonary veins implies marked mitral valvular insufficiency.

**Table 7.2** Hemodynamic patterns

| | RA | RVS | RVD | PAS | PAD | PAW | CI | SVR |
|---|---|---|---|---|---|---|---|---|
| Normal values | <6 | <25 | 0–12 | <25 | 0–12 | <6–12 | ≥2.5 | (800–1600) |
| Pulmonary edema | ↔↑ | ↔↑ | ↔↑ | ↑ | ↑ | ↑ | ↔↓ | ↑ |
| Cardiogenic shock | | | | | | | | |
|   LV failure | ↔↑ | ↔↑ | ↔↑ | ↔↑ | ↑ | ↑ | ↓ | ↔↑ |
|   RV failure$^{\xi}$ | ↑ | ↓↔↑* | ↑ | ↓↔↑* | ↔↓↑* | ↓↔↑* | ↓ | ↑ |
| Acute mitral regurgitation | ↔↑ | ↑ | ↔↑ | ↑ | ↑ | ↑ | ↔↓ | ↔↑ |
| Ventricular septal rupture | ↑ | ↔↑ | ↑ | ↔↑ | ↔↑ | ↔↑ | ↑PBF ↓SBF | ↔↑ |

There is significant patient-to-patient variation. Pressures in RA = right atrium; RVS/D = right ventricular systolic/diastolic; PAS/D = pulmonary artery systolic/diastolic; PAW = pulmonary artery wedge is in mmHg. CI = cardiac index (L/min/m²) and SVR = systemic vascular resistance (dynes/sec/cm⁵). MI = myocardial infarction, P/SBF = pulmonary/systemic blood flow.
$\xi$ = "Isolated" or predominant RV failure.
‡Forrester et al. classified non-reperfused MI patients into four hemodynamic subsets (NEJM 1976;295:1356–1362). PAWP and CI in clinically stable subset 1 patients are shown. Values in parenthesis represent range. Reprinted with permission from Hochman JS and Ingbar D, Cardiogenic Shock and Pulmonary Edema in Fauci AS, Braunwald E, Kasper DL et al., Harrison's Principles of Internal Medicine 17th Edition, McGraw-Hill Medical, 2008.

If suspicion of severe MR exists, such as shock in the setting of first inferior MI or with modest ECG and wall motion abnormalities, despite the absence of confirmatory evidence by transthoracic echocardiography, transesophageal imaging should be performed to evaluate mitral valve morphology and regurgitant severity. Transesophageal echocardiography is often helpful to further delineate mitral anatomy and to direct surgical strategies for repair.

In aggregate, data obtained from echocardiography, along with other clinical information available to the clinician, should help to guide appropriate patient management. One should also be mindful of the need for serial or late echocardiographic examinations in patients with cardiogenic shock complicated by acute MR, as several studies have shown that these patients can often have considerable delays in the onset of hemodynamic deterioration following hospital admission [15,20].

### Treatment of acute ischemic mitral regurgitation in cardiogenic shock
Studies of therapeutic strategies for the management of cardiogenic shock associated with acute MR have largely been limited to observational and

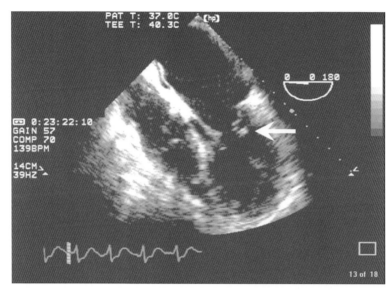

**Fig. 7.1** Two-dimensional echocardiographic image of a ruptured posterior papillary muscle (arrow).

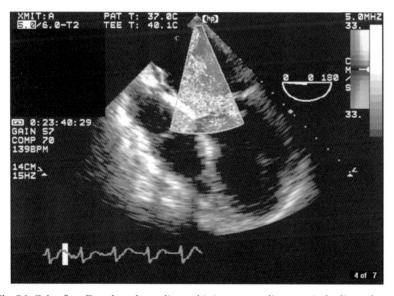

**Fig. 7.2** Color-flow Doppler echocardiographic image revealing anteriorly directed regurgitant jet with widened vena contracta consistent with severe mitral regurgitation from a ruptured posterior papillary muscle.

nonrandomized analyses. Most of these support a management approach focused on early mitral valve surgery [8–12,32], a finding corroborated by the SHOCK investigators who found unadjusted mortality rates favoring a surgical over medical management approach (40% vs. 71% mortality, respectively) [7]. However, a comparison of surgical and nonsurgical treatments in this registry also highlighted the significant selection bias, which has influenced all surgical series to date, as patients treated with an operative strategy tended to have smaller index infarctions, less hemodynamic compromise, and fewer medical comorbidities [7].

Whereas papillary muscle rupture or chordal tear is a clear indication for surgical repair, the proper management of those ischemic patients who have functional MR remains controversial. Although medical therapy has a well-defined role in the management of patients with stable or chronic disease, it has very limited efficacy in those with cardiogenic shock. In shock patients, medical management is most often employed as a strategy to achieve hemodynamic stabilization in preparation for surgery. However, decomposition can be rapid and unpredictable so surgery should not be delayed.

By improving cardiac output through reductions in systemic vascular resistance and improvements in mitral valve competence, intravenous sodium nitroprusside has been used in the acute setting to decrease MR [33]. The use of vasodilatory agents in this setting should be considered with extreme caution, as the hemodynamic effect of these therapies can often be unpredictable. Most authorities recommend invasive hemodynamic monitoring be employed if vasodilators are to be used. Furthermore, in the hypotensive patient with cardiogenic shock, vasodilators should not be used in isolation, but rather only as an adjunct to inotropic agents and intra-aortic balloon counterpulsation.

For those with ischemic functional MR, there has been at least some suggestion that percutaneous revascularization may help to reduce the MR burden [34–36]. In these individuals, medical therapy and intra-aortic balloon pump support may be effective until coronary blood flow is restored. Definitive surgical repair or mitral valve replacement should be considered for those individuals refractory to more conservative care. For patients with structural MR, as well as those with acute, severe MR resulting from infection or trauma, prompt surgical therapy is warranted. When amenable from an anatomic standpoint, valve repair is the option of choice; however, most patients with papillary muscle rupture or chordal disruption ultimately require valve replacement due to the presence of significant myocardial necrosis.

## Mitral stenosis

Although MR is a more common cause of cardiogenic shock, mitral valve stenosis can also result in similar hemodynamic perturbations if left untreated. In the vast majority of cases, mitral stenosis (MS) results from rheumatic heart disease [37,38] but can also be caused by congenital defects, infective

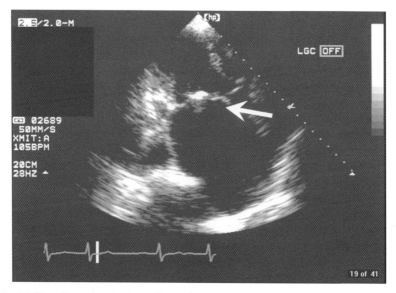

**Fig. 7.3** Two-dimensional echocardiographic image of severe rheumatic mitral valve stenosis (arrow).

endocarditis, and severe annular calcification. Although the incidence of rheumatic fever has been markedly reduced in most developed countries [39], it remains a major health concern in developing nations (Fig. 7.3) [40].

Rheumatic MS has an asymptomatic latent period ranging from 16 to 40 years following the initial episode of rheumatic fever, but accelerates rapidly to a more severe phenotype once symptoms begin to develop [38,41]. In a study by Olesen [42], who followed 271 patients with rheumatic MS prospectively, 10-year survival rates were dramatically influenced by functional class. The survival rates for patients with functional class I–IV symptoms were approximately 80%, 69%, 33%, and 0%, respectively.

From a pathophysiologic perspective, the key hemodynamic consequence of MS is the development of a pressure gradient between the left atrium and left ventricle. As this pressure gradient increases, the elevation in left atrial pressure is transmitted to the pulmonary circulation resulting in increases in both pulmonary pressures as well as pulmonary vascular resistance (Figs. 7.4 and 7.5). This, in turn, can manifest as pulmonary edema, right ventricular failure, and even shock. Once clinical MS develops, valve area decreases by an average of 0.1 cm$^2$ per year [43,44]. Whereas symptom development is a protracted process in those with MS, patients with more advanced disease can deteriorate acutely in functional class with even mild changes in hemodynamics. Any situation that either increases transmitral flow, such as third trimester pregnancy, decreases diastolic filling time, such as atrial fibrillation, can cause

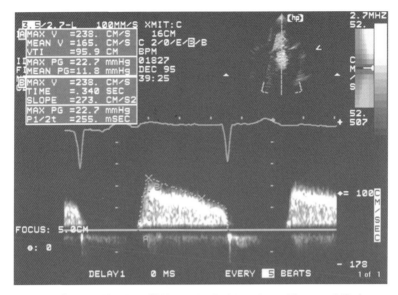

**Fig. 7.4** Doppler quantification of MS severity. In this patient with severe MS, the calculated pressure half-time is 255 ms.

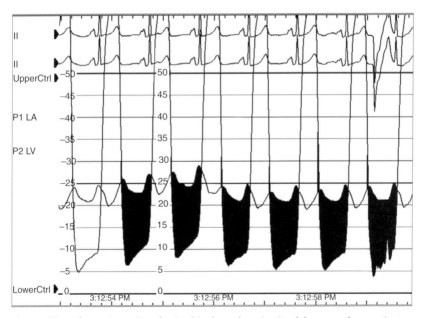

**Fig. 7.5** Hemodynamic tracing obtained in the catheterization laboratory for a patient with severe mitral stenosis, revealing significant gradient between the left atrium (LA) and left ventricle (LV).

patients with apparently stable disease to abruptly deteriorate and develop clinical shock.

Relief of mechanical obstruction in MS can, however, often dramatically and immediately improve hemodynamics. Reyes and colleagues [45], in a randomized comparison of percutaneous and open surgical valvotomy for patients with MS, demonstrated the potential for complete reversibility in pulmonary hypertension with definitive therapy.

Since its introduction in the mid-1980s [46,47], balloon mitral valvuloplasty has proven to be a reliable and effective method for treating advanced MS and, in many cases, has become the preferred therapeutic modality for these patients. Currently, percutaneous balloon mitral valvuloplasty (PBMV) is advocated by the American Heart Association/American College of Cardiology [48], provided the patient has favorable valvular morphology, has mild or no MR, and has no evidence of left atrial thrombus.

Only one study has evaluated the use of emergent PBMV in patients with MS and cardiogenic shock. Assessing an end-stage population in India, Likhandwala and others performed an observational study of balloon valvuloplasty for patients with shock, cardiac arrest, or refractory heart failure who were not surgical candidates due to advanced disease and marked hemodynamic instability [49]. Although the short-term mortality was 40% in this study, results did suggest the potential feasibility of PBMV in this very high-risk patient population. Additionally, several baseline variables were found to be predictive of mortality, including systolic blood pressure <80 mm Hg, $PO_2$ <60, pulmonary arterial systolic pressure >65 mm Hg, and mitral valve score ≥8 [50].

Further study comparing various modalities of mitral valvuloplasty in patients presenting with cardiogenic shock is clearly warranted. If tolerated, many of these patients will undergo left heart catheterization, coronary angiography, and right heart catheterization in anticipation of definitive repair. Invasive hemodynamic variables obtained in the catheterization laboratory have been shown to closely mirror less invasive echocardiographic-derived gradients, but the presence of concomitant obstructive coronary artery disease may influence the decision to pursue surgical intervention.

# Aortic valve disease

## Acute aortic insufficiency

Due to the ventricle's inability to adapt to rapid increases in end-diastolic volume, acute aortic insufficiency (AI) may result in cardiogenic shock. Common causes of acute AI include infective endocarditis with valve destruction and/or abscess formation, aortic dissection, traumatic valve leaflet rupture, and iatrogenic injury. In a case series of 268 adults referred to a single institution for aortic valve replacement for isolated AI, Roberts and colleagues noted that approximately 18% of patients had acute AI, all resulting from endocarditis or dissection [51].

## Diagnosis of acute aortic insufficiency

Like the patient with acute MR, patients with acute AI usually do not manifest the characteristic findings of chronic AI. This is due to the fact that LV stroke volume and diastolic filling volume are not increased in acute disease. In these patients, manifestations of cardiogenic shock and hemodynamic instability often dominate. The presence of concomitant aortic dissection may be suggested by inequality in upper extremity pulse and blood pressures, but other physical examination findings are largely unreliable. Even this finding may be difficult to discern in patients with tenuous hemodynamic status.

Transthoracic echocardiography is often sufficient to make the diagnosis of acute AI. Doppler criteria suggestive of severe AI include vena contracta width greater than 6 mm, pressure half-time less than 200 ms, and holodiastolic flow reversal in the descending thoracic aorta [52]. When dissection is suspected, computed tomography imaging, magnetic resonance imaging or transesophageal echocardiography should be used as an adjunctive diagnostic tool. Additionally, transesophageal echocardiography, which is preferred in unstable intubated shock, can help further define the abnormal aortic valve anatomy and may guide surgical planning.

## Treatment of acute aortic insufficiency in cardiogenic shock

For any patient with acute, severe AI, the therapeutic strategy should focus on eventual valve replacement. The use of vasodilators, such as nitroprusside, in conjunction with inotropic therapy may help with hemodynamic stabilization, but surgery should not be delayed [48]. Aortic counterpulsation is contraindicated due to the exacerbation in aortic regurgitation which can result from diastolic balloon inflation, and the future application of percutaneous valve replacement techniques in these patients is, as of yet, unstudied.

## Aortic stenosis

Although LV dysfunction and overt heart failure are uncommon findings among contemporary patients with aortic stenosis (AS), end-stage patients who have not received adequate medical care may present to the hospital with hemodynamic compromise (Fig. 7.6). There are three primary causes of valvular AS in adults: congenital bicuspid valvular disease with superimposed calcification, calcific disease of a normal tricuspid valve, and rheumatic heart disease. Although calcific disease is more common in North America and Europe [53,54], it is suspected that rheumatic disease remains the most common primary etiology of valvular AS worldwide.

When AS patients present with cardiogenic shock and/or multisystem organ failure, their outcomes are usually catastrophic. For appropriate surgical candidates, emergent operative aortic valve replacement (AVR) can be life saving. However, in many cases, these patients may be considered too ill and too unstable for traditional therapy. The current temporizing or palliative alternative to operative care is percutaneous balloon aortic valvuloplasty; eventually, it may include percutaneous AVR.

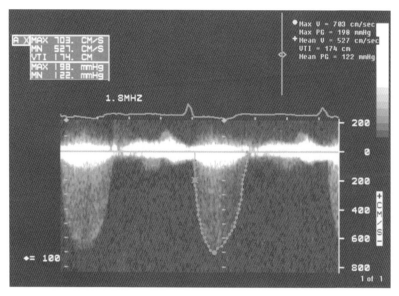

**Fig. 7.6** Continuous-wave Doppler velocities in a patient with severe aortic valve stenosis.

Balloon valvuloplasty for nonemergent patients with AS is uncommonly used, due to the significant morbidity and mortality associated with the procedure and the lack of sustainable hemodynamic results. In fact, rates of valvular restenosis have been estimated to approach 60% per year [55]. Other reasons for poor outcomes following catheter balloon valvuloplasty include the high incidence of concomitant obstructive coronary disease and the numerous significant medical comorbidities affecting these patients [56–58].

In the NHLBI registry data of catheter balloon valvuloplasty for AS [59], approximately 6% of patients presented with cardiogenic shock, with an associated 30-day mortality rate of nearly 50%. Although case series have shown that balloon valvuloplasty can be performed in AS patients considered to be too high risk for surgery [60–62], there are high rates of potentially catastrophic complications associated with this technique (including fatal cerebral embolism, ventricular perforation, acute AI, and cardiac arrest) [63]. In addition, patients with advanced AS and cardiogenic shock are exquisitely sensitive to the hemodynamic perturbations that can occur with balloon valvuloplasty; hence, periprocedural ischemia is very likely to precipitate a vicious cycle of ventricular dysfunction, ischemia/infarction, and hemodynamic collapse (Fig. 7.7) [58]. Most authorities suggest that, if balloon valvuloplasty is performed for severe symptomatic AS, it should be done with the explicit goal of "bridging" patients to more definitive operative valve replacement.

The feasibility of percutaneous AVR in high-risk patients with AS was first described by Cribier and colleagues using a transvenous, transseptal approach

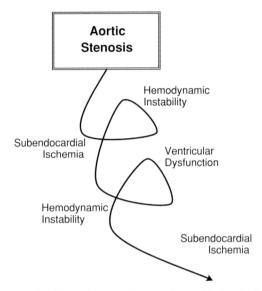

**Fig. 7.7** Pathologic cycle of hemodynamic deterioration and ischemia that may result from balloon valvuloplasty in patients with severe, symptomatic aortic stenosis.

[64,65]. More recently, Webb and colleagues reported their initial experience with a retrograde AVR procedure using percutaneous femoral arterial access [66]. Procedural success was achieved in 86% of their 50-patient cohort, with a 30-day mortality rate of 12%. As experience grows with the use of percutaneous AVR, it may become a viable option for nonsurgical patients with advanced AS and shock.

For critically ill patients with advanced AS who are too hemodynamically unstable to undergo surgery, medical therapy, although limited in its efficacy, has been shown to help stabilize such patients. In a recent study of twenty-five patients with LV dysfunction (cardiac index $\leq 2.2$ L/min/m$^2$ by Fick method and EF $\leq 35\%$) complicating severe AS who were not in shock, Khot and colleagues showed that the use of nitroprusside could significantly improve cardiac index and stroke volume [67]. Starting at a mean nitroprusside dose of $14 \pm 10$ mcg/min, and increasing to a mean dose of $103 \pm 67$ mcg/min at six hours and $128 \pm 96$ mcg/min at twenty-four hours, these investigators showed that vasodilator therapy was relatively safe and could significantly improve patient hemodynamics (cardiac increased to $2.22 \pm 0.44$ L/min/m$^2$ at 6h and $2.52 \pm 0.55$ L/min/m$^2$ at 24 hours; $p < 0.001$ for each increase compared with baseline). However, in some circumstances, vasodilator therapy can also further exacerbate hemodynamic instability; careful hemodynamic monitoring is essential, and plans for immediate, definitive relief of the valvular obstruction should be pursued. Nitroprusside has not been studied in those with cardiogenic shock and systemic hypotension and is not recommended.

Aortic counterpulsation may also be of benefit in the stabilization of patients with decompensated AS, especially when concomitant obstructive coronary disease and myocardial ischemia may be contributing to the hemodynamic compromise. There has even been recent suggestion that an intra-aortic balloon pump may be useful when employing a combined approach of percutaneous coronary revascularization followed by operative valve replacement in patients with complex, unstable aortic valve stenosis [68], although this remains to be corroborated in larger case series.

# Mechanical valve thrombosis

The incidence of mechanical prosthetic valve thrombosis ranges from 0.2% to 6% per year in those with aortic or mitral valve prostheses and as high as 13% in those with prostheses in the tricuspid valve position [69,70]. Thrombosis resulting in valvular obstruction is an extremely rare finding. When present, however, the hemodynamic consequences can be abrupt and life-threatening [71,72].

Results from several small case series suggest that most patients with thrombosed mechanical valves present with advanced heart failure or cardiogenic shock [71–73]. In a study of 29 patients admitted with mechanical valve obstruction and critical hemodynamic compromise, Buttard and colleagues found that nearly half of the patients had inadequate levels of systemic anticoagulation at presentation, many of whom had discontinued their chronic oral anticoagulation in anticipation of elective noncardiac surgery [73]. Additionally, many patients had concomitant atrial fibrillation. Over 40% of the patients died, with over one-quarter of the cohort dying in the preoperative period.

Diagnosing mechanical prosthetic valve thrombosis can be challenging, with only a minority of patients exhibiting classic signs of attenuated valvular auscultatory findings or appearance of new cardiac murmurs. In fact, it has been suggested that nearly 50% of obstructed valves may be diagnosed only at autopsy [74]. Ancillary diagnostic tools, such as cinefluoroscopy and transthoracic or transesophageal echocardiography, can improve the detection of partial or completely obstructive thrombi.

Cinefluorscopy can be used to directly visualize mechanical prosthetic valves. Most often, multiple views are necessary to adequately assess valve mobility. In the mitral position, imaging is usually performed with the camera in a shallow right-anterior oblique (RAO) and steep cranial position (e.g. 10–15 degrees RAO, 40–45 degrees cranial), as well as left-anterior oblique (LAO) with cranial angulation (e.g. 55–60 degrees LAO, 5–10 degrees cranial). For valves in the aortic position, an LAO-cranial image is often obtained (e.g. 75 degrees LAO, 25–30 degrees cranial), with en-face visualization in the RAO-cranial position

(a) Thrombosed mechanical valve

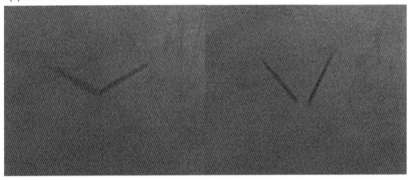

(b) Normal mechanical valve

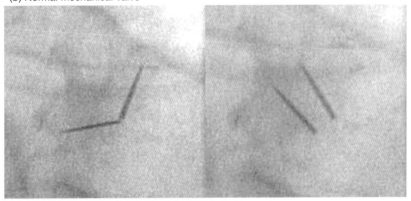

**Fig. 7.8** (a) Cinefluoroscopic views of a partially thrombosed bileaflet mechanical aortic valve. The left panel shows the valve completely closed, while the right panel reveals incomplete opening of the valve due to thrombosis. (b) Cinefluoroscopic view of a normal mechanical aortic valve. The left panel shows the valve in the closed position while the right panel shows the same valve in the open position.

(e.g. 40–45 degrees RAO, 40–45 degree cranial). Figure 7.8(a)&(b) shows typical fluoroscopic imaging of a partially obstructed and a normal mechanical aortic valve.

Measurement of Doppler echocardiographic variables is also essential for the assessment of suspected obstruction, and evaluation of valvular gradients and valve areas can assist in the diagnosis. Clinicians, however, must be cautious of overinterpreting these gradients in light of potential confounding mechanisms unrelated to malfunction of the prosthetic valve (e.g. tachycardia, increased cardiac output, subvalvular hypertrophy). Additionally, transesophageal echocardiography is the procedure of choice for visualizing leaflet motion and elucidating the etiology of valvular obstruction [75,76].

Until recently, the traditional treatment for prosthetic valve thrombosis has been emergent surgery, and reported operative mortality rates have ranged from 0% to 70%, largely depending on the patient's functional class at the time of surgery [70,71,77]. Lately, there has been increasing enthusiasm for the use of systemic fibrinolysis in the treatment of prosthetic valve thrombosis. It is currently considered the treatment of choice for tricuspid valve thrombosis [78,79], but its use in left-sided valvular obstruction is less clear due to the high-risk of cerebral thromboembolism. The role of fibrinolysis in these patients seems best applied to those with hemodynamic instability and cardiogenic shock, conditions that might otherwise preclude the use of conventional surgery. Several case reports have fueled contemporary interest in using fibrinolytics for high-risk patients with thrombotic valvular obstruction [78,79], and current consensus suggests that fibrinolytic therapy should be considered in critically ill patients with advanced symptoms in whom surgical intervention is either contraindicated or likely to be fatal [80]. Other potential circumstances which may favor fibrinolytic therapy consideration include lower-risk patients with small thrombus burden and no contraindications ($<0.8$ cm$^2$) [81], and those with substantial surgical risk. Aggregate findings from case series suggest that fibrinolytic therapy success ranges from 85–90%, with mortality rates on the order of 5–10%. In addition, embolic events ranged from 6–19%, hemorrhagic events were seen in 2–8% of patients, and recurrent thrombosis occurred in up to a quarter of patients [82–84].

When fibrinolysis is employed, streptokinase or urokinase have been the most commonly used agents, although successful lysis with recombinant tissue-type plasminogen activator (rt-PA) has been reported [83]. The recommended dosage of streptokinase is a 250,000 unit bolus over 30 minutes, followed by an infusion of 100,000 units/hour, while urokinase is usually given as an infusion at a dose of 4,400 units/kg/hour. The ideal duration of therapy is uncertain and infusion durations have ranged from 2 to 120 hours in limited case series [85,86]. Most authorities suggest dictating fibrinolytic therapy duration based upon clinical criteria, including resolution of hemodynamic instability and restoration of normal valvular Doppler echocardiographic velocities. In the absence of significant clinical improvement after 24 hours of fibrinolytic therapy, high-risk surgery should be entertained [80].

## Conclusion

Although much of the attention in cardiogenic shock has been directed toward emergent coronary revascularization for the acutely ischemic patient, there is a significant proportion of individuals whose hemodynamic instability is due, at least in part, to advanced valvular heart disease. In the majority of such cases, prompt surgical therapy is the treatment of choice. However, the presence of substantial comorbidities, end-organ dysfunction, and hemodynamic compromise often precludes attempts at any surgical intervention. Percutaneous treatments have been shown to have variable success, largely dependent on the underlying valvular pathology, but in many cases, they may provide enough clinical stability to effectively bridge a patient to more definitive operative care. It is clear from the limited evidence-based literature that more rigorous study of these high-risk patients is needed. At the same time, through larger prospective investigation, there is significant opportunity to improve the care and lives of patients with hemodynamically unstable valvular heart disease.

# References

1. Nichol G, Karmy-Jones R, Salerno C, Cantore L, Becker L. Systematic review of percutaneous cardiopulmonary bypass for cardiac arrest or cardiogenic shock states. *Resuscitation* 2006;70:381–94.
2. Goldberg RJ, Samad NA, Yarzebski J, Gurwitz J, Bigelow C, Gore JM. Temporal trends in cardiogenic shock complicating acute myocardial infarction. *N Engl J Med* 1999;340:1162–8.
3. Hochman JS, Sleeper LA, Webb JG, et al. Early revascularization in acute myocardial infarction complicated by cardiogenic shock. *N Engl J Med* 1999;341:625–34.
4. Hochman JS, Sleeper LA, Webb JG, et al. Early revascularization and long-term survival in cardiogenic shock complicating acute myocardial infarction. *J Am Med Assoc* 2006;295:2511–5.
5. Hochman JS, Buller CE, Sleeper LA, et al., for the shock study group. Cardiogenic shock complicating acute myocardial infarcation—etiologies, management and outcome: Overall findings of the shock trial registry. *J Am Coll Cardiol* 2000;1063–70.
6. Thompson CR, Buller CE, Sleeper LA, et al. Cardiogenic shock due to acute severe mitral regurgitation complicating acute myocardial infarction: a report from the SHOCK Trial Registry. *J Am Coll Cardiol* 2000;36:1104–9.
7. Fox AC, Glassman E, Isom OW. Surgically remediable complications of myocardial infarction. *Prog Cardiovasc Dis* 1979;21:461–84.
8. Nishimura RA, Schaff HV, Gersh BJ, Holmes DR Jr, Tajik AJ. Early repair of mechanical complications after acute myocardial infarction. *J Am Med Assoc* 1986;256:47–50.
9. Bolooki H. Emergency cardiac procedures in patients in cardiogenic shock due to complications of coronary artery disease. *Circulation* 1989;79:I137–48.
10. Bolooki H. Surgical treatment of complications of acute myocardial infarction. *J Am Med Assoc* 1990;263:1237–40.
11. Cercek B, Shah PK. Complicated acute myocardial infarction. Heart failure, shock, mechanical complications. *Cardiol Clin* 1991;9:569–93.
12. Yamanishi H, Izumoto H, Kitahara H, Kamata J, Tasai K, Kawazoe K. Clinical experiences of surgical repair for mitral regurgitation secondary to papillary muscle rupture complicating acute myocardial infarction. *Ann Thorac Cardiovasc Surg* 1998;4:83–6.
13. Maisel AS, Gilpin EA, Klein L, Le Winter M, Henning H, Collins D. The murmur of papillary muscle dysfunction in acute myocardial infarction: clinical features and prognostic implications. *Am Heart J* 1986;112:705–11.

14. Heikkila J. Mitral incompetence complicating acute myocardial infarction. *Br Heart J* 1967;29:162–9.

15. Wei J, Hutchins GM, Bulkley BH. Papillary muscle rupture in fatal acute myocardial infarction. A potentially treatable form of cardiogenic shock. *Ann Intern Med* 1979;90: 149–53.

16. Sharma SK, Seckler J, Israel DH, Borrico S, Ambrose JA. Clinical, angiographic and anatomic findings in acute severe ischemic mitral regurgitation. *Am J Cardiol* 1992;70: 277–80.

17. Nishimura RA, Schaff HV, Shub C, Gersh BJ, Edwards WD, Tajik AJ. Papillary muscle rupture complicating acute myocardial infarction: analysis of 17 patients. *Am J Cardiol* 1983;53:373–7.

18. Barbour DJ, Roberts WC. Rupture of left ventricular papillary muscle during acute myocardial infarction. Analysis of 22 necropsy cases. *J Am Coll Cardiol* 1986;8:138–53.

19. Llanera MR, Nance ML, Streicher JT, et al. Large animal model of ischemic mitral regurgitation. *Ann Thorac Surg* 1994;57:432–9.

20. Calvo FE, Figueras J, Coradellas J, Soler-Soler J. Severe mitral regurgitation complicating acute myocardial infarction. Clinical and angiographic differences between patients with and without papillary muscle rupture. *Eur Heart J* 1997;18:1606–10.

21. Kishon Y, Oh JK, Schaff HV, Mullany CJ, Tajik AJ, Gersh BJ. Mitral valve operation in postinfarction rupture of a papillary muscle: immediate results and long-term follow-up of 22 patients. *Mayo Clin Proc* 1992;67:1023–30.

22. Hackel DB, Wagner GS. Acute myocrdial infarction with papillary muscle rupture. *Clin Cardiol* 1993;16:59–64.

23. Cederqvist L, Soederstroem J. Papillary muscle rupture in myocardial infarction. A study based upon an autopsy material. *Acta Med Scand* 1964;176:287–92.

24. Pierard LA. Functional mitral regurgitation in acute coronary syndrome: what determines its prognostic impact? *Eur Heart J* 2006;27:2615–6.

25. He S, Fontaine AA, Schwammenthal E, Yoganathan AP, Levine RA. Integrated mechanism for functional mitral regurgitation. Leaflet restriction versus coapting force: in vitro studies. *Circulation* 1997;96:1826–34.

26. Coma-Canella I, Gamallo C, Onsurbe PM, Jadraque LM. Anatomic findings in acute papillary muscle necrosis. *Am Heart J* 1989;118:1188–92.

27. Grigioni F, Enriquez-Sarano M, Zehr KJ, Bailey KR, Tajik AJ. Ischemic mitral regurgitation: long-term outcome and prognostic implications with quantitative Doppler assessment. *Circulation* 2001;103:1759–64.

28. Tcheng JE, Jackman JD, Nelson CL, et al. Outcome of patients sustaining acute ischaemic mitral regurgitation during myocardial infarction. *Ann Intern Med* 1992;117: 18–24.

29. Douglas PS, Khandheria B, Stainback RF, et al. ACCF/ASE/ACEP/ASNC/SCAI/ SCCT/SCMR 2007 appropriateness criteria for transthoracic and transesophageal echocardiography: a report of the American College of Cardiology Foundation Quality Strategic Directions Committee Appropriateness Criteria Working Group, American Society of Echocardiography, American College of Emergency Physicians, American Society of Nuclear Cardiology, Society for Cardiovascular Angiography and Interventions, Society of Cardiovascular Computed Tomography, and the Society for Cardiovascular Magnetic Resonance endorsed by the American College of Chest

Physicians and the Society of Critical Care Medicine. *J Am Coll Cardiol* 2007;50: 187–204.

30. Enriquez-Sarano M, Avierinos JF, Messika-Zeitoun D, et al. Quantitative determinants of the outcome of asymptomatic mitral regurgitation. *N Engl J Med* 2005;352:875–83.

31. Amigoni M, Meris A, Thune JJ, et al. Mitral regurgitation in myocardial infarction complicated by heart failure, left ventricular dysfunction, or both: prognostic significance and relation to ventricular size and function. *Eur Heart J* 2007;28:326–33.

32. Gorman III JH, Jackson BM, Kolansky DM, Gorman RC. Emergency mitral valve replacement in the octogenarian. *Ann Thorac Surg* 2003;76:269–71.

33. Chatterjee K, Parmley WW, Swan HJ, Berman G, Forrester J, Marcus HS. Beneficial effects of vasodilator agents in severe mitral regurgitation due to dysfunction of subvalvular apparatus. *Circulation* 1973;48:684–90.

34. Reinfeld HB, Samet P, Hildner FJ. Resolution of congestive failure, mitral regurgitation, and angina after percutaneous transluminal coronary angioplasty of triple vessel disease. *Cathet Cardiovasc Diagn* 1985;11:273–7.

35. Heuser RR, Maddoux GL, Goss JE, Ramo BW, Raff GL, Shadoff N. Coronary angioplasty for acute mitral regurgitation due to myocardial infarction. *Ann Intern Med* 1987;107:852–5.

36. Shawl FA, Forman MB, Punja S, Goldbaum TS. Emergent coronary angioplasty in the treatment of acute ischemic mitral regurgitation: long-term results in five cases. *J Am Coll Cardiol* 1989;14:986–91.

37. Olson LJ, Subramanian R, Ackermann DM, et al. Surgical pathology of the mitral valve: a study of 712 cases spanning 21 years. *Mayo Clin Proc* 1987;62:22–34.

38. Horstkotte D, Niehues R, Strauer BE. Pathomorphological aspects, aetiology and natural history of acquired mitral valve stenosis. *Eur Heart J* 1991;12 (Suppl B):55–60.

39. Gordis L. The virtual disappearance of rheumatic fever in the United States: lessons in the rise and fall of disease. *Circulation* 1985;72:1155–62.

40. Marcus RH, Sareli P, Pocock WA, et al. The spectrum of severe rheumatic valve disease in a developing country. *Ann Intern Med* 1994;120:177–83.

41. Wood P. An appreciation of mitral stenosis. I. Clinical features. *Br Med J* 1954;4870: 1051–63.

42. Olesen KH. The natural history of 271 patients with mitral stenosis under medical treatment. *Br Heart J* 1962;24:349–57.

43. Gordon SP, Douglas PS, Come PC, Manning WJ. Two-dimensional and Doppler echocardiographic determinants of the natural history of mitral valve narrowing in patients with rheumatic mitral stenosis: implications for follow-up. *J Am Coll Cardiol* 1992;19:968–73.

44. Sagie A, Freitas N, Padial LR, et al. Doppler echocardiographic assessment of long-term progression of mitral stenosis in 103 patients: valve area and right heart disease. *J Am Coll Cardiol* 1996;28:472–9.

45. Reyes VP, Raju BS, Wynne J, et al. Percutaneous balloon valvuloplasty compared with open surgical commissurotomy for mitral stenosis. *N Engl J Med* 1994;331:961–7.

46. Inoue K, Owaki T, Nakamura T, et al. Clinical application of transvenous mitral commissurotomy by a new balloon catheter. *J Thorac Cardiovasc Surg* 1984;87: 394–402.

47. Lock JE, Khalilullah M, Shrivastava S, et al. Percutaneous catheter commissurotomy in rheumatic mitral stenosis. *N Engl J Med* 1985;313:1515–8.

48. Bonow RO, Carabello BA, Chatterjee K, et al. ACC/AHA 2006 guidelines for the management of patients with valvular heart disease. A report of the American College of Cardiology/American Heart Association Task Force on Practice Guidelines. *J Am Coll Cardiol* 2006;48:e1–148.

49. Likhandwala YY, Banker D, Vora AM, et al. Emergent balloon mitral valvotomy in patients with cardiac arrest, cardiogenic shock or refractory pulmonary edema. *J Am Coll Cardiol* 1998;32:154–8.

50. Wilkins GT, Weyman AE, Abascal VM, et al. Percutaneous balloon dilatation of the mitral valve: an analysis of echocardiographic variables related to outcome and mechanism of dilatation. *Br Heart J* 1988;60:299–308.

51. Roberts WC, Ko JM, Moore TR, Jones WH 3rd. Causes of pure aortic regurgitation in patients having isolated aortic valve replacement at a single US tertiary hospital (1993 to 2005). *Circulation* 2006;114:422–9.

52. Zoghbi WA, Enriquez-Sarano M, Foster E, et al. Recommendations for evaluation of the severity of native valvular regurgitation with two-dimensional and Doppler echocardiography. *J Am Soc Echocardiogr* 2003;16:777–802.

53. Passik CS, Ackermann DM, Pluth JR, Edwards WD. Temporal changes in the causes of aortic stenosis: a surgical pathologic study of 646 cases. *Mayo Clin Proc* 1987;62:119–23.

54. Roberts WC, Ko JM. Frequency by decades of unicuspid, bicuspid, and tricuspid aortic valves in adults having isolated aortic valve replacement for aortic stenosis, with or without associated aortic regurgitation. *Circulation* 2005;111:920–5.

55. Rahimtoola SH. Perspective on valvular heart disease: update II. In: Knoebel S, Dack S, eds. *An Era in Cardiovascular Medicine.* New York: Elsevier, 1991:45–70.

56. Sethi GK, Miller DC, Souchek J, et al. Clinical, hemodynamic and angiographic predictors of operative mortality in patients undergoing single valve replacement. *J Thorac Cardiovasc Surg* 1987;93:884–7.

57. Mullany CJ, Elveback ER, Frye RL, et al. Coronary artery disease and its management: influence on survival in patients undergoing aortic valve replacement. *J Am Coll Cardiol* 1987;10:66–72.

58. Rahimtoola SH. Catheter balloon valvuloplasty for severe calcific aortic stenosis: a limited role. *J Am Coll Cardiol* 1994;23:1076–8.

59. Otto CM, Mickel MC, Kennedy JW, et al. Three-year outcome after balloon aortic valvuloplasty: insights into prognosis of valvular aortic stenosis. *Circulation* 1994;89:642–50.

60. Safian RD, Berma AD, Diver DJ, et al. Balloon aortic valvuloplasty in 170 consecutive patients. *N Engl J Med* 1988;319:125–30.

61. Letac B, Cribier A, Koning R, et al. Results of percutaneous transluminal valvuloplasty in 218 adults with valvular aortic stenosis. *Am J Cardiol* 1988;62:598–605.

62. Moreno PR, Jang I, Newell JB, Block PC, Palacios IF. The role of percutaneous aortic valvuloplasty in patients with cardiogenic shock and critical aortic stenosis. *J Am Coll Cardiol* 1994;23:1071–5.

63. Isner JM, and the Mansfield Scientific Aortic Valvuloplasty Registry Investigators. Acute catastrophic complications of balloon aortic valvuloplasty. *J Am Coll Cardiol* 1991;17:1436–44.

64. Cribier A, Eltchaninoff H, Bash A, et al. Percutaneous transcatheter implantation of an aortic valve prosthesis for calcific aortic stenosis: first human case description. *Circulation* 2002;106:3006–8.

65. Cribier A, Eltchaninoff H, Tron C, et al. Early experience with percutaneous transcatheter implantation of heart valve prosthesis for the treatment of end-stage inoperable patients with calcific aortic stenosis. *J Am Coll Cardiol* 2004;43:698–703.

66. Webb JG, Pasupati S, Humphries K, et al. Percutaneous transarterial aortic valve replacement in selected high-risk patients with aortic stenosis. *Circulation* 2007;116: 755–63.

67. Khot UN, Novaro GM, Popovic ZB, et al. Nitroprusside in critically ill patients with left ventricular dysfunction and aortic stenosis. *N Engl J Med* 2003;348:1756–63.

68. Gu YL, Lessurun GAJ, van den Merkhof LFM, Zijlstra F. Intra-aortic balloon counterpulsation for complex aortic stenosis in hybrid strategy. *Int J Cardiol* 2007;117:e46–8.

69. Thorburn CW, Morgan JJ, Shanahan MX, Chang VP. Long-term results of tricuspid valve replacement and the problem of the prosthetic valve thrombosis. *Am J Cardiol* 1983;51:1128–32.

70. Roudaut R, Labbe T, Lorient Roudaut MF, et al. Mechanical cardiac valve thrombosis: is fibrinolysis justified? *Circulation* 1992;86(Suppl II):II-8–15.

71. Horstkotte D, Burckhardt D. Prosthetic valve thrombosis. *J Heart Valve Dis* 1995;4: 141–53.

72. Cannegieter SC, Rosendaal FR, Briet E. Thromboembolic and bleeding complications in patients with mechanical heart valve prostheses. *Circulation* 1994;89:635–41.

73. Buttard P, Bonnefoy E, Chevalier P, et al. Mechanical cardiac valve thrombosis in patients in critical hemodynamic compromise. *Eur J Cardiothorac Surg* 1997;11:710–3.

74. Kontos GH, Schaf HV, Orzulak TA, Puga FJ, Pluth JR, Danielson GK. Thrombotic obstruction of disc valves: clinical recognition and surgical management. *Ann Thorac Surg* 1989;48:60–5.

75. Miller FA, Khandheria BK, Tajik AJ. Echocardiographic assessment of prosthetic heart valves. In: Freeman WK, Seward JB, Khandheria BK, Tajik AJ, eds. *Transesophageal Echocardiography*. Boston: Little Brown, 1994;243–306.

76. Azevedo JE, Garcia-Fernandez MA, San Roman D, et al. Transesophageal echocardiography study of mitral valve prosthesis. *Rev Port Cardiol* 1992;11:759–67.

77. Sato N, Miura M, Itoh T, et al. Sound spectral analysis of prosthetic valvular clicks for diagnosis of thrombosed Bjork-Shiley tilting standard disc valve prostheses. *J Thorac Cardiovasc Surg* 1993;105:313–20.

78. Peterfly A, Henze A, Savidge GF, Landon C, Bjork VO. Late thrombotic malfunction of the Bjork-Shiley tilting disc valve in the tricuspid position. *Scan J Thorac Cardiovasc Surg* 1980:14:33–8.

79. Villanyi J, Wladika ZS, Bartek I, Lengyel M. Diagnosis and treatment of tricuspid mechanical valve dysfunction [abstract]. *Eur Heart J* 1992;13(Suppl):374.

80. Lengyel M, Fuster V, Keltai M, et al. Guidelines for management of left-sided prosthetic valve thrombosis: a role for thrombolytic therapy. *J Am Coll Cardiol* 1997;30: 1521–6.

81. Tong AT, Roudaut R, Ozkan M, et al. Transesophageal echocardiography improves risk assessment of thrombolysis of prosthetic valve thrombosis: results of the international PRO-TEE registry. *J Am Coll Cardiol* 2004;43:77–84.

82. Caceras-Loriga FM, Perez-Lopez H, Morlans-Hernandez K, et al. Thrombolysis as first choice therapy in prosthetic heart valve thrombosis. A study of 68 patients. *J Thromb Thrombolysis* 2006;21:185–90.

83. Roudaut R, Lafitte S, Roudaut MF, et al. Fibrinolysis of mechanical prosthetic valve thrombosis: a single-center study of 127 cases. *J Am Coll Cardiol* 2003;41:653–8.

84. Das M, Twomey D, Al Khaddour AA, Dunning J. Is thrombolysis or surgery the best option for acute prosthetic valve thrombosis? *Interact CardioVasc Thorac Surg* 2007;6:806–11.

85. Vasan RS, Kaul U, Sangvis XX, et al. Thrombolytic therapy for prosthetic valve thrombosis: a study based on serial Doppler echocardiographic evaluation. *Am Heart J* 1992;123:1575–80.

86. Graver LM, Gelber PM, Tyras DH. The risk and benefits of thrombolytic therapy in acute aortic and mitral prosthetic valve dysfunction: report of a case and review of the literature. *Ann Thorac Surg* 1988;46:85–8.

# Chapter 8

# Cardiogenic shock in other heart diseases: Acute decompensation of chronic heart failure, myocarditis, transient apical ballooning syndrome, peripartum cardiomyopathy, hypertrophic cardiomyopathy, restrictive cardiomyopathies, and thyrotoxicosis

Fredric Ginsberg and Joseph E. Parrillo

## Introduction

Cardiogenic shock is defined as persistent hypotension and tissue hypoperfusion due to cardiac dysfunction in the presence of adequate left ventricular filling pressure and intravascular volume. The most common cause of cardiogenic shock is acute myocardial infarction (AMI), with extensive myocardial injury and necrosis leading to left ventricular failure. Other complications of AMI that lead to cardiogenic shock include papillary muscle rupture with acute, severe mitral regurgitation, ventricular septal rupture, left ventricular free wall rupture with cardiac tamponade, and right ventricular infarction [1].

Cardiogenic shock is less often caused by conditions leading to acute, severe left ventricular or right ventricular failure not related to unstable coronary artery disease. These conditions include decompensation of chronic left ventricular systolic dysfunction, acute myocarditis, transient apical ballooning syndrome, left ventricular outflow tract obstruction as in hypertrophic cardiomyopathy (HCM), acute valvular regurgitation, severe mitral or aortic stenosis, or acute right ventricular failure syndromes such as acute, massive pulmonary embolism or cardiac tamponade [2]. It is of utmost importance to be able to quickly diagnose these conditions because most of them are reversible, and urgent and

*Cardiogenic Shock.* Edited by Judith S. Hochman and E. Magnus Ohman.
© 2009 American Heart Association, ISBN: 978-1-4051-7926-3

appropriate management differs from the management of cardiogenic shock due to AMI and can be life-saving.

## Acute decompensation of chronic heart failure

Acute worsening of chronic heart failure is among the most common causes of hospitalization in the U.S., accounting for over one million cases annually [3]. Up to 70% of all acute heart failure hospitalizations occur in patients with known chronic heart failure [4]. The majority of these patients will demonstrate congestion, manifested as dyspnea, edema, pulmonary rales, and elevated jugular venous pressure on physical examination, with adequate blood pressure and tissue perfusion. A significant minority, however, will show signs of decreased tissue perfusion, including confusion, cool extremities, narrow pulse pressure, hypotension with systolic blood pressure <90 mm Hg, and oliguria. A small percentage of patients will manifest overt signs of cardiogenic shock. In one study, among 486 patients admitted with decompensated heart failure, 28% showed signs of decreased tissue perfusion and congestion, and 5% had reduced perfusion without overt congestion [5]. In the EuroHeart Failure Survey II, 10.4% of acute decompensated heart failure patients presented in pulmonary edema and 2.2% had cardiogenic shock [6]. Other authors estimate that cardiogenic shock is present in 2–8% of patients hospitalized with acute decompensated heart failure [4]. In the ADHERE database of over 150,000 heart failure hospitalizations in the U.S., <3% of patients presented with systolic blood pressure <90 mm Hg [7]. In another study, almost 30% of patients with acute decompensated heart failure with cardiogenic shock had been hospitalized for heart failure during the previous 12 months [6].

Cardiogenic shock is the clinical factor that most directly impacts short-term prognosis in acute heart failure. In all patients admitted with acute heart failure and cardiogenic shock, 1-year mortality was 68.2%, compared with 37.9% in patients with acute heart failure without shock [8]. A multivariate analysis of the ADHERE data demonstrated that admission systolic blood pressure under 115 mm Hg and diastolic blood pressure under 55 mm Hg were both independent risk factors for in-hospital mortality, increasing the risk of mortality threefold [9], as well as increasing 1-year mortality [8]. In-hospital mortality in the EuroHeart Failure Survey II was 39.6% in patients with acute heart failure and cardiogenic shock (Fig. 8.1) [6].

In patients with acute decompensated heart failure and decreased perfusion or shock, potentially reversible causes of deterioration should be investigated. Acute myocardial ischemia and infarction should be evaluated using the ECG and cardiac biomarkers. In patients with acute ischemia, revascularization therapies such as percutaneous coronary intervention or coronary artery bypass surgery should be considered. Other reversible conditions include cardiac arrhythmia. Rapid atrial fibrillation is very common in patients with acute

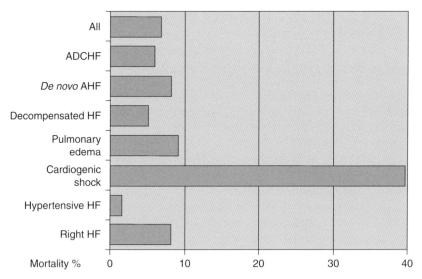

**Fig. 8.1** In-hospital mortality in EuroHeart Failure Survey II by history of HF and clinical class. ADCHF, acute decompensated heart failure; HF, heart failure; AHF, acute heart failure. (Reprinted with permission from Nieminen MS, Brutsaert D, Dickstein K, et al. *Eur Heart J* 2006;27:2725–36.)

decompensated heart failure, and it can lead to hypotension and low cardiac output due to the loss of the atrial contribution to left ventricular filling and cardiac output. Sustained tachycardia can directly impair myocardial function (tachycardia-induced cardiomyopathy) and can aggravate ischemia. Paroxysmal ventricular tachycardia is less common but can also seriously aggravate the heart failure syndrome. Worsening valve lesions, most commonly mitral regurgitation, need to be assessed and treated appropriately.

Other treatable factors that may seriously aggravate heart failure and lead to hypotension include adverse effects of medications, such as class I antiarrhythmic medications and calcium channel blockers such as diltiazem or verapamil. Serious acute comorbid conditions, such as sepsis, pneumonia, chronic obstructive pulmonary disease, pulmonary embolism, respiratory failure, anemia, renal failure, and thyroid disease, need to be identified and treated aggressively.

Patients with acute heart failure and signs of decreased perfusion, hypotension or shock, need rapid diagnostic assessments and institution of therapy simultaneously. Echocardiography needs to be performed urgently to assess left ventricular systolic and diastolic function, right ventricular function and pericardial and valvular abnormalities. Echo-Doppler can also assist with hemodynamic assessments. The use of a pulmonary artery catheter, although not always necessary, is often very useful for defining hemodynamic parameters more precisely, as well as assessing response to therapy. Specific indications for the use of a pulmonary artery catheter in acute heart failure include: (1) when clinical assessment of hemodynamic status is uncertain; (2) when coexistent serious pulmonary or renal disease makes clinical assessment of hemodynamics less reliable; (3) when patients are not improving with initial management; (4) to guide use of potent vasodilator therapy; (5) when persistent hypotension occurs as inotropes are being weaned; (6) during assessment for definitive therapies such as cardiac transplantation or ventricular assist devices (VADs) [5,10].

The medical management of cardiogenic shock is discussed in Chapter 3. A brief discussion follows here. Intravenous diuretics are used to relieve symptoms of congestion. However, diuretics may aggravate hypotension and hypoperfusion or shock. The choice of medical management in these patients is between parenteral vasodilator therapy, using nitroprusside or nitroglycerin, and sympathomimetic amines, which have both inotropic and vasopressor properties such as dopamine or norepinephrine, or using inotropes which also have vasodilating properties such as dobutamine or milrinone. Goals of therapy in patients with acute heart failure and hypotension or shock are to restore adequate cardiac output, to perfuse vital organs, improve peripheral tissue oxygenation, maintain adequate renal function and alleviate symptoms, without worsening myocardial function by causing arrhythmias, myocardial ischemia, or necrosis [4].

Vasodilator therapy can improve cardiac output and filling pressures with resultant reduction in subendocardial ischemia. Vasodilators can be used judiciously in patients with acute heart failure and hypoperfusion as long as there is not frank hypotension. Their use has not been associated with aggravation of arrhythmia or worsening of prognosis. However, nitroprusside and nitroglycerin often worsen hypotension, and this limits their usefulness in patients with hypoperfusion and precludes their use in patients with cardiogenic shock. The inotropic agents dobutamine and milrinone work by increasing intracellular myocyte cyclic AMP, which increases intracellular calcium release leading to increased contractile force. Dobutamine accomplishes this by stimulating the myocyte beta-receptor. Milrinone works by inhibiting the enzyme phosphodiesterase III, which breaks down cyclic AMP. This action in vascular smooth muscle is responsible for vasodilation with milrinone, which can aggravate hypotension.

The use of inotropic therapy for acute decompensated heart failure with hypoperfusion is controversial. Although these agents provide short-term benefit with improved blood pressure and improved end-organ perfusion, dobutamine and milrinone are associated with adverse effects, such as increasing heart rate, more frequent tachyarrhythmias, increased myocardial oxygen consumption, and worsening myocardial ischemia (Table 8.1) [4]. Even short-term use of inotropic drugs has been associated with increased mortality. In the ADHERE observational database, use of inotropes was associated with a 12.3–13.9% in-hospital mortality; mortality in patients who received nitroprusside or nitroglycerin was 4.7–7.1% [9]. These differences were felt to be significant even

**Table 8.1** Drawbacks of dobutamine and milrinone.

A. Dobutamine
(i)   Increased myocardial oxygen consumption
(ii)  Myocardial injury
(iii) Tolerance/tachyphylaxis
(iv)  Interaction with beta-blockers
(v)   Arrhythmogenesis
(vi)  Increased mortality

B. Milrinone
(i)   Hypotension
(ii)  Arrhythmogenesis
(iii) Worsening prognosis in ischemic disease

after adjusting for important concomitant variables. Short-term use of inotropic drugs for acute decompensated heart failure is also associated with worse survival after hospital discharge (Fig. 8.2) [3] and there are no convincing data that they improve quality of life in heart failure patients.

Because inotropic drugs are associated with worse survival, their use is reserved for patients with severe hemodynamic compromise, who demonstrate obtundation, oliguria, lactic acidosis, and impending hemodynamic collapse. In this situation, patients must receive short-term, life-saving hemodynamic

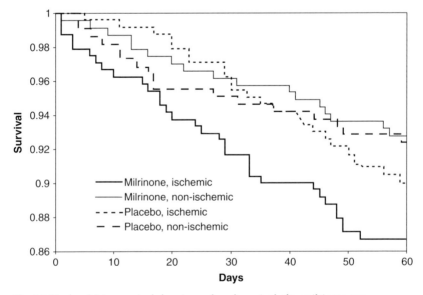

**Fig. 8.2** Kaplan–Meier survival showing reduced survival after milrinone use, especially in patients with ischemic cardiomyopathy. (Reprinted with permission from Felker GM, Benza RL, Chandler AB, et al. *J Am Coll Cardiol* 2003;41:997–1003.)

benefit, despite potential worsening of the longer term heart failure [11]. Dobutamine is preferred over milrinone because of the latter agent's potent vasodilator effects and resultant hypotension, although high doses of dobutamine can also lead to vasodilation and worsening hypotension. Dopamine can be used, as it has dose-related vasoconstrictor as well as inotropic properties and can improve end-organ perfusion acutely. Norepinephrine is reserved for the most severe cases of hypotension and shock.

Inotropic vasopressor drugs can be used as a "bridge" to stabilize patients prior to initiating mechanical support with intra-aortic balloon counterpulsation (IABP) or a VAD. They can also be used short-term prior to revascularization for ischemic heart failure or while patients are awaiting cardiac transplantation [11,12]. Once patients have been stabilized, the dose of inotropic therapy should be rapidly reduced as tolerated, with transition to long-term oral therapy with agents that improve the long-term prognosis of heart failure, such as angiotensin-converting enzyme inhibitors and beta-blockers [11].

Levosimendan is a newer inotropic agent that acts not by increasing intracellular calcium, but by binding to troponin C, sensitizing the cardiac myofilaments to calcium. It is available for use in Europe, but in the U.S. it is an investigational agent. It was hoped that this agent could provide effective inotropic therapy in acute decompensated heart failure without worsening mortality, as has been consistently demonstrated with dobutamine and milrinone. However, a randomized, prospective, double-blind, multicenter study was performed comparing levosimendan with dobutamine in 1,327 patients with acute decompensated heart failure, oliguria, and low cardiac index, but without overt shock. It showed no survival difference between the two agents, with 31-day and 180-day all cause mortality rates of 12–14% and 26–28% with each drug. Levosimendan was associated with lower blood pressure, a slight rise in heart rate, more atrial arrhythmias, and hypokalemia [13].

Stage D heart failure, that is, symptomatic heart failure at rest despite appropriate medical therapy, is associated with a >50% 1-year mortality [14]. Patients with severe heart failure who are dependent on intravenous inotropic therapy have an extremely poor prognosis, with only 24% survival at 1 year [15]. Cardiac transplantation is an option for patients with end-stage heart failure who are inotrope-dependent. Cardiac transplantation offers the best survival benefit for these patients, but is available for only a very few. It is estimated that 80,000–150,000 patients in the U.S. could benefit from cardiac transplantation in terms of improved quality of life and longevity [16]. However, only 2,200 donor hearts per year are currently available.

VADs are mechanical pumps inserted most commonly via a thoracotomy and are used to support the function of the failing heart. These devices are discussed in Chapter 9 and have been most commonly used to "bridge" patients with functional class IV heart failure, who are inotrope-dependent, to help them survive to cardiac transplantation. They can also be used as permanent support in patients who have severe comorbidities or end-organ dysfunction that preclude transplantation ("destination therapy"). VADs can also be used to support patients while therapies are being administered to attempt to reverse the myocardial cellular processes associated with the progressive worsening of heart failure [17]. A minority of patients can experience improvement in myocardial function ("reverse remodeling") while supported with a VAD, so that the VAD can eventually be removed ("bridge to recovery"). Lastly, VAD therapy can be used in patients with end-stage heart failure, who initially are not candidates for transplantation due to conditions such as malnutrition or end-organ dysfunction. Improved hemodynamics with VAD therapy can result in improvements in end-organ function and in patients' overall status so that transplantation becomes feasible ("bridge to eligibility") [17]. (VAD therapy [18–21] is discussed further in Chapter 9.)

The operative risk of VAD implantation is determined not by the severity of heart failure, but by comorbidities such as clotting system derangements, renal failure, right ventricular dysfunction, and nutritional status (Fig. 8.3). Patient selection and timing of VAD implantation in the course of a patient's heart failure illness are the critical factors governing the success and utility of VAD therapy. Placing VADs too late in the course of severe irreversible heart failure

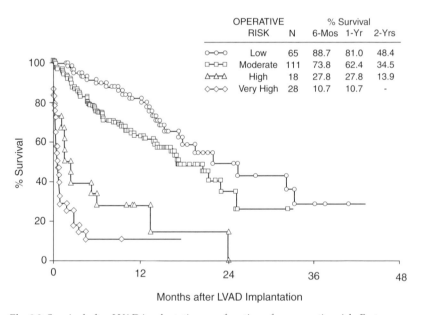

**Fig. 8.3** Survival after LVAD implantation as a function of preoperative risk. Factors which increase operative risk are renal and hepatic dysfunction, coagulation abnormalities, poor nutritional status, right ventricular dysfunction and lack of inotrope use preoperatively. (Reprinted with permission from Lietz K, Long JW, Kfoury AG, et al. *Circulation* 2007;116:497–505.)

is associated with high operative mortality and poor survival. When in the course of chronic severe heart failure VAD support provides survival benefit over medical therapy has yet to be defined [18].

## Myocarditis

Myocarditis is defined as inflammation of heart muscle [22]. Clinical illness caused by myocarditis varies widely. Patients may have very mild symptoms and recover quickly without specific therapy. Other patients may develop more severe illness, characterized by left ventricular dysfunction, heart failure, and chronic cardiomyopathy. A smaller number of patients with acute myocarditis can progress to critical illness, with cardiogenic shock.

The most common etiology of myocarditis is believed to be a viral infection [22]. Other infectious illnesses that can lead to myocarditis include Lyme disease, acute rheumatic fever, diphtheria, and Chagas' disease. Myocarditis has been reported in approximately 8% of patients with HIV, either due to opportunistic infection with Mycobacteria, fungi, or parasites, superimposed viral infections such as cytomegalovirus, or possibly due to HIV itself [23]. Autoimmune illnesses often associated with myocarditis include systemic lupus erythematosus, polymyositis, progressive systemic sclerosis, and mixed connective tissue disease [24]. Other specific forms of myocarditis include hypersensitivity or eosinophilic myocarditis [25] and giant cell myocarditis [26]. Pathogenesis of the most common form of myocarditis, lymphocytic myocarditis, involves myocyte damage caused by viral proteases and cytokine activation, as well as secondary human host immune activation with persistent overactivation of cellular immunity. Activated T lymphocytes target myocardial antigens with subsequent release of cytokines. Myocardial biopsy specimens will show infiltration with lymphocytes. These processes may lead to left ventricular dilatation and remodeling, with left ventricular systolic dysfunction and clinical heart failure [4,27], or they may abate, with subsequent improvement in left ventricular size and function.

Patients ill with acute myocarditis most often present with chest pain, fever, dyspnea, palpitations and syncope. The presentation may be that of acute heart failure or may mimic AMI [28]. The diagnosis of acute myocarditis is made on clinical grounds. Laboratory findings include leukocytosis, eosinophilia, elevation of C-reactive protein, and elevation of the cardiac biomarkers CK-MB and troponin. ECG abnormalities include ST-segment elevation or depression, T-wave inversion, and pathologic Q-waves. More severe cases may demonstrate ventricular arrhythmias and heart block [22,29].

Urgent echocardiography is essential to diagnose and quantitate left ventricular wall motion abnormalities, left and right ventricular function and left ventricular wall thickness. Contrast enhanced cardiac magnetic resonance imaging (CMR), looking for early and late enhancement with gadolinium, offers great promise to diagnose myocarditis and to improve the diagnostic yield of endomyocardial biopsy (EMB) [30–32]. Cardiac catheterization and coronary angiography are often necessary to exclude severe coronary artery disease as the cause of chest pain, acute heart failure, and ECG and echocardiographic abnormalities.

Patients with suspected acute myocarditis often undergo EMB to aid in the diagnosis. The Dallas Histopathologic Criteria defined myocarditis as the presence of an active inflammatory infiltrate accompanied by myocyte necrosis. The term "borderline myocarditis" is defined as active inflammation without necrosis. Unfortunately, there are limitations to using EMB in the diagnosis of myocarditis. The myocardial inflammation is often patchy, and involves left ventricle more extensively than right ventricle. Therefore, random nontargeted right ventricular biopsies can miss affected areas. Various series have reported positive biopsy results in only 10–67% of patients with myocarditis suspected on clinical grounds. In addition, a high frequency of intra-observer variation has been noted among pathologists in applying the Dallas Criteria [33]. Performing EMB earlier in a patient's course, taking multiple biopsy specimens, biopsy of left ventricle, and targeting biopsies using CMR have been suggested as ways of improving the diagnostic yield of EMB [32–34]. A positive biopsy has a high positive predictive value for the diagnosis of myocarditis, but it is important to emphasize that a negative biopsy does not preclude the diagnosis.

EMB is necessary to diagnose specific myocardial disorders that have unique pathogeneses, prognoses, and therapies, which cannot be diagnosed with non-invasive testing. A recent AHA/ACC/ESC scientific statement offered recommendations concerning the appropriate use of EMB based on patients' clinical presentations. EMB was deemed useful, beneficial, and effective (class I recommendation) in patients with acute heart failure and hemodynamic compromise, when causes such as coronary artery disease are excluded. EMB in this setting is necessary to differentiate giant cell myocarditis and necrotizing eosinophilic myocarditis from lymphocytic myocarditis, as immunosuppressive therapy is mandated in the first two diseases (see below). EMB was also deemed a class I recommendation in patients with new onset, subacute heart failure, with duration of illness 2 weeks to 3 months, who demonstrate severe ventricular arrhythmia or advanced heart block, or who fail to respond to conventional medical therapy in 1–2 weeks [35].

The majority of patients with clinical manifestations of lymphocytic myocarditis will improve. Patients with heart failure and left ventricular dysfunction will experience spontaneous resolution of their illness in 6–12 months in up to 50% of cases, without long-term sequelae [36]. Recovery is more likely to occur in patients with less severe reductions of left ventricular function. One series reported 4-year survival of 87% in patients with myocarditis without heart failure, but 54% survival in patients with myocarditis and heart failure [36]. Patients with heart failure and myocarditis can recover normal left ventricular function or can progress to chronic dilated cardiomyopathy.

Roughly one-quarter of patients with acute myocarditis, severe heart failure, and an ejection fraction of <35% will improve, one-half will develop chronic cardiomyopathy and heart failure, and one-quarter will deteriorate and may be candidates for cardiac transplantation [37].

A small percentage of patients with acute myocarditis present critically ill with acute cardiogenic shock [5,38]. This has been termed fulminant myocarditis. In distinction to acute severe myocarditis, patients with fulminant myocarditis have hemodynamic compromise and require support with inotropic and/or vasopressor medication, IABP, or other forms of mechanical cardiac support. Most often these patients have a recent and distinct onset of illness, and rapid deterioration of heart failure symptoms, unlike patients with acute severe myocarditis, who have a less distinct onset of symptoms, with gradual development of heart failure followed by acute decompensation [39]. When patients present with acute heart failure due to myocarditis, it is difficult to predict those who will progress to fulminant myocarditis and require hemodynamic support. There are no specific criteria to assist in this prediction, but patients who developed fulminant myocarditis tended to have higher C-reactive protein levels and more often had wide QRS complexes on ECG [40]. Ejection fraction was slightly lower in patients who developed fulminant myocarditis (40% versus 50%) but this did not distinguish these two groups in multiple logistic regression analysis.

In a study of 147 patients presenting with heart failure due to biopsy-positive active myocarditis, with ejection fraction <40%, 15 (10%) were diagnosed with fulminant myocarditis. Thirteen of these patients required hemodynamic support with high-dose vasopressor therapy, and 2 required support with a mechanical assist device. Patients with fulminant myocarditis tended to be younger, but there was no discrimination between fulminant myocarditis and acute severe myocarditis based on hemodynamic profiles. With aggressive therapy, patients with fulminant myocarditis had a better survival; 1-year survival was 93% and 11-year survival was 93% (no late deaths) compared with 85% at 1 year and 45% at 11 years in patients with acute severe myocarditis (Fig. 8.4) [41].

There is a growing experience using VADs for treatment of fulminant myocarditis and cardiogenic shock, in patients not responding to inotropic drugs and IABP. The patients generally demonstrated biventricular failure, severely reduced cardiac index, and other end-organ dysfunction. Biventricular assist devices, percutaneous left ventricular devices, and percutaneous cardiopulmonary bypass have been used for 7–43 days. Almost all patients survived and recovered left ventricular function in these reports [39,42–44].

During the acute phase of myocarditis characterized by left ventricular systolic dysfunction and pulmonary congestion without hemodynamic instability, patients require treatment with standard therapies for dilated cardiomyopathy and heart failure. The use of multidrug regimens is indicated. Diuretics help to lower left ventricular filling pressures and improve dyspnea. Angiotensin-converting enzyme inhibitors and aldosterone antagonists should be initiated, with careful monitoring of cardiac rhythm, electrolytes, and renal function.

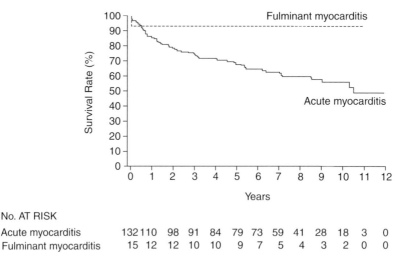

No. AT RISK

| | | | | | | | | | | | | |
|---|---|---|---|---|---|---|---|---|---|---|---|---|
| Acute myocarditis | 132 | 110 | 98 | 91 | 84 | 79 | 73 | 59 | 41 | 28 | 18 | 3 | 0 |
| Fulminant myocarditis | 15 | 12 | 12 | 10 | 10 | 9 | 7 | 5 | 4 | 3 | 2 | 0 | 0 |

**Fig. 8.4** Unadjusted transplantation-free survival according to clinicopathological classification. Patients with fulminant myocarditis were significantly less likely to die or require heart transplantation during follow-up than were patients with acute myocarditis ($P = 0.05$ by the log-rank test). (Reprinted with permission from McCarthy III RE, Boehmer JP, Hruban RH, et al. *N Engl J Med* 2000;342:690–5.)

Beta-blockers can be initiated at a low dose and gradually increased after the patient is stable. It is felt that these measures will promote reverse remodeling and improvement of left ventricular function, often to normal.

The use of immunosuppressive therapy in patients with fulminant myocarditis is controversial, and there have been no clinical trials to assess this therapy in these patients. Randomized trials of immunosuppressive therapy in myocarditis have been limited by small numbers of patients, varied immunosuppressive regimens, and a high incidence of spontaneous recovery of normal left ventricular function [45–48]. There is no evidence that patients with lymphocytic myocarditis benefit from the routine use of immunosuppressive therapy. However, therapy with corticosteroids and other immune-modulating agents should be considered in patients with deteriorating clinical status, or in patients with myocarditis associated with connective tissue disease, eosinophilic or granulomatous forms of the disease, or in patients with giant cell myocarditis. We favor the use of prednisone and azathioprine for patients with biopsy-proven lymphocytic myocarditis who are not improving on conventional heart failure medications [33].

In summary, patients with fulminant myocarditis have an acute, severe illness, characterized by cardiogenic shock and severe heart failure. Short-term prognosis is poor without aggressive treatment of abnormal hemodynamics with pharmacologic therapy and mechanical support. With aggressive therapies, often involving VADs, healing of myocarditis injury and improvement of left ventricular function can be expected, and long-term survival is excellent after recovery from the acute illness.

## Transient apical ballooning syndrome

A distinctive acute cardiomyopathy was first described in patients in Japan in 1991 [49]. This syndrome has subsequently been described in the U.S. and Europe [50,51]. It is characterized by the acute onset of chest symptoms, ECG changes mimicking AMI, and mild elevation of cardiac markers. Symptoms are precipitated by extreme emotional or physical stress in >70% of cases [52]. The characteristic finding is a distinctive wall motion abnormality involving the left ventricular apex, in the absence of significant coronary artery stenosis (Fig. 8.5). This syndrome has been termed transient apical ballooning syndrome (TABS), stress cardiomyopathy, or Tako-tsubo cardiomyopathy, so named because the Tako-tsubo pot used by Japanese fishermen to trap octopus has a shape similar to the left ventricle in this condition ("short neck-round flask") [51–54]. There is a marked preponderance for older females to be affected by this condition, 86–100% in reported series, with a mean age of 63–67 years. A total of 66–90% of patients will present with chest pain, and 15–20% will present with dyspnea,

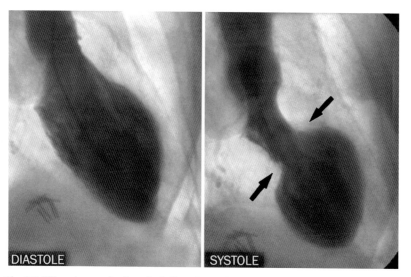

**Fig. 8.5** LV angiogram in diastole (left) and systole (right) in right anterior oblique projection demonstrating wall-motion abnormality characteristic of stress cardiomyopathy. At end systole, LV chamber adopts distinctive "short neck with round flask" configuration in which distal (apical) portion is dyskinetic/akinetic/hypokinetic, whereas in contrast, the remaining proximal (basal) segment is hypercontractile (sharp area of transition is shown by arrows). (Reprinted with permission from Sharkey SW, Lesser JR, Zenovich AG, et al. *Circulation* 2005;111:472–9.)

pulmonary edema, or shock. Most common ECG changes seen are ST-segment elevation or marked T-wave inversions in the precordial leads. These findings are indistinguishable from AMI. Elevation of CK-MB and troponin is seen in the majority of patients, but the enzyme rises are usually milder than would be expected given the marked ECG and left ventricular wall motion abnormalities.

Precipitators of TABS have included arguments with family members, the death of a loved one, or sudden financial setbacks. Physical stresses have included medical procedures such as thoracentesis or biopsy, institution of cancer chemotherapy or hemodialysis, and hip fracture and noncardiac surgeries and respiratory distress.

Echocardiography or left ventriculography shows moderate-to-severe left ventricular dysfunction in these patients, with characteristic hyperkinesis of inferior–basal and basal–septal segments, with severe hypokinesis, akinesis, or dyskinesis involving mid-anteroseptal, apical, and inferior–apical wall segments. Acutely, left ventricular ejection fraction is reduced to 20–40% [52,53]. Fewer than 20% of patients also demonstrate a left ventricular outflow tract gradient, due to basal septal hyperkinesis and transient systolic anterior motion of the anterior leaflet of the mitral valve [50,52,55].

Patients with TABS often present critically ill, with pulmonary edema, hypotension, and shock. Cardiogenic shock develops due to marked left ventricular systolic dysfunction and decreased stroke volume. Shock can also be exacerbated by the development of a left ventricular outflow tract gradient [56]. Cardiogenic shock has been reported in 5% of patients at presentation and has occurred during the course of the illness in 6–46% of patients in different series [50,52–54,57].

Suspicion of TABS and urgent diagnosis are important, as therapy and prognosis differ substantially from AMI. TABS should not be treated with thrombolytic therapy, as coronary occlusion is not involved in the pathogenesis. If cardiogenic shock develops, treatment with IABP is indicated. Inotropic therapy should be used judiciously. Dobutamine and other beta agonists may worsen cardiogenic shock by increasing hyperkinesis of the basal portion of the heart and causing or aggravating a left ventricular outflow tract gradient. There have been several case reports of patients with TABS with hypotension who develop frank cardiogenic shock after initiation of inotropic therapy. Because a hyperadrenergic state has been proposed to be a major pathogenic mechanism, empiric use of beta-blockers while patients are being supported with IABP has been recommended and has been used successfully. Echocardiography can be useful to guide therapy. For those with extensive wall motion abnormalities but no outflow obstruction, IABP support without beta-blockers is recommended. In the absence of an outflow tract gradient, inotropic therapy can be utilized, starting at low doses with careful monitoring of the response. Administration of the alpha agonist phenylephrine can also be considered in cases with a high left ventricular outflow tract gradient, as this drug increases afterload, causing left ventricular dilatation and a decrease in mitral valve systolic anterior motion and lowering of intraventricular gradients [55].

Although many patients with TABS are elderly with significant concomitant disease, aggressive therapy of hemodynamic compromise and cardiogenic shock is indicated because TABS is associated with a good prognosis. In almost all patients, the marked apical wall motion abnormalities begin to improve within days, and left ventricular function can be expected to recover to normal over several weeks. Follow-up of patients in various series has shown improvement of left ventricular ejection fraction to normal in the subacute phase. In-hospital mortality in larger series has been reported at 0–4% [50,52–54,57,58]. The large majority of survivors will recover completely with normal functional status.

The pathogenesis of TABS is unknown. Transient multivessel coronary spasm has been proposed, but this has not been demonstrated at the time of acute coronary angiography in the vast majority of patients. In most patients, the extent of left ventricular wall motion abnormality is larger than the distribution of a single coronary artery [50,51]. In our judgment, a hyperadrenergic state, precipitated by acute stress and causing myocardial stunning, is the most attractive hypothesis. Cardiac MRI has not shown evidence of infarction or myocarditis [59]. One study documented supraphysiologic levels of catecholamines and stress neuropeptides in patients during the acute phase of TABS, with levels higher than in patients with AMI. These levels remained markedly elevated 1 week later. Adrenal and sympathoneuronal hyperactivity has been proposed, and the apex of the left ventricle may be more sensitive than other left ventricular wall segments to the deleterious effects of adrenergic hyperstimulation [53].

TABS has been reported to occur in approximately 1.7–2.2% of admissions for acute coronary syndrome in Japan [57,59] and 2% of cases of acute heart failure due to acute coronary syndrome. TABS may be more common than currently recognized. Correct diagnosis is more likely to be made in centers where emergency coronary angiography is used in the treatment of acute coronary syndrome, and where primary percutaneous coronary intervention is the preferred treatment strategy for ST-segment elevation myocardial infarction.

In summary, TABS should be suspected in patients who present with symptoms and ECG findings consistent with AMI, who have a large apical wall motion abnormality seen on echocardiography or left ventriculography, and whose symptoms were precipitated by severe emotional or physical stress. Diagnosis is confirmed when urgent cardiac catheterization and coronary angiography demonstrate no significant coronary artery occlusion or stenosis.

The long-term prognosis is good. In one series, only 2 out of 72 patients had recurrence of TABS within 13 months [52]. In another series, the recurrence of TABS was calculated at 2.9% per year. Over a 4-year follow-up, long-term survival of patients who recovered from TABS was equivalent to sex-and age-matched control groups without a history of TABS [58].

# Peripartum cardiomyopathy

Peripartum cardiomyopathy is defined as left ventricular systolic dysfunction that occurs during the last month of pregnancy or within the first 5 months postpartum. No preexisting cause of heart failure is present and no other etiology of cardiomyopathy is evident [60]. Cardiomyopathy can occur earlier in the course of pregnancy, which does not meet the standard definition of this illness. However, the presentation and outcomes of patients with cardiomyopathy of earlier onset in pregnancy are similar to those who present later, and may actually be a continuum of pregnancy-associated cardiomyopathy [61]. The cause of peripartum cardiomyopathy is unknown. Myocarditis is evident on EMB in a minority of patients, and patients manifesting myocardial inflammatory cells should be treated for myocarditis as described earlier. Immune-mediated injury initiated by maternal reaction to fetal cells has been postulated [62].

The differential diagnosis of severe heart failure secondary to peripartum cardiomyopathy includes severe hypertension, sepsis, fluid overload, thromboembolic disease, acute spontaneous coronary artery dissection, amniotic fluid embolus, and heart failure secondary to preexisting rheumatic heart disease [62]. The incidence is estimated at approximately 1 in 5,000 deliveries in the U.S., but may be higher in Africa and Haiti [62,63]. Risks for developing peripartum cardiomyopathy include older age of the mother, multifetal pregnancy, and the presence of hypertension or pre-eclampsia [64].

Women with peripartum cardiomyopathy usually present with signs and symptoms of severe heart failure. Other presentations include cardiogenic shock, supraventricular and ventricular arrhythmia, and cardiac arrest [65]. With medical management, approximately 54% of patients will have resolution of cardiomyopathy, a rate of improvement better than that of other causes of dilated cardiomyopathy. In older literature, a 20–50% mortality rate was described. However, more recent studies report mortality in the range of 8–27% [61,62]. In a series of 55 patients with peripartum cardiomyopathy, 62% experienced improvement in left ventricular function and 45% had recovery to normal. Recovery was usually seen within 2 months of diagnosis and institution of therapy. However, 25% of patients had no improvement in left ventricular function, and 13% experienced deterioration. There were no deaths in this series [64]. Recovery of left ventricular function was more likely if left ventricular ejection fraction was >30% at diagnosis, or if left ventricular diameter was <5.6 cm [61,64]. The prognosis is not good for patients in whom left ventricular function does not improve.

The treatment of peripartum cardiomyopathy includes treatments shown to be effective in other forms of heart failure due to dilated cardiomyopathy. Sodium restriction, beta-blockers, diuretic therapy, and digoxin are used. The use of angiotensin-converting enzyme inhibitors and angiotensin-receptor blockers is contraindicated during pregnancy because of the risk of teratogenic effects, but they can be instituted in the postpartum period. The combination of hydralazine and nitrates can be used during and after pregnancy. The incidence of thromboembolic complications is high, and anticoagulation therapy should be prescribed in women with significant reduction in left ventricular ejection fraction. Heparin should be used during pregnancy, and warfarin can be instituted postpartum [60,66].

Although patients with peripartum cardiomyopathy often have severe heart failure, cardiogenic shock is rare. The use of aggressive vasodilator and inotropic therapy for heart failure is indicated. For patients who do not improve with aggressive pharmacologic therapy, IABP or VADs can be used [67,68]. In one series, VAD therapy was used in 4% of patients as a bridge to transplantation, and 10% of patients underwent cardiac transplantation [64]. Favorable outcomes after cardiac transplantation for patients with peripartum cardiomyopathy have been reported [69,70].

# Hypertrophic cardiomyopathy

HCM is a genetic cardiac disease, present in approximately 0.2% of the general U.S. population. It is the most common genetic cardiac disease. HCM is defined as left ventricular hypertrophy, with wall thickness >15 mm, with a nondilated left ventricle, in the absence of other disorders capable of producing similar degrees of left ventricular wall thickening [71]. It is caused by a genetic mutation that affects sarcomeric proteins. It is often inherited in an autosomal dominant pattern, with incomplete penetrance. Sporadic cases also occur. Many different genetic mutations have been identified. The phenotypic expression of the disease varies widely [72].

HCM is diagnosed by echocardiography. Typical features include left ventricular hypertrophy, which may be either concentric or asymmetric. Left ventricular chamber size is normal, and systolic function is normal or hyperdynamic. There often is obstruction to flow at the level of the left ventricular outflow tract, resulting in left ventricular outflow gradients. This is caused by abnormal anterior motion of the anterior mitral valve leaflet in systole, with abnormal coaptation of the leaflet with the basal portion of intraventricular septum. A left ventricular outflow tract gradient is present at rest in approximately 25–40% of patients and can be provoked by exercise in another 33% [71,73].

MRI can be used to assess the location and extent of left ventricular hypertrophy in HCM. Patchy gadolinium hyperenhancement correlates with areas of increased wall thickness and decreased contraction. A greater extent of hyperenhancement is seen in patients with left ventricular dilatation and lower ejection fraction, and increased collagen is seen in these areas histologically [74].

HCM usually becomes clinically apparent after childhood, sometimes not until middle or older age. HCM can manifest itself at any age and may worsen or improve with time. Many patients have no clinical manifestations and their cardiomyopathy may go undetected [72]. Patients with HCM can present with symptoms of chest pain, dyspnea, or syncope. The overall annual mortality is 1%. Up to 20–25% of patients with HCM may develop NYHA class III–IV heart failure, and heart failure is more common in elderly patients with HCM. Sudden cardiac death can occur [71,72].

Different mechanisms can be responsible for the development of heart failure in patients with HCM. Ischemia can occur without atherosclerotic coronary obstruction, due to marked left ventricular wall thickening and abnormal thickening and narrowing of intramural coronary arteries. Marked left ventricular outflow tract obstruction and high outflow tract gradients increase left ventricular wall tension and afterload. The presence of a left ventricular outflow tract gradient at rest is associated with a four-fold increased risk of developing heart failure [71]. Diastolic dysfunction is also common. Atrial fibrillation can precipitate heart failure, due to the loss of the contribution of atrial systole to cardiac output, especially in hypertrophied ventricles with abnormal filling patterns. Over time, a minority of patients experience ventricular remodeling and develop findings typical of a dilated cardiomyopathy with diffuse hypokinesis, left ventricular chamber dilatation, and reduced systolic function [72].

Cardiogenic shock can occur in patients with HCM due to acute worsening of left ventricular outflow tract obstruction. Five patients were reported who developed cardiogenic shock, either after physical stresses (hip surgery, barium enema) or administration of nitrate medication. All five patients had left ventricular hypertrophy and high outflow tract gradients (60–144 mm Hg) and hyperdynamic wall motion, although two patients also had apical wall motion abnormalities [75]. Another report described an elderly woman with echocardiographic features of HCM with left ventricular outflow tract obstruction and severe mitral regurgitation, who presented with shortness of breath and cardiogenic shock, also worsened by nitrate administration [76]. These patients did not improve or even worsened with standard inotropic therapy of cardiogenic shock. Shock resolved in all patients after cessation of inotropic agents and institution of intravenous fluids and beta-blockers. Another case report described cardiogenic shock in an elderly man after major surgery, in the presence of hyperdynamic left ventricular motion and a left ventricular outflow tract gradient, who recovered with intravenous administration of verapamil [77]. Administration of the alpha-agonist phenylephrine may be useful in cases of profound hypotension to relieve left ventricular outflow tract obstruction. Thus, complications of HCM in elderly patients, who were previously asymptomatic, can be precipitated by acute changes in left ventricular loading conditions. The occurrence and severity of left ventricular outflow tract obstruction is a dynamic process in HCM and can be aggravated by inotropic drugs, which increase contractility and worsen outflow tract gradients. Nitrates can also worsen the gradient by reducing preload and afterload and reducing left ventricular chamber size. Beta-blockers decrease contractility and heart rate,

increase stroke volume and left ventricular filling, and effectively treat this etiology of cardiogenic shock. Verapamil also decreases contractility and heart
rate, but there is a risk of excessive systemic vasodilation and hypotension.

Severe heart failure can also occur in HCM due to extensive left ventricular
remodeling, termed the "end-stage" or "dilated-hypokinetic" phase of HCM
[78]. Rather than hyperdynamic left ventricular systolic function, these patients
develop global systolic dysfunction with ejection fraction <50%. Half of these
patients show decreasing left ventricular wall thickness and increased left ventricular chamber size. Other morphologic patterns include a dilated, hypoki-
netic left ventricle with persistent hypertrophy, and left ventricular hypokinesis
with normal chamber size with varying degrees of wall thickness [78]. Left
ventricular outflow tract gradients are not present in this stage of the condition. Pathology shows evidence for septal and left ventricular free wall fibrosis
[79,80].

This end-stage phase of HCM develops gradually. A more prolonged time
from initial diagnosis of HCM to the development of the dilated phase was
noted (average time 14 years), in comparison to HCM patients without left ventricular dilatation. Only a minority of patients with HCM, reported at 3.5–5%,
will develop this phase. It is estimated to occur at a rate of 0.5–0.9% per year
[73,78,79].

As left ventricular ejection fraction falls, patients are at high risk for developing atrial fibrillation, class III–IV heart failure, and sudden cardiac death. The
prognosis of patients with end-stage phase of HCM is poor, with average time
to death or cardiac transplantation of 2.7–5 years. Annual mortality is reported
at 11%, and 5-year survival without transplantation is 75% after diagnosis of the
dilated phase of HCM [78–81]. These patients have severe heart failure, often at
higher left ventricular ejection fractions compared with patients with primary
dilated cardiomyopathy who have a similar clinical severity of heart failure.

When patients evolve from typical structural and clinical manifestations of HCM to the end-stage, dilated phase, medical therapy should be
altered. Beta-blockers should be continued, but calcium channel blockers and
disopyramide should be discontinued. Therapy with angiotensin-converting
enzyme inhibitors, angiotensin receptor blockers, aldosterone antagonists, and
hydralazine-nitrate combinations should be used as indicated. Atrial fibrillation should be aggressively controlled with restoration of sinus rhythm when
possible. The development of the end-stage phase of HCM is the most common
indication for transplantation in patients with this cardiomyopathy [78].

## Restrictive cardiomyopathies

The restrictive cardiomyopathies are disorders of heart muscle with a primary
abnormality of diastolic filling. In these conditions, ventricular relaxation and
compliance are abnormal, and small increases in ventricular volume in diastole

result in abnormally rapid and marked rises in pressure. Ventricular chamber sizes are normal and wall motion and systolic function are usually preserved. The atria are dilated [82,83]. Signs and symptoms of right or left ventricular failure may predominate. Cardiogenic shock is an uncommon mode of presentation in these cardiomyopathies, usually occurring at the end-stage of chronic heart failure.

A variety of conditions can cause restrictive cardiomyopathy. Infiltrative diseases include amyloidosis, sarcoidosis, and Gaucher's disease. Storage diseases that can affect the heart include hemochromatosis and Fabry's disease. Endomyocardial diseases, such as the cardiomyopathy of the hypereosinophilic syndrome, endomyocardial fibrosis, and carcinoid heart disease, can cause restriction. Idiopathic, familial restrictive cardiomyopathy has also been described.

## Amyloidosis

Amyloidosis is an illness characterized by extracellular deposition of insoluble abnormal proteins that lead to organ dysfunction [84]. More than 24 different amyloid proteins have been identified; these are indistinguishable by light microscopy [85]. Normal myocardial contractile elements are replaced by amyloid protein resulting in restrictive cardiomyopathy. Left ventricular systolic dysfunction may occur late in the course of the disease [86].

Amyloidosis is classified into systemic AL amyloidosis, hereditary systemic amyloidosis (ATTR), and senile systemic amyloidosis. Cardiac involvement is common in these three types. Systemic AA amyloidosis, which occurs as a complication of inflammatory diseases, rarely results in cardiac illness [84].

AL amyloidosis accounts for 85% of newly diagnosed cases. Fifty percent of AL cases have clinical evidence of heart involvement, and two-thirds show abnormalities on echocardiography. The amyloid protein in AL is derived from monoclonal immunoglobulin light chains, either from a B cell dyscrasia or a benign monoclonal gammopathy [84]. The prognosis of AL amyloidosis with cardiac involvement is poor, with 40% survival at 2 years after cardiac involvement is identified and <6 months in patients with heart failure [86].

In ATTR amyloidosis, the amyloid protein is made up of a genetically mutated transport protein, transthyretin, which is produced by the liver. Cardiac involvement is common and may predominantly affect the conduction system. The prognosis of cardiac ATTR amyloidosis is better than AL amyloidosis [87].

Senile systemic amyloid (SSA) most often occurs in patients over age 70 years and is associated with a better prognosis than AL or ATTR forms. The median survival is 5 years [88]. It represents 2% of diagnosed cases of cardiac amyloid, but mild forms are more common and may not be recognized clinically. In SSA, the amyloid protein is a nonmutant transthyretin.

Cardiac amyloidosis most often presents with heart failure, and signs of right ventricular failure often predominate. Dizziness and syncope are common, due to autonomic dysfunction with orthostatic hypotension or heart block. ECG classically shows low voltage and pseudo-infarction patterns. Atrial fibrillation and flutter are seen in 7–25% of cases [84]. Characteristic findings on echocardiography include marked thickening of the left ventricle with a speckled, granular appearance. Diastolic dysfunction is seen on Doppler evaluation. The left ventricle is not dilated, and both atria are dilated. Thickening of cardiac valves and interatrial septum and small pericardial effusions are seen. The combination of marked left ventricular wall thickening and low voltage on ECG should strongly suggest this diagnosis [84].

The diagnosis of AL amyloidosis is made by demonstrating monoclonal light chains in serum or urine. All forms of systemic amyloidosis require tissue biopsy for diagnosis, and the amyloid protein can be found in biopsies of abdominal fat, buccal mucosa, kidney, or rectum. EMB may be required in cases with only cardiac involvement [89].

Medical therapy of heart failure due to cardiac amyloidosis is limited. Diuretics are used for edema and pulmonary congestion [83]. Large doses may be needed if patients also have edema due to kidney involvement and nephrotic syndrome. Because patients with amyloid cardiomyopathy frequently have hypotension and orthostasis, ACE-inhibitors and nitrates need to be used judiciously and are often poorly tolerated [87,89]. The use of beta-blockers is also problematic due to bradycardia and hypotension. Calcium channel blockers and digoxin are contraindicated, as digoxin is bound to amyloid protein and can result in digoxin toxicity despite therapeutic serum levels of the drug. Low-dose dopamine may be used to aid diuresis. There are no data available on the use of inotropic agents in amyloid cardiomyopathy with shock [87]. Patients in atrial fibrillation require anticoagulation. Pacemaker therapy is indicated to treat persistent bradycardia or heart block, although pacing likely does not prolong survival [85]. There are no data available on the use of biventricular pacemakers or implantable cardioverter defibrillators (ICDs).

In patients with AL cardiomyopathy, heart transplantation combined with chemotherapy and stem cell therapy can prolong survival in selected patients, with reported 60% survival at 2 years. ATTR cardiac amyloidosis has been treated with cardiac transplantation with or without liver transplantation [86].

## Sarcoidosis

The myocardium is involved in >25% of cases of sarcoidosis in the U.S. and is the cause of death in 13–25% of these cases [90]. Myocardial sarcoidosis is a difficult diagnosis to make, as only 40–50% of patients with cardiac sarcoid at autopsy demonstrated clinical cardiac manifestations. Only 14% of patients will have abnormalities on echocardiography. Most patients with diagnosed cardiac sarcoidosis have conduction system disease or arrhythmia, including complete heart block in 23–30%, ventricular tachycardia in 23%, and supraventricular tachycardia in 15%. Sudden death accounts for two-thirds of patients who die from cardiac causes [91]. A 60% 5-year survival is reported [92].

Heart failure accounts for 25% of deaths from cardiac sarcoidosis [90]. Myocardial infiltration with noncaseating granulomas and myocardial fibrosis results in dilated cardiomyopathy, left ventricular aneurysms, restrictive cardiomyopathy, or valve regurgitation [93]. EMB offers a diagnostic sensitivity of only 20–30% due to patchy involvement. Diagnosis of cardiac sarcoidosis using noninvasive testing is difficult, although preliminary results with PET scanning and CMR are promising [90,93].

The treatment of heart failure includes standard medical therapies, including diuretics, beta-blockers, and ACE-inhibitors. For patients with serious arrhythmias, amiodarone and ICDs are indicated. Cardiac surgery is often indicated for treatment of left ventricular aneurysms or severe valve disease. Expert opinion favors the use of corticosteroids, although this may not be effective in reducing arrhythmias [90,93].

## Hypereosinophilic syndrome

Hypereosinophilic syndrome (HES) is a lymphoproliferative disease of unknown cause. Infiltration with eosinophils occurs in many organs, and cardiac involvement is most common and is the major determinant of morbidity and mortality [94]. Patients with cardiac involvement present with heart failure, chest pain, and systemic emboli, including stroke.

Cardiac pathologic findings in HES are endocardial fibrosis, myocarditis with eosinophil infiltration, and mural thrombus in right and left ventricles [95,96]. Heart failure occurs due to restrictive cardiomyopathy. Severe mitral regurgitation may also occur as a result of fibrosis of papillary muscles and subleaflet structures. Echocardiographic findings include left ventricular wall thickening, right ventricular and left ventricular apical thrombosis, restricted mitral valve leaflet motion, and pericardial effusion. Left ventricular ejection fraction is usually normal [97]. Serial echocardiograms at 6-month intervals are recommended as the heart may become involved after the initial diagnosis of HES is made, and cardiac abnormalities will worsen.

Therapy with corticosteroids is indicated in patients with myocardial disease [98]. Hydroxyurea and other chemotherapies can also be used. Anticoagulation is indicated in the presence of cardiac mural thrombosis or if an embolic event has occurred. Emboli may not be effectively prevented with warfarin, and the addition of antiplatelet agents should be considered [95].

Cardiac surgery has been performed in patients with severe mitral or tricuspid valve regurgitation. There is a high incidence of thrombosis of mechanical prostheses and valve repair, so the use of a bioprosthesis is recommended [95].

## Primary restrictive cardiomyopathy

In a series of ninety-four patients with idiopathic restrictive cardiomyopathy seventy-two percent were over age 60 years. Patients presented with heart failure most commonly, and 28% were in functional class III or IV. Atrial fibrillation was present in 74%. EMB revealed cardiac fibrosis in 80% [82].

Five-year survival was 64%, with heart failure accounting for 47% of deaths. Treatment is not well defined. Careful use of diuretics, maintenance of sinus rhythm, and optimal control of atrial fibrillation are important. Four patients underwent cardiac transplantation.

## Thyrotoxicosis

Hyperthyroidism is associated with significant alterations in hemodynamics. Increases of heart rate, blood volume, stroke volume, and left ventricular ejection fraction are seen. Cardiac output may be two to three times above normal. Vasodilation occurs and systemic vascular resistance may be as low as 50% of normal. Absence of left ventricular contractile reserve during exercise has been reported [99]. These physiologic changes rarely result in the development of heart failure, which has been reported in 6% of thyrotoxic patients.

Thyrotoxicosis can cause a true cardiomyopathy with decreased left ventricular contractility, left ventricular enlargement, and reduced ejection fraction [100–102]. The pathophysiology of this cardiomyopathy is not clear. Proposed mechanisms are prolonged tachycardia (tachycardia-induced cardiomyopathy), decreased renal blood flow resulting in overactivation of the renin-angiotensin system, or aggravation of pre-existing hypertensive or coronary heart disease.

Thyrotoxic cardiomyopathy is usually reversible and the prognosis is favorable. Beta-blockers are started early to control tachycardia and to treat the systemic effects of hyperthyroidism. Control of rapid heart rates is essential. Diuretics and ACE-inhibitors are also recommended. Anti-thyroid medications such as propylthiouracil or methimazole are indicated to treat the primary disorder. Electrical cardioversion of atrial fibrillation or flutter should be performed once patients are euthyroid.

## Conclusion

Although severe acute heart failure and cardiogenic shock are most often caused by AMI, recognition of less common etiologies is important. These conditions have unique pathophysiologies and often have characteristic presentations that can aid in proper diagnosis. Many of these noninfarction causes of cardiogenic shock are reversible. Rapid institution of specific therapies is often life-saving, and the longer term prognosis may be quite favorable after recovery from the acute, severe phase of the disease.

# References

1. Topalian S, Ginsberg F, Parrillo JE. Cardiogenic shock. *Crit Care Med* 2008;36(Suppl); S66–74.
2. Reynolds HR, Hochman JS. Cardiogenic shock. Current concepts and improving outcome. *Circulation* 2008;117:686–97.
3. Dec GW. Acute decompensated heart failure: the shrinking role of inotropic therapy. *J Am Coll Cardiol* 2005;46(1):65–7.
4. Parissis JT, Farmakis D, Nieminen M. Classical inotropes and new cardiac enhancers. *Heart Fail Rev* 2007;12:149–56.
5. Nohria A, Lewis E, Stevenson LW. Medical management of advanced heart failure. *JAMA* 2002;287(5):628–40.
6. Nieminen MS, Brutsaert D, Dickstein K, et al. EuroHeart Failure Survey II (EHFS II): a survey on hospitalized acute heart failure patients: description of population. *Eur Heart J* 2006;27:2725–36.
7. Bayram M, DeLuca L, Massie MB, et al. Reassessment of dobutamine, dopamine, and milrinone in the management of acute heart failure syndromes. *Am J Cardiol* 2005;96(Suppl):47G–58G.
8. Alla F, Zannad F, Filippatos G. Epidemiology of acute heart failure syndromes. *Heart Fail Rev* 2007;12:91–5.
9. Abraham WT, Adams KF, Fonarow GC, et al. In-hospital mortality in patients with acute decompensated heart failure requiring intravenous vasoactive medications. *J Am Coll Cardiol* 2005;46(1):57–64.
10. Wu AH. Management of patients with non-ischaemic cardiomyopathy. *Heart* 2007;93:403–8.
11. Felker GM, O'Connor CM. Inotropic therapy for heart failure: an evidence-based approach. *Am Heart J* 2001;142:393–401.
12. Chatti R, Fradj NB, Trabelsi W, et al. Algorithm for therapeutic management of acute heart failure syndromes. *Heart Fail Rev* 2007;12:113–7.
13. Mebazaa A, Nieminen MS, Packer M, et al. Levosimendan vs dobutamine for patients with acute decompensated heart failure. The SURVIVE Randomized Trial. *JAMA* 2007;297(17):1883–91.
14. Renlund DG, Kfoury AG. When the failing, end-stage heart is not end-stage. *N Engl J Med* 2006;355(18):1922–5.
15. Rose EA, Gelijns AC, Moscowitz AJ, et al. For the randomized evaluation of mechanical assistance for the Treatment of Congestive Heart Failure (REMATCH) Group. Long-term use of a left ventricular assist device for end-stage heart failure. *N Engl J Med* 2001;345:1435–43.
16. Stevenson LW, Couper G. On the fledgling field of mechanical circulatory support. *J Am Coll Cardiol* 2007;50(8):748–51.
17. Hunt SA. Mechanical circulatory support. New data, old problems. *Circulation* 2007;116:461–2.
18. Lietz K, Long JW, Kfoury AG, et al. Outcomes of left ventricular assist device implantation as destination therapy in the post-REMATCH era. Implications for patient selection. *Circulation* 2007;116:497–505.
19. Rogers JG, Butler J, Lansman SI, et al. Chronic mechanical circulatory support for inotrope-dependent heart failure patients who are not transplant candidates. Results of the INTrEPID Trial. *J Am Coll Cardiol* 2007;50(8):741–7.

20. Birks EJ, Tansley PD, Hardy J, et al. Left ventricular assist device and drug therapy for the reversal of heart failure. *N Engl J Med* 2006;355(18):1873–84.

21. Simon MA, Kormos RL, Murali S, et al. Myocardial recovery using ventricular assist devices. Prevalence, clinical characteristics, and outcomes. *Circulation* 2005;112(Suppl I):I-32-36.

22. Feldman A, McNamara D. Myocarditis. *N Engl J Med* 2000;343:1388–98.

23. Barbaro G, Fisher SD, Lipshultz SE. Pathogenesis of HIV-associated cardiovascular complications. *Lancet Infect Dis* 2001;1:115–24.

24. Liu P, Mason J. Advances in the understanding of myocarditis. *Circulation* 2001;104:1076–82.

25. Ginsberg FL, Parrillo JE. Eosinophilic myocarditis. In: Dec GW, ed. *Heart Failure Clinics, Myocarditis*. Philadelphia: W.B. Saunders, 2005;1(3):419–29.

26. Cooper L, Berry G, Shabetai R. Idiopathic giant cell myocarditis: natural history and treatment. *N Engl J Med* 1997;336:1860–6.

27. Kavinsky CJ, Parrillo JE. Rheumatic fever and cardiovascular diseases. *Samter's Immunological Disease* 1995;5:823–40.

28. Haas G. Etiology, evaluation and management of acute myocarditis. *Cardiol Rev* 2001;9:88–95.

29. Lauer B, Niederan C, Kuhl U, et al. Cardiac troponin T in patients with clinically suspected myocarditis. *J Am Coll Cardiol* 2003;42:466–72.

30. Liu PP, Yan AT. Cardiovascular magnetic resonance for the diagnosis of acute myocarditis: prospects for detecting myocardial inflammation. *J Am Coll Cardiol* 2005;45:1923–5.

31. Abdel-Aty H, Boye P, Zagrosek A, et al. Diagnostic performance of cardiovascular magnetic resonance in patients with suspected acute myocarditis. *J Am Coll Cardiol* 2005;45:1815–22.

32. Mahrholdt H, Goedecke C, Wagner A, et al. Cardiovascular magnetic resonance assessment of human myocarditis. *Circulation* 2004;109:1250–8.

33. Parrillo JE. Inflammatory cardiomyopathy (myocarditis): which patients should be treated with anti-inflammatory therapy? *Circulation* 2001;104:4–6.

34. McKenna W, Davies M. Immunosuppression for myocarditis. *N Engl J Med* 1995;333:312–13.

35. Cooper T, Baughman K, Feldman AM, et al. The role of endomyocardial biopsy in the management of cardiovascular disease: a scientific statement from the American Heart Association, the American College of Cardiology and the European Society of Cardiology. *Circulation* 2007;116:2216–33.

36. D'Ambrosio A, Patti G, Manzoli A, et al. The fate of acute myocarditis between spontaneous improvement and evolution to dilated cardiomyopathy: a review. *Heart* 2001;85:499–504.

37. Dec GW. Introduction to clinical myocarditis. In: Cooper LT, ed . *Myocarditis: From Bench to Bedside*. Totowa, NJ: Humana Press, 2003:257–81.

38. Ginsberg F, Parrillo JE. Acute heart failure and myocarditis. In: Mebazza A, Gheorghiade M, Zanad F, Parrillo JE, eds. *Textbook of Severe Acute Heart Failure Syndromes*. London: Springer Science, 2008:183–99.

39. Grinda JM, Chevalier P, D'Attellis N, et al. Fulminant myocarditis in adults and children: bi-ventricular assist device for recovery. *Eur J Cardiothorac Surg* 2004;26: 1169–73.

40. Kato S, Morimoto S, Hiramitsu S, et al. Risk factors for patients developing a fulminant course with acute myocarditis. *Circ J* 2004;68:734–9.

41. McCarthy III RE, Boehmer JP, Hruban RH, et al. Long-term outcome of fulminant myocarditis as compared with acute (nonfulminant) myocarditis. *N Engl J Med* 2000;342:690–5.

42. Leprince P, Combes A, Bonnet N, et al. Circulatory support for fulminant myocarditis: consideration for implantation, weaning and explantation. *Eur J Cardiothoracic Surg* 2003;24:399–403.

43. Kato S, Morimoto S, Hiramitsu S, et al. Use of percutaneous cardiopulmonary support of patients with fulminant myocarditis and cardiogenic shock for improving prognosis. *Am J Cardiol* 1999;83(4):623–5.

44. Chandra D, Kar B, Idelchik G, et al. Usefulness of percutaneous left ventricular assist device as a bridge to recovery from myocarditis. *Am J Cardiol* 2007;99: 1755–6.

45. Parrillo JE, Cunnion R, Epstein S, et al. A prospective, randomized controlled trial of prednisone for dilated cardiomyopathy. *N Engl J Med* 1989;1061–8.

46. Mason J, O'Connell J, Herskowitz A, et al. A clinical trial of immunosuppressive therapy for myocarditis. *N Engl J Med* 1995;333:269–75.

47. Wojnicz R, Nowalany-Kozielska E, Wojcieckowska C, et al. Randomized placebo controlled study for immunosuppressive treatment of inflammatory dilated cardiomyopathy. Two year follow-up results. *Circulation* 2001;104:39–45.

48. Frustaci A, Chimenti C, Calabrese F, et al. Immunosuppressive therapy for active lymphocytic myocarditis. Virological and immunologic profile of responders versus nonresponders. *Circulation* 2003;107:857–63.

49. Dote I, Sato H, Tateishi H, et al. Myocardial stunning due to simultaneous multivessel spasm: a review of five cases. *J Cardiol* 1991;21:203–14.

50. Desmet WJR, Adriaenssens BFM, Dens JAY. Apical ballooning of the left ventricle: first series in white patients. *Heart* 2003;89:1027–31.

51. Sharkey SW, Lesser JR, Zenovich AG, et al. Acute and reversible cardiomyopathy provoked by stress in women from the United States. *Circulation* 2005;111: 472–9.

52. Tsuchihashi K, Ueshima K, Uchida T, et al. Transient left ventricular apical ballooning without coronary artery stenosis: a novel heart syndrome mimicking acute myocardial infarction. *J Am Coll Cardiol* 2001;38(1):11–18.

53. Wittstein IS, Thiemann DR, Lima JAC, et al. Neurohumoral features of myocardial stunning due to sudden emotional stress. *N Engl J Med* 2005;352(6): 539–48.

54. Donohue D, Movahed M. Clinical characteristics, demographics and prognosis of transient left ventricular apical ballooning syndrome. *Heart Fail Rev* 2005;10: 311–16.

55. Villareal RP, Achari A, Wilansky S, et al. Anteroapical stunning and left ventricular outflow tract obstruction. *Mayo Clin Proc* 2001;76(1):79–83.

56. Prasad A. Apical ballooning syndrome. An important differential diagnosis of acute myocardial infarction. *Circulation* 2007;115:e56–9.

57. Gianni M, Dentali F, Grandi AM, et al. Apical ballooning syndrome or takotsubo cardiomyopathy: a systematic review. *Eur Heart J* 2006;27:1523–9.

58. Elesber AA, Prasad A, Lennon RJ, et al. Four-year recurrence rate and prognosis of the apical ballooning syndrome. *J Am Coll Cardiol* 2007;50(5):448–52.

59. Dec GW. Recognition of the apical ballooning syndrome in the United States. *Circulation* 2005;111:388–90.

60. Pearson G, Veille J, Rahimtoola S, et al. Peripartum cardiomyopathy: National Heart, Lung, and Blood Institute and Office of Rare Diseases (National Institutes of Health) Workshop Recommendations and Review. *JAMA* 2000;83(9):1183–8.

61. Elkayam U, Akhter MW, Singh H, et al. Pregnancy-associated cardiomyopathy. Clinical characteristics and a comparison between early and late presentation. *Circulation* 2005;111:2050–5.

62. Tidswell M. Peripartum cardiomyopathy. *Crit Care Clin* 2004;20:777–88.

63. Reimold S, Rutherford JD. Peripartum cardiomyopathy, Editorial. *N Engl J Med* 2001;344(21):1629–30.

64. Amos AM, Jaber WA, Russell SD. Improved outcomes in peripartum cardiomyopathy with contemporary. *Am Heart J* 2006;152:509–13.

65. Ruiz-Bailen M, Lopez-Martinez A, Ramos-Cuadra JA, et al. Peripartum cardiomyopathy: a case series. *Intensive Care Med* 2001;27(1):306–9.

66. Lampert MB, Lang RM. Peripartum cardiomyopathy. *Am Heart J* 1995;130:860–70.

67. Murali S, Baldisseri MR. Peripartum cardiomyopathy. *Crit Care Med* 2005; 33(Suppl)S340–6.

68. Lewis R, Mabie W, Burlew B, et al. Biventricular assist device as a bridge to cardiac transplantation in the treatment of peripartum cardiomyopathy. *South Med J* 1997;90(9):955–8.

69. Aziz TM, Burgess MI, Acladious NN, et al. Heart transplantation for peripartum cardiomyopathy: a report of three cases and a literature review. *Cardiovasc Surg* 1999;7(5):565–7.

70. Keogh A, Macdonald P, Spratt P, et al. Outcome in peripartum cardiomyopathy after heart transplantation. *J Heart Lung Transplant* 1994;13:202–7.

71. Maron MS, Olivotto I, Betocchi S, et al. Effect of left ventricular outflow tract obstruction on clinical outcome in hypertrophic cardiomyopathy. *N Engl J Med* 2003;348(4):295–303.

72. Maron BJ. Hypertrophic cardiomyopathy. A systematic review. *JAMA* 2002;287(10): 1308–20.

73. Maron MS, Olivotto I, Zenovich AG, et al. Hypertrophic cardiomyopathy is predominantly a disease of left ventricular outflow tract obstruction. *Circulation* 2006;114:2232–9.

74. Nagueh SF, Mahmarian JJ. Noninvasive cardiac imaging in patients with hypertrophic cardiomyopathy. *J Am Coll Cardiol* 2006;48:2410–22.

75. Kirschner E, Berger M, Goldberg E. Hypertrophic obstructive cardiomyopathy presenting with profound hypotension. *Chest* 1992;101(3):711–4.

76. Rosen B, Kriwisky M, Rozenman Y, et al. Hypovolemia-induced reversible severe mitral regurgitation due to left ventricular outflow tract obstruction. *Echocardiography* 2002;19(8):679–82.

77. Tamborini G, Pepi M, Susini G, et al. Reversal of cardiogenic shock and severe mitral regurgitation through verapamil in hypertensive hypertrophic cardiomyopathy. *Chest* 1993;104(1):319–20.

78. Harris KM, Spirito P, Maron MS, et al. Prevalence, clinical profile, and significance of left ventricular remodeling in the end-stage phase of hypertrophic cardiomyopathy. *Circulation* 2006;114:216–25.
79. Biagini E, Coccolo F, Ferlito M, et al. Dilated-hypokinetic evolution of hypertrophic cardiomyopathy. *J Am Coll Cardiol* 2005;46(8):1543–50.
80. Ommen SR. Hypertrophic cardiomyopathy. There is much more to the recipe than just outflow obstruction. *J Am Coll Cardiol* 2005;46(8):1551–2.
81. Thaman R, Gimeno JR, Murphy RT, et al. Prevalence and clinical significance of systolic impairment in hypertrophic cardiomyopathy. *Heart* 2005;91:920–5.
82. Ammash NM, Seward JB, Bailey KR, et al. Clinical profile and outcome of idiopathic restrictive cardiomyopathy. *Circulation* 2000;101:2490–6.
83. Kushwaha SS, Fallon JT, Fuster V. Restrictive cardiomyopathy. *N Engl J Med* 1997;336(4):267–76.
84. Selvanayagam JB, Hawkins PN, Paul B, et al. Evaluation and management of the cardiac amyloidosis. *J Am Coll Cardiol* 2007;50:2101–10.
85. Shah KB, Inoue Y, Mehra M. Amyloidosis and the heart: a comprehensive review. *Arch Intern Med* 2006;166:1805–13.
86. Sack F, Kristen A, Goldschmidt H, et al. Treatment options for severe cardiac amyloidosis: heart transplantation combined with chemotherapy and stem cell transplantation for patients with AL amyloidosis and heart and liver transplantation for patients with ATTR-amyloidosis. *Eur J Cardiothorac Surg* 2008;33: 257–62.
87. Falk RH. Diagnosis and management of the cardiac amyloidoses. *Circulation* 2005;112:2047–60.
88. Kyle RA, Spittell PC, Gertz MA, et al. The premortem recognition of systemic senile amyloidosis with cardiac involvement. *Am J Med* 1996;101(4):395–400.
89. Hassan W, Al-Sergani H, Mourad W, et al. Amyloid heart disease. New insights in pathophysiology diagnosis and management. *Tex Heart Inst J* 2005;32: 178–84.
90. Doughan AR, Williams BR. Cardiac sarcoidosis. *Heart* 2006;92:282–8.
91. Silverman KJ, Hutchins GM, Bulkley BH. Cardiac sarcoid: a clincopathologic study of 84 unselected patients with systemic sarcoidosis. *Circulation* 1978;58(6): 1204–11.
92. Okura Y, Dec GW, Hare JM, et al. A clinical and histopathological comparison of cardiac sarcoidosis and idiopathic giant cell myocarditis. *J Am Coll Cardiol* 2003;41: 322–9.
93. Cooper LT. Giant cell and granulomatous myocarditis. *Heart Fail Clin* 2005;1: 431–7.
94. Parrillo JE, Borer JS, Henry WL, et al. The cardiovascular manifestations of the hypereosinophilic syndrome. *Am J Med* 1979;67:572–82.
95. Ginsberg G, Parrillo JE. Eosinophilic myocarditis. *Heart Fail Clin* 2005;1:419–29.
96. Parrillo JE. Heart disease and the eosinophil. *N Engl J Med* 1990;323:1560–1.
97. Ommen S, Seward J, Tajik A. Clinical and echocardiographic features of hypereosinophilic syndrome. *Am J Cardiol* 2000;86:110–3.
98. Parrillo JE, Fauci AS, Wolff SM. Therapy of the hypereosinophilic syndrome. *Ann Intern Med* 1978;89(2):167–72.

99. Fodel BM, Ellahham S, Ringel M, et al. Hyperthyroid heart disease. *Clin Cardiol* 2000;23:402–8.

100. Ladensen PW. Recognition and management of cardiovascular disease related to thyroid dysfunction. *Am J Med* 1990;88:638–41.

101. Kelin I, Ojamaa K. Thyroid hormone and the cardiovascular system. *N Engl J Med* 2001;344(7):501–9.

102. Froeschl M, Haddad H, Commons AS, Veinot JP. Thyrotoxicosis – an uncommon cause of heart failure. *CV Pathol* 2005;14:24–7.

103. Felker GM, Benza RL, Chandler AB, et al. Heart failure etiology and response to milrinone in decompensated heart failure Results from the OPTIME-CHF study. *J Am Coll Cardiol* 2003;41:997–1003.

# Chapter 9

# The role for mechanical circulatory support for cardiogenic shock

Joseph G. Rogers and Carmelo A. Milano

Heart failure remains a common cause of cardiovascular death in industrialized countries, and the incidence will increase as the population ages and novel strategies are developed for managing ischemic heart disease, congenital heart disease, and left ventricular (LV) dysfunction [1–3]. With increasing frequency, patients survive devastating myocardial injury but are left with residual ventricular dysfunction and symptomatic heart failure. At the extreme end of this spectrum are individuals with both acute and chronic heart failure whose cardiac dysfunction precludes adequate end-organ perfusion, resulting in symptoms at rest and with trivial activity.

The chasm that exists between our recognition of cardiogenic shock and our ability to effectively manage it with standard therapies has led to the development of alternative mechanical therapies, including intraaortic balloon counterpulsation (IABP), temporary percutaneous mechanical circulatory support devices, extracorporeal membrane oxygenators (ECMOs), and implantable left ventricular assist devices (LVADs). Cardiac transplantation is another mechanical treatment for cardiogenic shock, but the shortage of suitable donor organs, prolonged waiting times, patient age, and the comorbidities associated with ischemic heart disease renders transplant an impractical treatment for the majority of patients with cardiogenic shock.

This chapter reviews the use of mechanical treatments to support the circulation in patients with acutely decompensated chronic heart failure as well as cardiogenic shock complicating acute myocardial infarction. At present, the dataset and guideline based recommendations supporting the role of mechanical circulatory support (MCS) in the management of cardiogenic shock is limited.

*Cardiogenic Shock*. Edited by Judith S. Hochman and E. Magnus Ohman.
© 2009 American Heart Association, ISBN: 978-1-4051-7926-3

Table 9.1 Clinical and hemodynamic characteristics of patients considered for mechanical circulatory support.

| Clinical Profile |
| --- |
| • Severe LV dysfunction with an ejection fraction $\leq 25\%$<br>• New York Heart Association Class IV symptoms<br>• End-organ hypoperfusion (particularly renal insufficiency)<br>• Treatment with intravenous inotropic support |
| Hemodynamic Profile |
| • Systemic hypotension (systolic blood pressure <90 mm Hg)<br>• Elevated right and left heart filling pressures<br>• Pulmonary arterial hypertension*<br>• Elevated systemic vascular resistance<br>• Cardiac index $\leq 2.0$ L/min/m$^2$ |

*In shock, with low cardiac output, pulmonary artery pressure may not be elevated.

## Patient selection for mechanical circulatory support

The profile of patients considered for MCS is shown in Table 9.1. In our experience, it has been useful to define patient-specific hemodynamics with invasive measurement to guide targeted pharmacotherapy before considering mechanical support. Aggressive attempts should be made to optimize the volume status and cardiac output using combinations of preload reducing agents (diuretics, nitroglycerin), afterload reducing agents (oral vasodilators such as ACE-inhibitors and hydralazine or intravenous preparations such as sodium nitroprusside), and inotropic support (milrinone and dobutamine). The hypotensive patient should be appropriately volume resuscitated. If hypotension persists despite euvolemia or evident volume overload, dopamine may provide sufficient vasoconstriction to maintain end-organ perfusion. The patient's response to these therapeutic maneuvers should be rapidly assessed, and individuals not responding should be referred for mechanical circulatory assistance (Fig. 9.1). The stepwise approach outlined uses less invasive devices, such as IABP and percutaneous VADs as first-line therapy. If the patient does not derive hemodynamic support sufficient to maintain end-organ function and a sustainable cardiac output, additional mechanical support should be employed based on the likelihood of recovery of ventricular function and the options for more advanced heart failure therapies.

If time permits, other critical issues should be addressed, including supplemental nutrition, particularly in the cachectic chronic heart failure population who frequently present with biochemical evidence of malnutrition including low serum levels of albumin, prealbumin, transferrin, and trace elements.

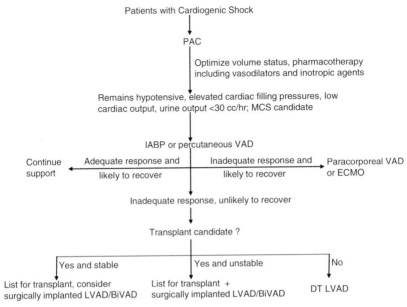

**Fig. 9.1** Approach to the patient in cardiogenic shock who requires mechanical support. Abbreviations: PAC, pulmonary artery catheter; IABP, intra-aortic balloon pump; VAD, ventricular assist device; ECMO, extracorporeal membrane oxygenator; LVAD, left ventricular assist device; BiVAD, biventricular assist device; DT, destination therapy (ineligible for transplantation); MCS, mechanical circulatory support.

A recent analysis of risk factors for mortality following LVAD implantation demonstrated that metrics of inadequate nutrition are strong predictors of early postoperative mortality [4].

# Mechanical therapies for heart failure

Multiple mechanical options exist for the patient with severe heart failure who is refractory to medical therapy [5]. One of the clinical challenges is matching the patient to the mechanical support strategy. Clinicians must make this decision based on several factors, including the anticipated duration of support, the possibility of myocardial recovery, the perceived need for single- or biventricular support, and the need for partial or complete replacement of ventricular function.

## Intra-aortic balloon pump

Since the conception and testing of the IABP nearly 50 years ago, use of this simple and effective device has grown and the results have improved [6,7]. The IABP is inserted via the femoral artery into the descending thoracic aorta just distal to the left subclavian artery and above the level of the renal arteries.

**Table 9.2** Physiologic effects of IABP support.

| Physiologic change | Mechanism | Reference |
|---|---|---|
| Enhanced coronary blood flow | • Balloon inflation during diastole increases intraaortic pressure and coronary perfusion | 8 |
| | • The mean arterial pressure increases as a result of a greater increase in the diastolic pressure than reduction of the systolic pressure | 9–11 |
| | • The absolute change in coronary perfusion is dependent on vasoregulation | 12 |
| Left ventricular unloading | • Displacement of blood into the peripheral circulation | 11 |
| | • Reduction of systolic blood pressure | 9,10 |
| | • Reduction of left ventricular end-diastolic pressure | 9,11 |
| | • Reduced left ventricular wall stress | 12 |
| | • Reduced left ventricular oxygen consumption | 9,12 |
| Improved cardiac output | • Preserved or increased stroke volume | 11 |
| | • Increased cardiac output as a result of afterload reduction | 13 |

It provides hemodynamic support via inflation during cardiac diastole and deflation during systole. Beneficial hemodynamic effects and improvements in coronary blood flow have been demonstrated with proper use (Table 9.2). The IABP must be correctly timed in the cardiac cycle to achieve maximal hemodynamic benefit. Early inflation or late deflation results in expansion of the balloon during systole, thereby increasing LV afterload, lowering cardiac output, and increasing myocardial oxygen consumption and cardiac work. Late inflation and early deflation of the balloon decrease the hemodynamic benefits of proper timing with a decrease in maximal afterload reduction (Fig. 9.2). Prior to insertion the patient should be assessed to ensure that no contraindications to IABP support are present, including severe femoral–iliac–aortic vascular disease, moderate–severe aortic insufficiency, or a significant bleeding diathesis. It is also important to prospectively consider the end-point for IABP therapy, including progression to LVAD or cardiac transplantation if the patient does not experience sufficient myocardial recovery to sustain hemodynamic stability and end-organ function.

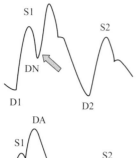

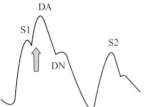

Normal timing of the IABP (arrow) with inflation at the dicrotic notch (DN) and good diastolic augmentation (DA). Unassisted end-diastolic pressure (D1) is higher than assisted end-diastolic pressure (D2). Assisted peak systolic pressure (S2) is lower than unassisted peak systolic pressure (S1).

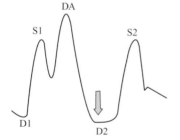

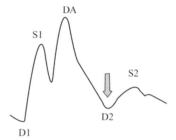

**Early inflation**—rapid rise in diastolic pressure with dicrotic notch after IABP inflation; causes increased afterload.

**Late inflation**—prolonged dip before a decreased diastolic augmentation reduces effectiveness.

**Early deflation**—prolonged dip of assisted end-diastolic pressure and no decrease in assisted systolic pressure; no afterload reduction.

**Late deflation**—the assisted end-diastolic pressure is higher than the unassisted end-diastolic pressure; causes increased afterload.

**Fig. 9.2** Timing the IABP. (Reprinted with permission from Santa-Cruz RA, Cohen MG, Ohman EM. *Cathet Cardiovasc Interv* 2006;67:68–77.)

The IABP is intended for short-term support (hours to days) and is most commonly used to support patients with cardiogenic shock due to acute myocardial infarction, as an adjunct to percutaneous coronary interventions, as a treatment for perioperative hemodynamic instability following cardiac surgery, and for the treatment of unstable angina [14]. The AHA/ACC Practice Guidelines on the management of ST elevation myocardial infarction support the use of IABP in patients with the following characteristics: persistent hypotension or a low-output state after appropriate pharmacotherapy has been employed, recurrent ischemic chest pain, hemodynamic instability, significantly depressed LV function, and a large amount of myocardium at risk [15]. These guidelines also recommend consideration of IABP support in acute myocardial infarction complicated by refractory polymorphic ventricular tachycardia and pulmonary congestion.

There is an extensive literature supporting the use of aortic counterpulsation in a variety of clinical settings. The use of the IABP as an adjunct to fibrinolytic therapy has been shown to improve infarct-related artery patency rates [16–18] and provide hemodynamic stability, although similar benefits may not be as pronounced in individuals undergoing percutaneous coronary intervention (PCI) [19]. Improvements in other outcomes, including mortality, appear to be strongly dependent on patient selection and concomitant therapies. Van't Hof randomized 238 patients who were primarily Killip class I undergoing primary PCI to receive adjunctive IABP or standard care [20]. The primary endpoint of death, nonfatal reinfarction, stroke, or ejection fraction of <30% at 6 months was equivalent in both groups. In contrast, Ohman recently demonstrated that patients with acute myocardial infarction complicated by hypotension and evidence of significant left ventricular dysfunction (Killip III/IV) treated with fibrinolytic therapy derived a survival advantage from early institution of IABP support compared with those treated with fibrinolysis alone (80% vs. 39%, $P$ = 0.05) [21]. The SHOCK registry reported the outcomes of 856 acute myocardial infarction patients treated with or without an IABP as an adjunct to fibrinolytic therapy [22]. Patients treated with an IABP had lower in-hospital mortality than those who did not (50% vs. 72%, $P < 0.001$); however, this improvement was confounded by a higher frequency of revascularization in those treated with an IABP. The SHOCK trial randomized 302 patients with an acute myocardial infarction to receive either early revascularization or a period of stabilization followed by revascularization [23]. An IABP was used in 86% of patients in both arms of the trial. There was no difference in 30-day mortality between these management strategies; 6-month mortality was lower in the patients treated with early revascularization (50.3% vs. 63.1%, RR = 0.80, $P = 0.027$), and the relatively low overall mortality rates in this critically ill population were attributed to advances in adjunctive therapies, including the aggressive use of the IABP. The recently published National Registry of Myocardial Infarction 2 (NRMI 2) assessed IABP efficacy in 23,180 patients with acute myocardial infarction complicated by cardiogenic shock [24]. The overall mortality of this population was 70%. The IABP reduced mortality of patients receiving thrombolytic therapy (OR 0.80, 95% CI 0.72–0.93, $P < 0.01$) but did not impact mortality in those treated with primary PCI. A separate analysis of the same dataset demonstrated a reduction in acute myocardial infarction mortality complicated by cardiogenic shock in high-volume IABP centers and that IABP use in selected patients independently predicted lower mortality, a relationship that persisted after correction for revascularization procedures [25]. A preliminary report of a small randomized trial that was not powered to examine outcomes did not demonstrate an improvement in the APACHE II score, which was the primary endpoint, when IABP was inserted after primary PCI in a cardiogenic shock cohort that had persistent shock despite PCI [26]. A recent meta-analysis of seven randomized trials ($N = 1009$) using IABP in ST-elevation myocardial infarction failed to demonstrate improvement in 30-day mortality or ejection fraction, although the majority of patients were not in cardiogenic shock in those trials [27]. Appropriately designed and powered randomized trials are needed to define the relative risks and benefits associated with IABP in the treatment of cardiogenic shock [28].

The risks of IABP support in a contemporary cohort were presented in the Benchmark Counter Pulsation Registry that included 16,909 patients at one of 203 hospitals worldwide [14]. Cardiogenic shock was the indication for IABP implantation in nearly 20%. Significant adverse events occurred in 2.6%, including major limb ischemia, balloon leak, and bleeding. Multivariate analysis identified peripheral vascular disease, female sex, a body surface area of $<1.65$ m$^2$, and age $\geq$75 years as risk factors for complications. Hemolysis and thrombocytopenia attributable to either the IABP or the concomitant use of heparin are also seen with IABP support.

In most instances, the IABP is used urgently to improve the hemodynamic status of a patient with acute myocardial ischemia or refractory heart failure. Clinicians are frequently faced with the subsequent challenge of determining the appropriate timing for IABP removal or escalation of therapy to more durable circulatory support. Hausmann developed a scoring system that predicted ability to wean from IABP support and then prospectively tested this in a cohort of patients with low-output states undergoing cardiac surgery [29]. High epinephrine requirements ($>0.5$ mcg/kg/min), a left atrial pressure $>15$ mm Hg, urine output $<100$ mL/hour, and a mixed venous oxygen saturation $<60\%$ predicted early mortality following IABP insertion. Assessment of the patient for IABP removal involves weaning of the assist ratio from 1:1 to 1:2 and then 1:3 over the course of several hours. During this period, careful evaluation of clinical parameters (chest pain, dyspnea, blood pressure, heart rate, arrhythmias, urine output) or invasive hemodynamics allow the clinician to make a decision regarding the appropriateness of IABP removal. Escalation of care to implantable LVAD or transplant should be considered in viable candidates who fail to wean from IABP support after 5–7 days, despite receiving appropriate adjunctive therapies including revascularization and treatment for LV dysfunction.

An important limitation of a femoral artery IABP is unstable insertion and the requirement for bedrest, which predisposes patients to complications associated with immobility such as atelectasis and pneumonia. Alternative surgical implantation strategies that allow ambulation include subclavian artery insertion or permanent aortic implantation have been used [30].

## Percutaneous left ventricular assist devices intended for short-term support

Development of several small centrifugal (nonpulsatile) pumps that can be implanted percutaneously and used for short-term support represents a major innovation in the field of mechanical circulatory support. The obvious utility of these devices is the management of acute cardiogenic shock related to myocardial infarction or myocarditis in which rapid application of circulatory support is required and there is a possibility of myocardial recovery. These devices may also be beneficial in supporting high-risk PCIs and electrophysiological procedures, percutaneous valve repair, and postcardiotomy shock.

## TandemHeart™ (CardiacAssist, Inc, Pittsburgh, PA)

The TandemHeart is an extracorporeal centrifugal pump capable of providing 3.5–4.0 L/min of nonpulsatile flow. Flow to the pump is obtained with a 21F venous catheter inserted in the femoral vein and passed into the left atrium via a transseptal puncture (Fig. 9.3A). The pump returns blood to the circulation via a 15F femoral arterial catheter. The system requires systemic anticoagulation and is approved for short-term (6 hours) use, although reports have described longer support duration [31,32]. In two randomized trials, TandemHeart provided superior improvements in cardiac output and reductions in filling pressures compared with IABP support, but neither trial demonstrated an improvement in survival [33,34]. Several centers use the TandemHeart as first-line therapy in critically ill cardiogenic shock patients as a means to achieve clinical stability prior to proceeding to more definitive mechanical support. Limitations of the

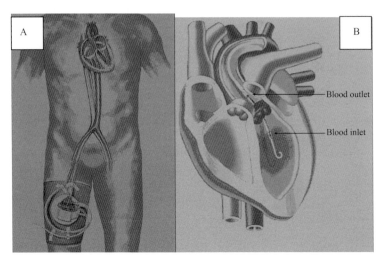

**Fig. 9.3** Temporary mechanical circulatory support devices. (A) The TandemHeart percutaneous VAD is a temporary device that accesses the vascular system via catheters in the femoral vessels. The femoral venous catheter is advanced into the left atrium via a transseptal puncture. The VAD is capable of providing flow of 3.5–4.0 L/min. (Courtesy of CardiacAssist, Inc, Pittsburgh, PA.) (B) The Impella is inserted retrograde across the aortic valve. An external electric motor drives the rotor in the catheter tip at speeds up to 50,000 rpm. (Courtesy of ABIOMED, Danvers, MA.)

Tandem Heart include the requirement for bedrest, the technical challenge of transseptal placement of the drainage catheter, bleeding and the potential for limb ischemia.

### Impella™ (ABIOMED, Danvers, MA)

This device is a small percutaneously implanted axial flow pump inserted retrograde across the aortic valve that draws blood from the LV and delivers it into the aorta (Fig. 9.3B). The catheter has been produced in two sizes. The smaller device is a 12F catheter intended for percutaneous insertion in the catheterization laboratory via the femoral artery that can deliver flows up to 2.5 L/min. The larger catheter is 21F, can provide 5.0 L/min, and is intended for surgical insertion through an aortotomy. This device has been primarily used in Europe, where studies have demonstrated increased cardiac output and reductions in filling pressures [35–37]. Limitations of this device include the requirement for bedrest and the transaortic valve placement; a structurally abnormal valve may preclude its use.

### Cancion™ (Orquis Medical, Lake Forest, CA)

This centrifugal flow device uses continuous aortic flow augmentation as a conceptual basis for the treatment of heart failure [38,39]. Blood flows into this pump via a catheter in the femoral artery and is returned to the circulation through a catheter positioned in the proximal descending aorta. Flow rates with the Cancion pump range from 1 to 1.5 L/min. Preliminary animal and human experiences suggest that this approach results in improved cardiac output, a reduction in cardiac filling pressures and systemic vascular resistance, and improved renal function. The mechanism(s) underlying these improvements are unknown but have been attributed to enhanced nitric oxide production resulting from alterations in aortic shear stress [40].

### Venoarterial extracorporeal membrane oxygenation (VA-ECMO)

ECMO is an important adjunctive device capable of providing circulatory support as well as oxygenation in the setting of respiratory failure. VA-ECMO uses a centrifugal pump to drain venous blood, oxygenate the blood using a membrane oxygenator, and return the blood to the systemic arterial system at physiologic perfusion pressure. VA-ECMO provides considerably greater support relative to the devices discussed above, in that it replaces both right and left ventricular function. Furthermore, it replaces pulmonary function providing complete gas exchange. Thus, VA-ECMO is the favored strategy for cases of profound biventricular failure, cardiac arrest, or combined cardiac–pulmonary failure. Continued improvements in the cannula design, oxygenator, and centrifugal pump have made use easier and safer.

Cannulation for VA-ECMO may be achieved either peripherally or centrally. Peripheral cannulation usually involves femoral vein or jugular vein drainage and inflow via a femoral artery. Central cannulation is preferred in cardiac surgical cases, using a right atrial drainage cannula and outflow via an ascending aortic cannula.

ECMO is effective for short-term support lasting up to a week and is particularly valuable in patients with severe biventricular failure in whom recovery is anticipated or a plan exists to move forward with more durable mechanical support or transplantation. It has been used to support high-risk coronary interventions, including patients with left main coronary disease and those with severe LV dysfunction. A registry experience with ECMO in this setting, which included 105 patients, demonstrated a 95% procedural success rate with an in-hospital mortality of 7.6% in the entire cohort and 2.6% in patients <75 years of age and those without a left main intervention [41]. Shawl and colleagues reported a single-center experience in 107 patients treated with ECMO-supported PCI [42]. The procedural success rate in this population was 98%. Survival free of cardiac death was 83% and 77% at 1 and 2 years, respectively. Further, the subset of patients who had serial measurement of ejection fraction showed an improvement from 20.6% to 29.3% ($P < 0.001$). ECMO is the treatment of choice at several institutions for patients with cardiogenic shock and severe pulmonary edema in whom oxygenation using mechanical ventilation is ineffective. In this application, survival rates of patients who require ECMO are lower than other methods of support, largely related to the patient selection. The University of Michigan reported a 43% 1-year survival rate in critically ill patients treated with ECMO as a bridge to transplantation or other mechanical support [43]. The Cleveland Clinic demonstrated 1-day, 30-day, and 1-year survival rates of 90%, 38%, and 29%, respectively, in an unselected cohort of adult patients treated for variable periods of time on ECMO [44].

Limitations of VA-ECMO include the need for relatively high levels of systemic anticoagulation, typically with heparin. In addition, since the left heart is not directly cannulated, LV distention can occur, leading to increased pulmonary venous pressures and further cardiac injury. This complication is averted with either atrial septostomy or placement of an LV vent. The use of peripheral cannulation is associated with a relatively high rate of local vascular complications related to the size of the cannulae [41]. An additional limitation is the general requirement that the ECMO circuit be monitored by a perfusionist.

## Surgically implanted mechanical circulatory support pumps intended for short-term support

Centrimag$^{TM}$ (Thoratec Corporation, Pleasanton, CA) is a magnetically driven centrifugal pump that can be used for uni- or biventricular support. This device provides continuous flow with outputs to 10 L/min. The primary application of the Centrimag to date is to support critically ill patients, many of whom have postcardiotomy shock. In addition to providing adequate circulatory support, moribund patients with evidence of significant end-organ dysfunction have been supported for days to weeks with demonstrable recovery of renal and hepatic function, allowing triage of the patient to more definitive therapy [45,46].

The **Abiomed AB 5000**$^{TM}$ (ABIOMED, Danvers, MA) is a pneumatically driven extracorporeal pulsatile device capable of uni- or biventricular support. This device typically requires direct cannulation of the heart with inflow cannulae placed in the atria and outflow cannuale attached to the great vessels. The cannulae exit the body just beneath the costal margins and connect to the pump placed on the anterior abdominal wall. An important advantage is that patients may be extubated and can ambulate with this device. This pump has been used for weeks to months, enabling prolonged recovery time. Anticoagulation is required, and thromboembolism remains a limitation of this device.

The **Thoratec pVAD**$^{TM}$ (Thoratec Corporation), like the AB 5000, is an extracorporeal pneumatically driven device that can be used for right ventricular, left ventricular, or biventricular support. The device has a stroke volume of 65 cc and can deliver a cardiac output of 6.5 L/min at a rate of 100 bpm. This pump requires direct cannulation of the heart and has been used for longer-term support as a bridge to transplant.

Many patients who receive a short-term VAD for cardiogenic shock have an underlying disease process from which ventricular recovery is possible. Thus, an important aspect of postimplantation management is a prospective plan to reassess native ventricular function and make decisions regarding the potential for device removal. The patient is first evaluated for evidence of physiologic recovery that includes resolution of metabolic abnormalities (electrolyte imbalance, correction of acidosis, stable renal function), demonstration of a stable cardiac rhythm, and evidence of adequate perfusion. Next, the adequacy of native heart function to support the circulation is assessed while the device support is reduced. Clinical signs, hemodynamic assessment (pulmonary artery catheter and systemic arterial catheter), and an echocardiogram are used to monitor the performance of native ventricular function as ventricular preload is increased. If systemic hypotension, an increased pulmonary artery wedge pressure (PAWP), an elevated central venous pressure, or ventricular dilation occurs during VAD weaning, the patient is not ready for device removal.

## Devices intended for long-term support

An important subset of patients with cardiogenic shock has profound ventricular injury that is unlikely to recover. In the absence of advanced age or comorbidities, these patients are eligible for long-term VAD support, most commonly as a bridge to transplantation. These surgically implanted pumps obtain blood via a cannula inserted into the LV apex and return the blood to the circulation through a conduit sewn to the ascending aorta (Fig. 9.4). Following recovery from the implant, patients are ambulatory and capable of independent

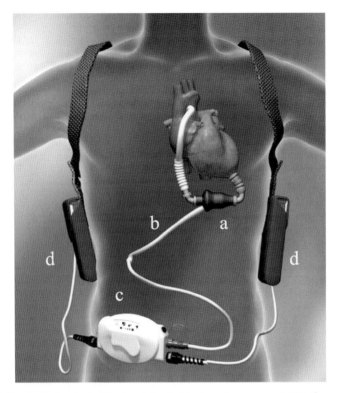

**Fig. 9.4** Surgically implanted devices intended for long-term support. This figure represents the basic configuration of surgically implanted VADs. The pump (a) is placed in an extraperitoneal pocket. The inflow conduit is inserted through a sewing ring into the left ventricle and the outflow graft is attached to the ascending aorta. A driveline (b), tunneled across the abdomen through the subcutaneous tissue, attaches to a small driver (c) and two batteries (d) capable of providing uninterrupted power for up to 4 hours. (Courtesy of Thoratec Corporation, Pleasanton, CA.)

living outside the hospital. The first-generation pumps (Thoratec HeartMate XVE, Novacor) are pulsatile, volume-displacement pumps capable of providing flows of up to 10 L/min. The second-generation pumps (Thoratec HeartMate II, Jarvik 2000, Micromed Debakey) are axial flow devices that house an impellar that rotates between 8000 and 12,000 RPM and provide continuous, nonpulsatile flow. The major advantages to these pumps are smaller size, quiet functioning mode, and fewer moving parts. It is anticipated that there will be fewer mechanical complications and adverse events with the second-generation devices. The third-generation pumps are centrifugal flow pumps that provide nonpulsatile flow at slower operating speeds but are still capable of flow up to 10 L/min. One intriguing aspect of these pumps is that the moving impellar is partially or

## A Volume-Displacement Pump

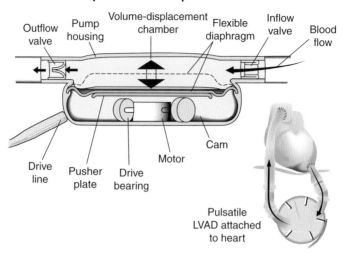

Pulsatile
LVAD attached
to heart

## B Axial-Flow Pump

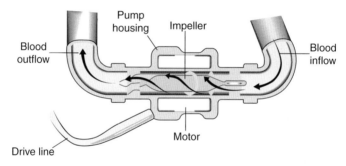

## C Centrifugal Pump

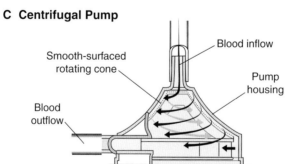

completely magnetically levitated, eliminating the need for a mechanical bearing. It is anticipated that these pumps will have an incremental improvement in durability. At present, the third-generation devices are experimental and none has FDA approval. A comparison of each of these pumps is shown in Fig. 9.5.

## First-generation devices

Both the HeartMate (HM) XVE™ (Thoratec Corporation, Pleasanton, CA) and the Novacor™ (WorldHeart, Oakland, CA) pumps have been used worldwide, and there is a rich dataset describing the outcomes of patients who have received them as a bridge to transplant or as "destination therapy" in non-transplant candidates. The original HM XVE bridge to transplant experience included 280 VAD patients and a historical control cohort of 48 patients managed medically [47]. Despite aggressive therapy with inotropes and IABP, medically supported patients had systemic hypotension, a mean cardiac index (CI) of 1.67 L/min/m², and a mean PAWP of 27 mm Hg. The mean duration of VAD support was 112 days, and 54 patients were effectively supported for >180 days. The device-treated patients had improved survival to transplant as well as superior posttransplant survival. The HM XVE was also the subject of the only randomized trial comparing VAD support with medical therapy in nontransplant patients [48]. Patients treated with the HM XVE had statistically better survival rates at 1 and 2 years with superior improvements in exercise time and quality of life measures. However, survival in the device-treated patients

---

**Fig. 9.5** Mechanism of action of the implantable mechanical circulatory support devices. The volume-displacement pump (A) consists of a chamber or sac that fills and empties cyclically. In the device shown here, an external drive line provides electrical power to a motor within the device. The motor drives a pusher plate up and down repeatedly, expanding and compressing the volume-displacement chamber. The direction of blood flow is maintained by inflow and outflow valves. The anatomical position of a typical volume-displacement pump is shown in the inset. The pump is placed in the abdomen; the inflow cannula is inserted into the left ventricular apex; and the outflow cannula is inserted into the ascending aorta. The total artificial heart is a type of volume-displacement pump, but the patient's own ventricles are removed and the pump is inserted orthotopically. The axial-flow pump (B) contains an impellar, a rotor with helical blades that curve around a central shaft. An external drive line provides electrical power to a motor that drives the rotation of the impellar by electromagnetic induction. Blood is drawn by the spinning impellar from the inflow cannula to the outflow cannula. Blood flow is nonpulsatile. The centrifugal pump (C) uses centrifugal force to drive nonpulsatile blood flow. The device shown here consists of a conical rotor contained within a housing. Blood flows into the apex of the cone and exits at the base. The spinning of the rotor creates a centrifugal force that generates nonpulsatile blood flow. (Reprinted with permission from Baughman KL, Jarcho JA. N Engl J Med 2007;357:846–9.)

was only 50% at 1 year and 22% at 2 years. Further analysis of REMATCH revealed that the most common causes of death in the device-treated patients were infection, neurologic injury, and device malfunction.

The Novacor VAD underwent a similar evaluation in the bridge to transplant application in a population of patients with advanced symptomatic heart failure and severe hemodynamic compromise and was approved for the support of patients awaiting transplantation. The Novacor pump was assessed as destination therapy in the nonrandomized INTrEPID trial [49]. Device-treated patients had a nearly 50% mortality reduction at 6 months. However, early postoperative mortality in both REMATCH and INTrEPID was excessive and is indicative of the moribund population undergoing VAD placement in the current era.

## Second-generation devices

Three axial flow devices are currently undergoing clinical trials. The HeartMate II$^{TM}$ (Thoratec Corporation) has been evaluated for bridge to transplant and destination therapy. The bridge to transplant trial enrolled 133 patients with clinical characteristics similar to those included in trials of first-generation pumps [50]. Nearly 90% of patients were treated with an inotropic agent, and 41% were on IABP support. There was evidence of end-organ dysfunction manifest as abnormal serum chemistries and hemodynamic compromise (mean PAWP = 26 mm Hg, CI = 2.0 l/min/m$^2$). The primary end-point of the trial was survival at 180 days, transplanted, or listed for transplant as a status 1A or 1B (i.e. actively listed and without a significant VAD complication that would preclude successful transplant). Seventy-nine percent of patients treated with the VAD successfully reached the primary endpoint (Fig. 9.6). Further, there was an important improvement in exercise performance and quality of life.

The Jarvik 2000$^{TM}$ (Jarvik Heart, Inc., New York, NY) is a small axial flow device inserted directly into the left ventricle. The outflow cannula can be sewn to the ascending aorta or, alternatively, the descending aorta. The latter may offer an advantage to patients with multiple prior sternotomies. This device is currently in trial in the United States Preliminary reports suggest bridge to transplant survival similar to other devices [51,52].

The third device in this category is the Micromed Debakey VAD$^{TM}$ (MicroMed Cardiovascular, Houston, TX). A recent trial demonstrated that 55% of patients were successfully bridged to transplant, recovered, or were still on support at the time of analysis [53]. Concern was raised during the conduct of this trial that there was a higher than desired risk of pump thrombus and thromboembolism. These concerns have limited the experimental use of this device.

## Third-generation devices

Several iterations of the next generation of mechanical circulatory support devices are beginning to undergo testing in the United States, and some are

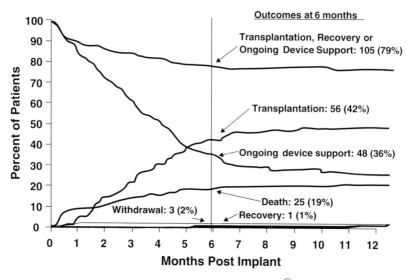

**Fig. 9.6** Competing outcomes analysis from the HeartMate II® Bridge to Transplant trial. The primary endpoint of the study was the number of patients transplanted, recovered with device removal or alive on the device and listed for transplant at a high priority status (1A or 1B) at 6 months. Kaplan–Meier curves are shown for the primary endpoint of the trial as well as the components. Additionally, 3 patients withdrew from the trial. (Adapted with permission from Miller LW, Pagani FD, Russell SD. *N Engl J Med* 2007;357:885–896.)

already approved in Europe and Australia. The fundamental difference from prior generations is that these pumps are implantable, relatively small centrifugal flow pumps. The sizes of the impellar and canister are larger, allowing reduced pump speeds to maintain outputs of up to 10 L/min. The other major design modification is that the impellars are suspended in an electromagnet, eliminating the need for a bearing, thus theoretically improving device durability. Similar to the axial flow devices, the centrifugal flow pumps provide nonpulsatile flow.

## Summary and conclusions

Failure of medical therapy to provide sufficient hemodynamic support for patients with cardiogenic shock, coupled with a shortage of suitable donor organs, provides the rationale for the continued development and use of mechanical circulatory support devices. The role of the cardiologist in selecting appropriate patients, and understanding and managing mechanical circulatory support devices will continue to grow as additional percutaneously placed devices become available. The experience to date has demonstrated that several implantable devices are capable of providing adequate support to bridge critically ill patients to cardiac transplantation. It also appears that mechanical support is superior to best medical therapy in selected patients who are inotrope-dependent but not candidates for transplantation. Arguably, the results of current LVAD trials have not demonstrated the full potential of mechanical circulatory support, which we believe is largely related to the inclusion of very high-risk patients in these studies. Further refinements in selection criteria focused on exclusion of patients too ill to likely derive a survival benefit will further enhance overall survival rates with this technology.

# References

1. Hunt SA, Abraham WT, Chin MH, et al. ACC/AHA 2005 guideline update for the diagnosis and management of chronic heart failure in the adult: a report of the American College of Cardiology/American Heart Association Task Force on Practice Guidelines (writing committee to update the 2001 guidelines for the evaluation and management of heart failure). *Circulation* 2005;112:e154–235.
2. Swedberg K, Cleland J, Dargie H, et al. Task Force for the Diagnosis and Treatment of Chronic Heart Failure of the European Society of Cardiology. *Eur Heart J* 2005;26:1115–50.
3. Rich MW. Epidemiology, pathophysiology, and etiology of congestive heart failure in older adults. *J Am Geriatr Soc* 1997;45:968–74.
4. Lietz K, Long JW, Kfoury AG, et al. Outcomes of left ventricular assist device implantation as destination therapy in the post-REMATCH era: implications for patient selection. *Circulation* 2007;116:497–505.
5. Nieminen M, Bohm M, Cowie MR, et al. Executive summary of the guidelines on the diagnosis and treatment of acute heart failure. *Eur Heart J* 2005;26:384–416.
6. Moulopoulos SD, Topaz S, Kolff WJ. Diastolic balloon pumping (with carbon dioxide) in the aorta—a mechanica assistance to the failing circulation. *Am Heart J* 1962;63:669–75.
7. Kantrowitz A, Tjonneland S, Freed PS, et al. Initial clinical experience with intraaortic balloon pumping in cardiogenic shock. *JAMA* 1968;203:113–8.
8. Kern MJ, Aguirre F, Bach R, et al. Augmentation of coronary blood flow by intra-aortic balloon pumping in patients after coronary angioplasty. *Circulation* 1993;87:500–11.
9. Williams DO, Korr KS, Gerwitz H, et al. The effect of intraaortic balloon couterpulsation on regional myocardial blood flow and oxygen consumption in the presence of coronary artery disease in patients with unstable angina. *Circulation* 1982;66:593–7.
10. Fuchs RM, Brin KP, Brinker JA, et al. Augmentation of regional coronary blood flow by intra-aortic balloon counterpulsation in patients with unstable angina. *Circulation* 1983;68:117–23.
11. Santa-Cruz RA, Cohen MG, Ohman EM. Aortic counterpulsation: a review of hemodynamic effects and indications for use. *Cathet Cardiovasc Interv* 2006;67:68–77.
12. Trost JC, Hillis LD. Intra-aortic balloon counterpulsation. *Am J Cardiol* 2006;97:1391–8.
13. Mueller H, Ayres SM, Conklin EF, et al. The effects of intra-aortic counterpulsation on cardiac performance and metabolism in shock associated with acute myocardial infarction. *J Clin Invest* 1971;50:1885–900.

14. Ferguson JJ, Cohen M, Freedman RJ, et al. The current practice of intra-aortic balloon counterpulsation: results from the Benchmark Registry. *J Am Coll Cardiol* 2001;38: 1456–62.

15. Antman EM, Anbe DT, Armstrong PW, et al. ACC/AHA Guidelines for the management of patients with ST-elevation myocardial infarction: a report of the American College of Cardiology/American Heart Association task force on practive guidelines (Committee to revise the 1999 guidelines for the management of patients with acute myocardial infarction). *Circulation* 2004;110:e82–293.

16. Ohman EM, George BS, White CJ, et al. Use of aortic counterpulsation to improve sustained coronary artery patency during acute myocardial infarction: results of a randomized trial. *Circulation* 1994;90:972–9.

17. Kono T, Morita H, Nishina T, et al. Aortic counterpulsation may improve late patency of the occluded coronary artery in patients with early failure of thrombolytic therapy. *J Am Coll Cardiol* 1996;28:876–81.

18. Ohman EM, Califf RM, George BS, et al. The use of intraaortic balloon pumping as an adjunct to reperfusion therapy in acute myocardial infarction. *Am Heart J* 1991;121:895–901.

19. Stone GW, Marsalese D, Brodie BR, et al. A prospective, randomized evaluation of prophylactic intraaortic balloon counterpulsation in high risk patients with acute myocardial infarction treated with primary angioplasty. *J Am Coll Cardiol* 1997;29:1459–67.

20. van't Hof AWJ, Liem AL, deBoer MJ, et al. A randomized comparison of intra-aortic balloon pumping after primary percutaneous coronary angioplasty in high risk patients with acute myocardial infarction. *Eur Heart J* 1999;20:659–65.

21. Ohman EM, Nanas J, Stomel RJ, et al. Thrombolysis and counterpulsation to improve survival in myocardial infarction complicated by hypotension and suspected cardiogenic shock or heart failure: results of the TACTICS trial. *J Thromb Thrombolysis* 2005;19:33–9.

22. Sanborn TA, Sleeper LA, Bates ER, et al. Impact of thrombolysis, intraaortic balloon pump counterpulsation and their combination in patients with cardiogenic shock complicating acute myocardial infarction: a report from the SHOCK trial registry. *J Am Coll Cardiol* 2000;36:1123–9.

23. Hochman JS, Sleeper LA, Webb JG, et al. Early revascularization in acute myocardial infarction complicated by cardiogenic shock. *N Engl J Med* 1999;341:625–34.

24. Barron HV, Every NR, Parsons LS, et al. The use of intra-aortic balloon counterpulsation in patients with cardiogenic shock complicating acute myocardial infarction: data from the National Registry of Myocardial Infarction. *Am Heart J* 2001;141: 933–9.

25. Chen EW, Canto JG, Parsons LS, et al. Relation between hospital intra-aortic balloon counterpulsation volume and mortality in acute myocardial infarction complicated by cardiogenic shock. *Circulation* 2003;108:951–7.

26. Prondzinsky R, Lemm H, Swyter M, Wegener N, et al. A Prospective, Randomized Evaluation of Intraaortic Balloon Counterpulsation for the Prevention of Multiorgan-Dysfunction and – Failure in Patients With Acute Myocardial Infarction complicated by Cardiogenic Shock *Circulation* 2006 Suppl.;114(18):II-555, 2668.

27. Sjauw KD, Engström AE, Vis MM, et al. A systematic review and meta-analysis of intra aortic balloon pump therapy in ST-elevation myocardial infarction: should we change the guidelines? *Eur Heart J* 2009;30:459–68.

28. Thiele H, Schuler G. Cardiogenic shock: to pump or not to pump? *Eur Heart J* 2009;30:389–90.

29. Hausmann H, Potapov EV, Koster A, et al. Prognosis after the implantation of an intra-aortic balloon pump in cardiac surgery calculated with a new score. *Circulation* 2002;106(Suppl I):I-203–6.

30. Jeevanandam V, Jayakar D, Anderson AS. Circulatory assistance with a permanent implantable IABP: initial human experience. *Circulation* 2002;106;I-183–8.

31. Kar B, Adkins LE, Civitello AB, et al. Clinical experience with the TandemHeart percutaneous ventricular assist device. *Tex Heart Inst J* 2006;33:111–5.

32. Chandra D, Kar B, Idelchik G, et al. Usefulness of percutaneous left ventricular assist device as a bridge to recovery from myocarditis. *Am J Cardiol* 2007;99:1755–6.

33. Burkhoff D, Cohen H, Brunckhorst C, et al. A randomized multicenter clinical study to evaluate the safety and efficacy of the TandemHeart percutaneous ventricular assist device versus conventional therapy with intraaortic balloon pumping for treatment of cardiogenic shock. *Am Heart J* 2006;152:469.e1–8.

34. Thiele H, Sick P, Boudriot E, et al. Randomized comparison of intra-aortic balloon support with a percutaneous left ventricular assist device in patients with revascularized acute myocardial infarction complicated by cardiogenic shock. *Eur Heart J* 2005;26:1276–83.

35. Jurmann MJ, Siniawski H, Erb M, et al. Initial experience with miniature axial flow ventricular assist devices for postcardiotomy heart failure. *Ann Thorac Surg* 2004;77:1642–7.

36. Garatti A, Colombo T, Russo C. Left ventricular mechanical support with the impella recover left direct microaxial blood pump: a single-center experience. *Artif Organs* 2006;30;523–8.

37. Siegenthaler MP, Brehm K, Strecker T, et al. The impella recover microaxial left ventricular assist device reduces mortality for postcardiotomy failure: a three-center experience. *J Thorac Cardiovasc Surg* 2004;127:812–22.

38. Haithcock BE, Morita H, Fanous NH, et al. Hemodynamic unloading of the failing left ventricle using an arterial-to-arterial extracorporeal flow circuit. *Ann Thorac Surg* 2004;77:158–63.

39. Konstam MA, Czerska B, Bohm M, et al. Continuous aortic flow augmentation: A pilow study of hemodynamic and renal responses to a novel percutaneous intervention in decompensated heart failure. *Circulation* 2005;112:3107–14.

40. Patten RD, DeNofrio D, El-Zaru M, et al. Ventricular assist device therapy normalizes inducible nitric oxide synthase expression and reduces cardiomyocyte apoptosis in the failing human heart. *J Am Coll Cardiol* 2005;45:1419–24.

41. Vogel RA, Shawl F, Tommaso C, et al. Initial report of a national registry of elective cardiopulmonary bypass supported coronary angioplasty. *J Am Coll Cardiol* 1990;15:23–9.

42. Shawl FA, Quyyumi AA, Bajaj, et al. Percutaneous cardiopulmonary bypass-supported coronary angioplasty in patients with unstable angina pectoris or myocardial infarction and a left ventricular ejection fraction of $\leq$ 25%. *Am J Cardiol* 1996;77: 14–19.

43. Pagani FD, Lynch W, Swaniker F, et al. Extracorporeal life support to left ventricular assist device bridge to heart transplant: a strategy to optimize survival and resource utilization. *Circulation* 1999;100:II-206–10.

44. Smedira NG, Moazami N, Golding CM, et al. Clinical experience with 202 adults receiving extrcorporeal membrane oxygenation for cardiac failure: survival at five years. *J Thorac Cardiovasc Surg* 2001;122:92–102.

45. John R, Lioa K, Lietz K, et al. Experience with the levitronix centrimag circulatory support system as a bridge to decision in patients with refractory acute cardiogenic shock and multisystem organ failure. *J Thorac Cardiovasc Surg* 2007;134:351–8.

46. Robertis FD, Birks EJ, Rogers P, et al. Clinical performance with the levitronix centrimag short-term ventricular assist device. *J Heart Lung Transplant* 2006;25:181–6.

47. Frazier OH, Rose EA, Ox MC, et al. Multicenter clinical evaluation of the HeartMate vented electric left ventricular assist system in patients awaiting heart transplantation. *J Thorac Cardiovasc Surg* 2001;122:1186–95.

48. Rose EA, Gelijns AC, Moskowitz AJ, et al. Long-term use of a left ventricular assist device for end-stage heart failure. *N Engl J Med* 2001;345:1435–43.

49. Rogers JG, Butler J, Lansman SL, et al. Chronic mechanical circulatory support for inotrope-dependent heart failure patients who are not transplant candidates. *J Am Coll Cardiol* 2007;50:741–7.

50. Miller LW, Pagani FD, Russell SD, et al. Use of a continuous-flow device in patients awaiting heart transplantation. *N Engl J Med* 2007;357:885–96.

51. Frazier OH, Myers TJ, Westaby S, et al. Use of the Jarvik 2000 left ventricular assist system as a bridge to heart transplantation or as destination therapy for patients with chronic heart failure. *Ann Surg* 2003;237:631–7.

52. Siegenthaler MP, Westaby S, Frazier OH, et al. Advanced heart failure: feasibility study of long-term continuous axial flow pump support. *Eur Heart J* 2005;26:1031–8.

53. Goldstein DJ. Worldwide experience with the MicroMed DeBakey ventricular assist device® as a bridge to transplantation. *Circulation* 2003;108:II-272–7.

54. Baughman KI, Jarcho JA. Bridge to life—cardiac mechanical support. *N Engl J Med* 2007;357:846–9.

# Chapter 10

# Percutaneous coronary intervention for cardiogenic shock

Eric R. Bates

## Introduction

Major milestones in reducing mortality from ST-elevation myocardial infarction (STEMI) include organization of coronary care units in the 1960s to treat lethal arrhythmias [1] and the development of fibrinolytic therapy in the 1980s to reduce infarct size [2–5]. Presently, the most common cause of death in patients hospitalized with myocardial infarction (MI) is cardiogenic shock, not arrhythmia. Cardiogenic shock is characterized by low cardiac output and organ hypoperfusion. The etiology is usually myocardial necrosis and ischemia due to infarct artery thrombosis that results in severe left ventricular dysfunction. Unfortunately, neither the incidence nor the mortality rate associated with cardiogenic shock has been reduced by modern cardiac intensive care unit interventions, including vasopressor and inotropic drug infusions [6], hemodynamic monitoring [7], and intra-aortic balloon pump (IABP) counterpulsation [8]. Several multicenter randomized megatrials [2–5] have demonstrated a survival advantage with fibrinolytic therapy in STEMI, with the greatest benefit in patients with the most jeopardized myocardium (e.g. anterior STEMI, new left bundle branch block). Therefore, it is paradoxical and disappointing that the survival benefit with fibrinolytic therapy for the subset of patients with cardiogenic shock is modest, perhaps because of low reperfusion rates due to hypotension [9]. Percutaneous coronary intervention (PCI), however, does achieve high infarct artery patency rates in patients with cardiogenic shock [10], and a survival advantage has been demonstrated [10–13].

*Cardiogenic Shock.* Edited by Judith S. Hochman and E. Magnus Ohman.
© 2009 American Heart Association, ISBN: 978-1-4051-7926-3

# Historical background

Mathey and colleagues [14] first reported that the shock state could be reversed with successful reperfusion with intracoronary streptokinase. Although a multi-center STEMI registry report [15] on 44 patients treated with intracoronary streptokinase documented a 66% in-hospital mortality rate, it suggested the importance of successful reperfusion on outcome. Only 43% of the shock patients had successful reperfusion (compared with 71% for the entire registry), but their mortality rate was 42% as opposed to 84% among those with unsuccessful reperfusion. Early trials of intravenous fibrinolytic therapy demonstrated substantially lower TIMI 2 and 3 grade perfusion among patients who later died from cardiogenic shock [16]. Interestingly, recent observations in acute heart failure patients have documented that hemodynamic alterations can diminish coronary perfusion, even among patients without significant coronary artery disease. These findings point to the importance of hypotension and hypoperfusion states leading to further clinical deterioration [17].

Andreas Gruentzig developed a percutaneous balloon catheter that was first used to dilate a human coronary artery stenosis on September 16, 1977 [18]. The initial reports on balloon angioplasty in patients with STEMI followed in the early 1980s [19,20], and in 1982, Meyer was the first to use PCI to treat cardiogenic shock [21]. In the first treatment series, reported in 1985, O'Neill and colleagues obtained successful reperfusion in 24 (88%) of 27 patients, with an in-hospital mortality rate of 25% [22]. Brown and coworkers had a 61% successful reperfusion rate, associated with a 42% mortality rate; the mortality rate was 82% when reperfusion was unsuccessful [23]. Multiple small observational reports since then have consistently shown a survival benefit for patients with successful PCI compared with those in whom PCI was unsuccessful or with historical controls [24].

# Clinical results

There have been a few large observational reports on reperfusion therapy for cardiogenic shock. The Global Utilization of Streptokinase and Tissue Plasminogen Activator for Occluded Coronary Arteries (GUSTO)-1 trial [25] included 2972 patients with cardiogenic shock treated with fibrinolytic therapy. There was a lower 30-day mortality rate for the 22% of patients who were subsequently treated with PCI compared with those receiving only medical therapy (43% vs. 61% with shock on arrival, 32% vs. 61% for those who developed shock after arrival). Another GUSTO-1 analysis included 2200 patients with cardiogenic shock [26]. Compared with a delayed strategy, angiography within 24 hours of shock onset with revascularization by PCI or coronary artery bypass graft surgery when deemed appropriate was independently associated with reduced 30-day mortality (38% vs. 62%).

A recent large registry evaluated the outcome of 1333 patients undergoing primary PCI for cardiogenic shock [27]. The in-hospital mortality in this cohort was 46%. The independent predictors of mortality were left main disease, TIMI flow <3 after PCI, older age, three-vessel disease, and longer time between symptom onset and PCI.

Unfortunately, none of these reports represent randomized, controlled studies of PCI. A selection bias favoring PCI over historical controls could easily have resulted from excluding the elderly or patients in extremis or with comorbid disease. Hochman and colleagues have documented that patients with cardiogenic shock who are selected for cardiac catheterization are younger and less likely to die (51% vs. 85%), even when not revascularized [28]. Nevertheless, several studies and clinical experience clearly demonstrate the favorable impact a patent infarct artery can have on reversing the shock state.

Two small randomized trials have been performed. The Swiss Multicenter trial of Angioplasty SHock (SMASH) [29] randomized 55 patients to undergo either emergency angiography and revascularization when indicated or initial medical management, but the trial was terminated prematurely because of poor enrollment. Mortality at 30 days was 69% in the invasive arm versus 78% in the medical arm. At 1 year, the mortality figures were 74% and 83%, respectively. Although the study failed to reach statistical significance because of the small sample size, the trend was clinically important. The Should We Emergently Revascularize Occluded Coronaries for Cardiogenic Shock (SHOCK) trial [11–13] randomized 302 patients to emergent revascularization or initial medical stabilization followed by late revascularization for selected patients. Concurrently, the 30 participating sites collected registry data on 1190 patients presenting with cardiogenic shock who were not randomized [30]. Medical stabilization included fibrinolytic therapy in over half the patients as well as inotropic and vasopressor agents. IABP counterpulsation was used in 86% of the patients. In the revascularization arm, 97% of patients underwent early angiography; of those who were revascularized, 64% underwent PCI, and 36% had coronary artery bypass graft surgery. Half of the revascularization group had received fibrinolytic therapy, so PCI was often rescue, not primary PCI. There was no statistically significant difference in 30-day mortality between the revascularization and medical therapy groups (46.7% vs. 56.0%; $P = 0.11$), but by the 6-month endpoint, a significant survival advantage had emerged for patients randomized to revascularization (50.3% vs. 63.1%, $P = 0.027$) that was maintained at 1 year (53.3% vs. 66.4%) (Fig. 10.1).

## Patient selection

Emergency PCI is recommended by the ACC/AHA STEMI guidelines for those less than 75 years old who develop shock within 36 hours of MI and who are

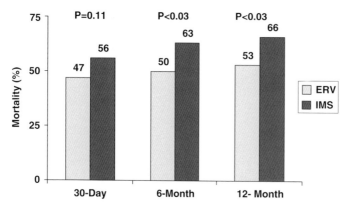

**Fig. 10.1** Mortality rates in the SHOCK trial [11,12] for those assigned to early revascularization (ERV) vs. initial medical stabilization (IMS) followed by late or no revascularization.

suitable for revascularization that can be performed within 18 hours of shock, unless further support is deemed futile (Fig. 10.2) [31]. The best candidates for PCI are patients without prior MI who are younger than 70 years of age with fewer comorbidities and symptom duration less than 12 hours. The severity, distribution, and diffuseness of coronary artery disease and the degree of left ventricular dysfunction also influence outcome. Poor candidates because of very high mortality risk are those with rapidly progressive hemodynamic deterioration despite therapeutic interventions and elderly patients with comorbid disease. Additionally, patients with life-shortening illnesses, no vascular access, previously defined coronary anatomy that was unsuitable for revascularization, anoxic brain damage, and prior cardiomyopathy are poor candidates. Except for the elderly, all other subgroups had treatment benefit with revascularization in the SHOCK trial (Fig. 10.3) [11]. The apparent lack of benefit for the elderly may have been due to the chance finding that baseline ejection fraction in the elderly was lower in those assigned to the early revascularization group.

The elderly patient subgroup in the SHOCK registry [32] was analyzed to gain further insight into patients at least 75 years of age. Whereas the randomized trial included only 56 patients in that age group, the registry included 277 patients. Overall, in-hospital mortality in the elderly was 76% versus 55% in the younger age group ($P < 0.001$). The 44 elderly patients selected for early revascularization, however, had a significantly lower mortality rate than those who did not undergo early revascularization (48% vs. 81%; $P = 0.0002$). Other reports [33–35] also support the use of primary PCI in selected elderly patients with cardiogenic shock complicating MI, so age alone should not be an exclusion

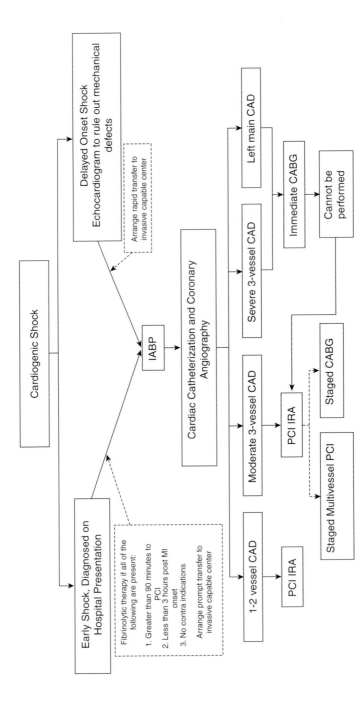

**Fig. 10.2** Recommendations for initial reperfusion therapy. Abbreviations: CABG, coronary artery bypass graft surgery; CAD, coronary artery disease; IABP, intra-aortic balloon counterpulsation; IRA, infarct-related artery; LBBB, left bundle branch block; MI, myocardial infarction; PCI, percutaneous coronary intervention. (Reprinted with permission from Antman EM, Anbe DT, Armstrong PW, et al. *Circulation* 2004;110:e82–293.)

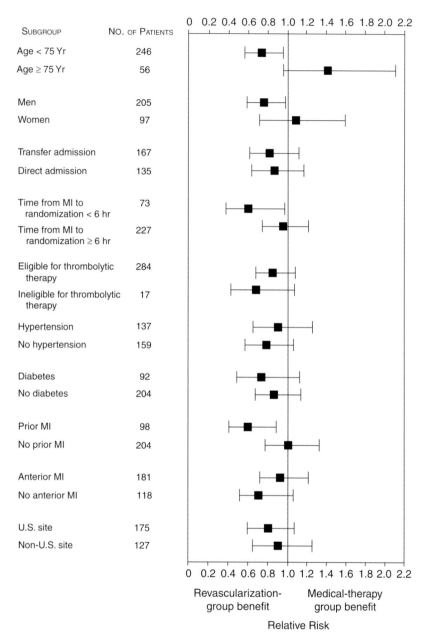

**Fig. 10.3** Relative risk of 30-day mortality in those assigned to early revascularization (revascularization group) versus initial medical stabilization (medical-therapy group) for subgroups in the SHOCK trial. (Reprinted with permission from Hochman JS, Sleeper LA, Webb JG, et al. *N Engl J Med* 1999;341:625–34.)

criterion when selecting patients for cardiac catheterization. Prior functional status, comorbidity, and patient and family preferences are important selection criteria.

The majority of STEMI patients are admitted to hospitals without revascularization capability. Data from the National Registry of Myocardial Infarction (NRMI) show that mortality in patients with cardiogenic shock not transferred for revascularization remains unacceptably high [36]. In STEMI complicated by cardiogenic shock, inter-hospital transfer of patients is more challenging than in uncomplicated STEMI because of hemodynamic instability and increased complication rates. Small retrospective series showed that inter-hospital transfer of selected shock patients was safe and led to improved survival when both fibrinolysis and IABP support were employed [37,38]. Among the SHOCK registry's 1190 patients, 44% were transferred to tertiary care centers [39]. Despite delayed time-to-treatment, transfer patients had a similar mortality benefit with early revascularization as direct admit patients, probably because of survivor selection bias. Selected STEMI patients with cardiogenic shock admitted to hospitals without revascularization capability should be transferred to centers with revascularization capability for immediate angiography [31].

Over the last several years there has been a strong focus on bringing patients to the cath lab within 90 minutes of arrival to hospital. Although early arrival and timely reperfusion prevent cardiogenic shock, patients who develop shock will also benefit from later reperfusion. In the SHOCK trial, the mortality benefit with an early invasive strategy was equal among patients who were direct admits as among those transferred from other hospitals. The average time from shock onset to randomization was about 6 hours, which meant that many patients had PCI >12 hours after MI onset. Thus, an important aspect of the management of cardiogenic shock is that even late reperfusion with primary PCI has something to offer [11].

Patients with large MI may go through a period of pre-shock with nonhypotensive peripheral hypoperfusion before they develop cardiogenic shock. The clinical manifestations are oliguria (urine output <30 cc/hr) and/or cold extremities despite a systolic blood pressure >90 mm Hg. In the SHOCK registry [40], these patients had an in-hospital mortality rate of 43% compared with a rate of 66% in patients with classic cardiogenic shock. Early recognition and treatment may prevent the onset of hypotension and tissue hypoperfusion.

## Pre-procedure care

Before PCI can be performed, several other interventions must be pursued. Initial patient resuscitation is aimed at stabilizing oxygenation and perfusion (Table 10.1). A careful fluid challenge should be used to exclude hypovolemic shock, unless the patient is in obvious pulmonary edema. In right ventricular

**Table 10.1** Stabilization before PCI for cardiogenic shock.

| |
|---|
| 1. Maximize volume (RAP 10–14 mm Hg, PAWP 18–20 mm Hg) |
| 2. Maximize oxygenation (e.g. ventilator) |
| 3. Control rhythm (e.g. pacemaker, cardioversion) |
| 4. Correct electrolyte and acid-base imbalances |
| 5. Sympathomimetic amines (e.g. dobutamine, dopamine, norepinephrine, phenylephrine) |
| 6. Diuretics (e.g. furosemide) |
| 7. Antiarrhythmics (e.g. amiodarone) |
| 8. IABP counterpulsation |

Abbreviations: PAWP, pulmonary artery wedge pressure; RAP, right atrial pressure; IABP, intra-aortic ballon pump.

shock, where preload is critical, fluid support and avoidance of nitrates and morphine are indicated.

Oxygenation and airway support usually require tracheal intubation and mechanical ventilation. Positive end-expiratory pressure decreases preload and afterload. Muscular paralysis (in addition to sedation) improves procedural safety and decreases oxygen demand. If there is a concern about airway support and oxygenation, intubation should be carried out before cardiac catheterization as intubation on the table can represent a challenge, particularly when patients are having multiple devices in both groins.

Urine output needs to be monitored hourly. An arterial catheter allows constant monitoring of blood pressure. Central hemodynamic monitoring using a pulmonary artery catheter can provide valuable information and aid in the titration of fluids and medications. Although use of the pulmonary artery catheter has not been associated with mortality benefit, it is very helpful in managing cardiogenic shock.

Sustained atrial and ventricular tachyarrhythmias should be electrically converted to sinus rhythm to maximize cardiac output. Often, agents such as amiodarone are required to maintain sinus rhythm. Likewise, bradycardia and high-degree heart block should be treated with atropine or temporary pacing. AV pacing may be preferable, especially in the setting of RV failure [41].

Hypokalemia and hypomagnesemia predispose to ventricular arrhythmias and should be corrected. Hyperventilation may be required to correct metabolic acidosis, but sodium bicarbonate should be avoided given a short half-life and the large sodium load. Aspirin 325 mg and unfractionated heparin should be administered to facilitate further invasive care and to prevent reinfarction, ventricular mural thrombus formation, or deep venous thrombosis. Clopidogrel is best withheld until cardiac catheterization has determined whether there is a need for emergency surgery because of its prolonged action and increased risk for perioperative bleeding. Morphine sulfate decreases pain, excessive sympathetic activity, preload, and afterload, but should only be administered in small increments. Diuretics decrease filling pressures and should be used to control volume. Beta-blockers and calcium channel blockers should be avoided because they are negative inotropic agents.

Inotropic and vasopressor drugs are the major initial interventions for reversing hypotension and improving vital organ perfusion. The choice of sympathomimetic agents should be dictated by hemodynamic parameters and will often change as the clinical condition evolves and complications develop. Beta agonists enhance contractility and can provide support until stunned and reperfused myocardium recovers. However, they also induce tachycardia, can worsen myocardial ischemia in the peri-infarct zone, and enhance arrhythmogenicity. The lowest dose needed to support the circulation should be used and, as the patient's condition improves or as other means of support are instituted, the dose should be titrated down to the minimum dose required to provide circulatory support. Further discussion of agents used in the medical management of cardiogenic shock is provided in Chapter 3.

When pharmacological therapy provides insufficient hemodynamic support, mechanical circulatory assistance can be instituted. IABP counterpulsaton augments diastolic coronary flow, decreases afterload, improves systemic perfusion, and decreases infarct artery reocclusion rates. The best use of IABP counterpulsation is in patients with ischemic, viable, but nonfunctioning myocardium that can be revascularized. IABP counterpulsation offers little support to shock patients with extensively scarred ventricles or after late presentation. Contraindications for IABP counterpulsation include aortic regurgitation, aortic dissection, and peripheral vascular disease.

The timing of IABP insertion has not been well studied. In many cardiac catheterization laboratories, the IABP is inserted in most patients with shock prior to PCI to stabilize them during the angiography and subsequent PCI. An observational study suggested that there was lower mortality when IABP counterpulsation was initiated prior to PCI. However, the study was nonrandomized and the patients with IABP counterpulsation prior to PCI tended to have substantially lower blood pressure [42]. Interestingly, recent studies in large anterior MIs in a canine model found substantial reduction in infarct size when IABP counterpulsation was initiated prior to reperfusion [43].

Devices that offer greater circulatory support than IABP counterpulsation are available and have been used in cardiogenic shock (Chapter 9). These include percutaneous cardiopulmonary bypass [44], extracorporeal life support [45], and percutaneous ventricular assist devices [46].

## Procedure

Vascular sheaths are percutaneously placed in both femoral arteries and veins. An IABP catheter is initially inserted through one femoral artery for counterpulsation support, and a pulmonary artery catheter is inserted through a femoral vein for hemodynamic diagnosis and monitoring of therapy. The other venous sheath is used for blood draws, drug administration, and placement of a temporary pacemaker, if necessary. Angiography and PCI are performed through the second arterial sheath only after the patient is maximally supported.

The hemodynamic profile of left ventricular shock, as defined by Forrester and coworkers [7], includes pulmonary artery wedge pressure greater than 18 mm Hg and a cardiac index less than 2.2 L/min/m$^2$. Others definitions include a pulmonary artery wedge pressure of at least 15 or 12 mm Hg and a cardiac index of less than 2.0 or 1.8 L/min/m$^2$. The hemodynamic profile of right ventricular shock includes right atrial pressure of 85% or more of the pulmonary artery wedge pressure, steep Y descent in the right atrial pressure tracing, and the dip and plateau (i.e. square root sign) in the right ventricular wave form. Large V waves in the pulmonary artery wedge tracing suggest the presence of severe mitral regurgitation. An oxygen saturation step-up (>5%) from the right atrium to the right ventricle confirms the diagnosis of ventricular septal rupture. Equalization of right atrial, right ventricular end-diastolic, pulmonary artery diastolic, and pulmonary artery wedge pressures occurs with severe right ventricular infarction or pericardial tamponade due to free wall rupture or hemorrhagic effusion.

Admitting labs should be obtained, if not previously performed. An arterial blood gas should be measured to evaluate oxygenation and acid-base status. A low osmolar ionic contrast agent is preferable to minimize hemodynamic complications and prothrombotic effects associated with other contrast agents. The activated clotting time should be checked if PCI is to be performed and supplemental heparin titrated to prolong the activated clotting time >300 seconds [or >200 seconds if a platelet glycoprotein (GP) IIb/IIIa inhibitor is used].

Two angiograms of the left coronary artery in orthogonal projections and one left anterior oblique injection of the right coronary artery are made in an attempt to identify the infarct artery. Left ventriculography is usually not performed because of the contrast load, as the end-diastolic pressure is usually too high, but measurement of the left ventricular end-diastolic pressure at the end of the procedure could be helpful. However, it should be recognized that a left ventriculogram is the quickest way to diagnose mitral regurgitation and ventricular septal rupture, if suspicion is high and an adequate quality echocardiogram has not been obtained. When PCI is to be attempted, it should be performed as quickly and efficiently as possible with limited contrast injections.

Angiographic exclusions for PCI include infarct artery stenosis <70% with TIMI-3 flow, or lesion morphology that is high-risk for no-reflow or other complications. Emergency coronary artery bypass graft surgery may be considered for patients with left main disease, severe coronary anatomy unsuitable for PCI, multivessel disease, mechanical complications, or failed PCI if there is ongoing myocardial ischemia (Chapter 11). In some cases, it is desirable to perform balloon angioplasty alone or thrombus extraction only to restore reperfusion while waiting for the surgical team to be assembled.

The use of GP IIb/IIIa inhibitors has been demonstrated to improve outcome in patients undergoing primary PCI [47]. Observational studies suggest a benefit of abciximab in primary stenting for cardiogenic shock [48–51]. Although there are no randomized controlled trials evaluating use of abciximab or other GP IIb/IIIa inhibitors in cardiogenic shock, they are commonly used as adjunctive therapy. Their use appears to be particularly beneficial among patients who receive stents. From the Cleveland Clinic experience, it appears that patients who had stent placement with abciximab had 33% mortality at 2.5 years versus 43% for those without abciximab and 68% mortality for those with neither stents nor abciximab [49]. Although the majority of studies have used abciximab, it is noteworthy that in the randomized PURSUIT trial there was a significant mortality benefit among patients who randomized to eptifibatide (vs. placebo) among the small cohort who had cardiogenic shock complicating NSTEMI [52].

An appropriate 6F or 7F PCI guide catheter is placed in position. Coronary flow will occasionally be reestablished in the infarct artery once the lesion is crossed with a soft or floppy-tipped, 0.014-inch, steerable guidewire. The soft tip is less traumatic than stiffer wires, which are seldom needed. The guidewire is then advanced distally in the true lumen and not in a small side branch or under an intimal dissection. No role has been demonstrated for routine use of thrombectomy devices or distal protection devices. Recently, one study in noncardiogenic shock patients has shown that thrombus aspiration with an extraction device improved 1-year mortality [53]. This should be considered if there is a high clot burden. If the infarct artery remains occluded after crossing with the guidewire, it may be preferable to cross the occlusion with a balloon catheter and then withdraw it without inflating the balloon to establish reperfusion. The more gradual reperfusion provided with the wire or balloon catheter may result in less reperfusion arrhythmias than rapidly inflating the balloon immediately after crossing the lesion. It is then often possible to have a first impression of the infarct lesion and the distal artery with a small injection of contrast medium. PCI is performed with an appropriately sized balloon using an approximately 1:1 or 1.1:1 balloon-to-artery ratio, usually followed by stent implantation. An optimal result after stenting is obtained with <20% post-procedural diameter stenosis, TIMI-3 flow, and ECG evidence of myocardial reperfusion. Procedural success was 77% in the SHOCK trial [11] and 79% in the National Cardiovascular Data Registry (NCDR) [54].

Coronary stents decrease restenosis rates by 50% in elective PCI compared with balloon angioplasty, but they have not reduced mortality rates in primary PCI [55]. Some observational studies in cardiogenic shock that have not completely corrected for confounding variables suggest lower mortality rates with stents than percutaneous transluminal coronary angioplasty [49,51,56], but others show no benefit [57] or higher mortality rates [50]. Randomized studies have not been performed. Most patients undergoing primary PCI for cardiogenic shock will receive stents because they improve the immediate angiographic result and decrease subsequent target vessel revascularization in survivors. Although drug-eluting stents have been shown to decrease target vessel revascularization rates in STEMI [58], many operators will choose bare metal stents for this indication. Both thrombus burden and the inability to confirm in advance because of the urgency of the procedure that the patient will comply with clopidogrel therapy for up to 1 year may increase the risk for late stent thrombosis with drug-eluting stents.

Although PCI for STEMI is usually limited to the infarct artery, patients in cardiogenic shock with multivessel disease may have the best survival chance with PCI of all proximal discrete lesions. Early resolution of arrhythmias, conduction blocks, or hypotension suggest an important therapeutic benefit. Conversely, failure to improve within the first 24 hours usually predicts mortality.

## Procedural complications

Sustained ventricular tachycardia should be promptly cardioverted, and ventricular fibrillation requires defibrillation. Lidocaine or amiodarone may be required to suppress ventricular arrhythmias. Accelerated idioventricular rhythm is usually benign and self-limited. Asystole, bradycardia, and atrioventricular block may require immediate intravenous therapy with atropine or epinephrine or longer treatment with a temporary pacemaker, but usually resolve with successful reperfusion. The cardiodepressor Bezold-Jarisch reflex (bradycardia, vasodilation, hypotension) should be anticipated when primary PCI is performed for a proximal or mid-right coronary artery occlusion. In the SHOCK trial, the following complications occurred: acute renal failure (13%), severe hemorrhage (28%), sepsis (19%), and vascular complications (11%) [11].

Contrast medium reactions are rare. Benadryl is usually sufficient for urticaria. Bronchospasm should be treated with bronchodilators, although epinephrine may be required.

Coronary artery dissection can usually be successfully treated by placement of a stent. Coronary perforation is poorly tolerated in these patients, who do not respond well to prolonged balloon inflations and who do poorly with implantation of a polytetrafluoroethylene-covered stent.

Despite all of the interventions described above, PCI success rates in these patients are 10–20% lower than the >95% success rates with primary PCI in patients without cardiogenic shock. With improved equipment and operator experience, the main limitation in the current era is the ability to restore normal coronary blood flow in the infarct artery. The no-reflow phenomenon (TIMI 0–1 flow) or slow reflow (TIMI 2 flow) may occur transiently or may persist. This is usually due to microvascular dysfunction from coronary spasm, distal embolization, endothelial injury, or interstitial edema and is associated with poorer recovery of left ventricular function and a higher incidence of post-procedural complications [59]. Treatment options include 100 mcg boluses of intracoronary adenosine or nitroprusside given as frequently as tolerated through the guiding catheter or through an infusion catheter or the distal lumen of the balloon catheter. Intracoronary verapamil is used to treat no-reflow during elective PCI, but should be avoided in patients with cardiogenic shock because it is a negative inotrope. Caution should be used in stenting lesions with no-reflow, because poor run-off may increase the likelihood of stent thrombosis.

Access site bleeding and retroperitoneal hematoma are concerns, given the antithrombotic medications received by these patients. Meticulous access technique, proper dosing of drugs based on renal function, and early sheath removal decrease bleeding complication rates. Off-label use of bivalirudin instead of unfractionated heparin and abbreviated infusions of GP IIb/IIIa inhibitors are used by some physicians, but have not been tested for efficacy. Protamine can be used to reverse heparin anticoagulation. Platelet transfusions can reverse the antiplatelet effect of abciximab, but not eptifibatide or tirofiban. The threshold for administering red blood cells in these patients is lower than in elective PCI because of their unstable hemodynamic state.

Patients with cardiogenic shock are at increased risk for contrast nephropathy, so the lowest possible volume of contrast medium should be used. Other risk factors include age, diabetes, pre-existing renal dysfunction, and use of nonsteroidal anti-inflammatory agents.

## Post-procedure care

Patients will be treated in the coronary care unit. Early cessation of anticoagulation therapy and early femoral sheath removal are recommended, if possible. Prolonged use of IABP counterpulsation is associated with complications in 10% to 30% of patients. These include limb ischemia, infection, hemolysis, thrombocytopenia, thrombosis, and embolism. In the largest registry for IABP complications in the setting of acute MI, the rate of limb ischemia was 2.3%, serious access bleeding 1.4%, vascular surgery 0.7%, and deep vein thrombosis 0.1% [60]. The risk-to-benefit ratio of pulmonary artery catheters from the GUSTO trial suggested no increased risk among patients with cardiogenic shock [61], but the pulmonary artery catheter should be removed as soon as possible to avoid the risk of catheter sepsis. When removing vascular sheaths, the activating clotting time should be <170 seconds to minimize the risk of bleeding. Anticoagulation may be resumed 4–6 hours after sheath removal for other indications (atrial fibrillation, prosthetic valves, large anterior MI, mural thrombus, IABP, persistent shock).

Cardiac auscultation should be serially performed to monitor for a new murmur suggestive of mitral regurgitation or ventricular septal rupture. The signs and symptoms for retroperitoneal hematoma include hypotension, marked suprainguinal tenderness, and severe back or lower quadrant abdominal pain. The groin should be inspected for hematoma, pseudoaneurysm, or arteriovenous fistula. Glucose control may require an insulin drip. Inotropic and vasopressor agents should be titrated to hemodynamics and clinical indices of systemic perfusion. The hematocrit and creatinine should be monitored. Anticoagulation levels should be carefully adjusted. Renal or liver dysfunction, which often change over time in this population, may require adjustment of other drug doses.

Patients should be treated with daily aspirin 75–162 mg indefinitely after daily doses of 325 mg for 1 month for bare metal stent, 3 months after sirolimus drug-eluting stent implantation, and 6 months after paclitaxel drug-eluting stent implantation. Daily clopidogrel 75 mg should be administered for a minimum 1 month and ideally 12 months after bare metal stent implantation, and for at least 12 months following drug-eluting stent implantation if patients are not at high risk for bleeding [62]. Beta-blockers, angiotensin-converting enzyme inhibitors, and aldosterone inhibitors should be introduced only after the patient has become hemodynamically stable and gradually titrated as in chronic heart failure patients. Patients who develop symptoms or electrocardiographic changes of recurrent ischemia or reinfarction should undergo repeat cardiac catheterization and intervention when indicated.

## Prognosis

Cardiac power (mean arterial pressure × cardiac output/451) may be the strongest hemodynamic predictor of in-hospital mortality [63]. In the SHOCK registry [64], in-hospital mortality rates rose from 34% to 51% as the number of diseased arteries increased from one to three. After PCI, the mortality rate was 86% with absent reperfusion (TIMI 0/1 flow), 50% with incomplete reperfusion (TIMI 2 flow), and 33% with complete reperfusion (TIMI 3 flow). Similarly, final TIMI flow was a major predictor of outcome in the ALKK registry

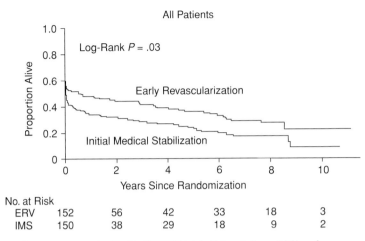

**Fig. 10.4** Long-term survival in the SHOCK trial. Abbreviations: ERV, early revascularization; IMS, initial medical stabilization. (Reprinted with permission from Hochman JS, Sleeper LA, Webb JG, et al. *JAMA* 2006;295:2511–15.)

with mortality rates of 78%, 66%, and 37% for TIMI 0/1, TIMI 2, and TIMI 3 flow, respectively [27]. The American College of Cardiology–National Cardiovascular Data Registry evaluated 483 consecutive patients who underwent emergency PCI for cardiogenic shock [54]. Predictors of in-hospital mortality included age, female sex, baseline renal insufficiency, and total occlusion in the left anterior descending artery.

Eighty-seven percent of the 1-year survivors in the SHOCK trial were in NYHA functional class I or II [65]. The 13 lives saved per 100 patients treated with early revascularization in the SHOCK trial at 6 months and 1 year were maintained at 3 and 6 years [13]. Overall survival rates at 6 years were 32.8% in the early revascularization group and 19.6% in the initial medical stabilization group (Fig. 10.4). The 6-year survival rates for the hospital survivors were 62.4% versus 44.4%, respectively.

At 30 days in the GUSTO-1 trial [66], 20,360 patients without shock (88.9%) and 953 (50.4%) patients with shock were alive. After a median of 11 years, 69.4% without and 55.2% with shock remained alive. Patients receiving PCI were less likely to die (24.1% vs. 34.6%). Beginning in the second year, mortality rates were 2% to 4% per year for all patients regardless of shock status (Fig. 10.5).

## Conclusion

Patients with cardiogenic shock complicating STEMI have a substantial survival benefit with PCI compared with no or late in-hospital revascularization. These patients need to be directly admitted or transferred to tertiary care centers

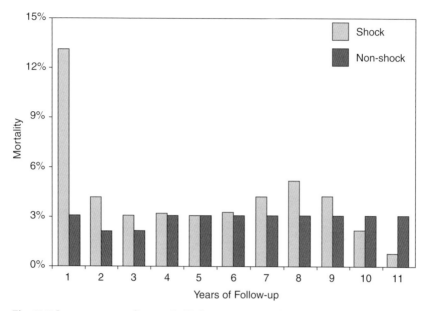

**Fig. 10.5** Long-term mortality rate in 30-day survivors in the GUSTO-I trial. (Reprinted with permission from Singh M, White J, Hasdai D, et al. *J Am Coll Cardiol* 2007;50:1752–8.)

with expertise in acute revascularization and advanced intensive care, unless further care is deemed futile. Coronary artery revascularization is the only intervention that improves survival in these patients. Importantly, recent emphasis on time-to-treatment and the increasing use of primary PCI as the reperfusion modality have decreased the number of patients developing cardiogenic shock as a complication of STEMI.

# References

1. Killip T, Kimball T. Treatment of myocardial infarction in a coronary care unit. *Am J Cardiol* 1967;20:457–64.
2. Gruppo Italiano per lo Studio della Streptochinasi nell'Infarto Miocardico (GISSI). Effectiveness of intravenous thrombolytic treatment in acute myocardial infarction. *Lancet* 1986;1:397–402.
3. AIMS Trial Study Group. Effect of intravenous APSAC on mortality after acute myocardial infarction: preliminary report of a placebo controlled clinical trial. *Lancet* 1988;1:545–9.
4. Wilcox RG, Olsson CG, Skene AM, et al. Trial of tissue plasminogen activator for mortality reduction in acute myocardial infarction: Anglo-Scandinavian Study of Early Thrombolysis (ASSET). *Lancet* 1988;2:525–30.
5. ISIS-2 (Second International Study of Infarct Survival) Collaborative Group. Randomized trial of intravenous streptokinase, oral aspirin, both or neither among 17,187 cases of suspected acute myocardial infarction. *Lancet* 1988;2:349–60.

6. Griffith GC, Wallace WB, Cochran B, et al. The treatment of shock associated with myocardial infarction. *Circulation* 1954;9:527–32.

7. Forrester JS, Diamond G, Chatterjee K, et al. Medical therapy of acute myocardial infarction by application of hemodynamic subsets. *N Engl J Med* 1976;195:1356–62.

8. Scheidt S, Wilner G, Mueller H, et al. Intra-aortic balloon counterpulsation in cardiogenic shock: report of a cooperative clinical trial. *N Engl J Med* 1973;188:979–84.

9. Bates ER, Topol EJ. Limitations of thrombolytic therapy for acute myocardial infarction complicated by congestive heart failure and cardiogenic shock. *J Am Coll Cardiol* 1991;18:1077–84.

10. Lee L, Bates ER, Pitt B, et al. Percutaneous transluminal coronary angioplasty improves survival in acute myocardial infarction complicated by cardiogenic shock. *Circulation* 1988;78:1345–51.

11. Hochman JS, Sleeper LA, Webb JG, et al. Early revascularization in acute myocardial infarction complicated by cardiogenic shock. SHOCK Investigators. Should We Emergently Revascularize Occluded Coronaries for Cardiogenic Shock. *N Engl J Med* 1999;341:625–34.

12. Hochman JS, Sleeper LA, White HD, et al. One-year survival following early revascularization for cardiogenic shock. *JAMA* 2001;285:190–2.

13. Hochman JS, Sleeper LA, Webb JG, et al. Early revascularization and long-term survival in cardiogenic shock complicating acute myocardial infarction. *JAMA* 2006;295:2511–15.

14. Mathey D, Kuck KH, Remmecke J, et al. Transluminal recanalization of coronary artery thrombosis: a preliminary report of its application in cardiogenic shock. *Eur Heart J* 1980;1:207–12.

15. Kennedy J, Gensini G, Timmis G, et al. Acute myocardial infarction treated with intracoronary streptokinase: a report of the Society for Cardiac Angiography. *Am J Cardiol* 1985;55:871–7.

16. Ohman EM, Topol EJ, Califf RM, et al. An analysis of the cause of early mortality after administration of thrombolytic therapy. *Coron Artery Dis* 1993;4:957–64.

17. Beohar N, Erdogan AK, Lee DC, et al. Acute heart failure syndromes and coronary perfusion. *J Am Coll Cardiol* 2008;52:13–16.

18. Gruentzig A. Transluminal dilatation of coronary-artery stenosis. *Lancet* 1978:1:263.

19. Mathey DG, Kuck KH, Tilsner V, et al. Nonsurgical coronary artery recanalization in acute transmural myocardial infarction. *Circulation* 1981;63:489–97.

20. Hartzler GO, Rutherford BD, McConahay DR, et al. Percutaneous transluminal coronary angioplasty with and without thrombolytic therapy for treatment of acute myocardial infarction. *Am Heart J* 1983;106:965–73.

21. Meyer J, Merx W, Dörr R, et al. Successful treatment of acute myocardial infarction shock by combined percutaneous transluminal coronary recanalization (PTCR) and percutaneous transluminal coronary angioplasty (PTCA). *Am Heart J* 1982;103: 132–4.

22. O'Neill WW, Erbel R, Laufer N, et al. Coronary angioplasty therapy of cardiogenic shock complicating acute myocardial infarction (abstract). *Circulation* 1985;72 (Suppl II):309.

23. Brown TM, Jannone LA, Gordon DF, et al. Percutaneous myocardial reperfusion reduces mortality in acute myocardial infarction complicated by cardiogenic shock (abstract). *Circulation* 1985;72(Suppl III):309.

24. Bates ER, Moscucci M. Post-myocardial infarction cardiogenic shock. In: Brown DL, ed. *Cardiac Intensive Care.* Philadelphia: WB Saunders, 1998:215–27.

25. Holmes DR Jr, Bates ER, Kleiman NS, et al. Contemporary reperfusion therapy for cardiogenic shock: the GUSTO-1 trial experience. *J Am Coll Cardiol* 1995;26:668–74.

26. Berger PB, Holmes DR Jr, Stebbins A, et al. Impact of an aggressive invasive catheterization and revascularization strategy on mortality in patients with cardiogenic shock in the Global Utilization of Streptokinase and Tissue Plasminogen Activator for Occluded Coronary Arteries (GUSTO-1) Trial. *Circulation* 1997;96:122–7.

27. Zeymer U, Vogt A, Zahn R, et al. Predictors of in-hospital mortality in 1333 patients with acute myocardial infarction complicated by cardiogenic shock treated with primary percutaneous coronary intervention (PCI); Results of the primary PCI registry of the Arbeitsgemeinschaft Leitende Kardiologische Krankenhausarzte (ALKK). *Eur Heart J* 2004;25:322–8.

28. Hochman JS, Boland J, Sleeper AL, et al. Current spectrum of cardiogenic shock and effect of early revascularization on mortality. Results of an international registry. *Circulation* 1995;91:873–81.

29. Urban P, Stauffer JC, Bleed D, et al. A randomized evaluation of early revascularization to treat shock complicating acute myocardial infarction. The (Swiss) Multicenter Trial of Angioplasty for Shock-(S)MASH. *Eur Heart J* 1999;20:1030–8.

30. Hochman JS, Buller CE, Sleeper LA, et al. Cardiogenic shock complicating acute myocardial infarction – etiologies, management and outcome: a report from the SHOCK trial registry. *J Am Coll Cardiol* 2000;336:1063–70.

31. Antman EM, Anbe DT, Armstrong PW, et al. ACC/AHA guidelines for the management of patients with ST-elevation myocardial infarction – executive summary. *Circulation* 2004;110:e82–293.

32. Dzavik V, Sleeper LA, Cocke TP, et al. Early revascularization is associated with improved survival in elderly patients with acute myocardial infarction complicated by cardiogenic shock: a report from the SHOCK Trial Registry. *Eur Heart J* 2003;24: 828–37.

33. Antoniucci D, Valenti R, Migliorini A, et al. Comparison of impact of emergency percutaneous revascularization on outcome of patients ≥75 to those <75 years of age with acute myocardial infarction complicated by cardiogenic shock. *Am J Cardiol* 2003;91:1458–61.

34. Dauerman HL, Ryan TJ Jr. Piper WD, et al. Outcomes of percutaneous coronary intervention among elderly patients in cardiogenic shock: a multicenter, decade-long experience. *J Invasive Cardiol* 2003;15:380–4.

35. Prasad A, Lennon RJ, Rihal CS, et al. Outcomes of elderly patients with cardiogenic shock treated with early percutaneous revascularization. *Am Heart J* 2004;147:1066–70.

36. Babaev A, Every NR, Frederick P, et al. Trends in revascularization and mortality in patients with cardiogenic shock complicating acute myocardial infarction. Observations from the National Registry of Myocardial Infarction (abstract). *Circulation* 2002;106(Suppl II):II–364.

37. Stomel RJ, Rasak M, Bates ER. Treatment strategies for acute myocardial infarction complicated by cardiogenic shock in a community hospital. *Chest* 1994:105:997–1002.

38. Kovack PJ, Rasak MA, Bates ER, et al. Thrombolysis plus aortic counterpulsation: improved survival in patients who present to community hospitals with cardiogenic shock. *J Am Coll Cardiol* 1997;29:1454–8.

39. Jeger RV, Tseng C-H, Hochman JS, Bates ER. Inter-hospital transfer for emergency revascularization in patients with ST-elevation myocardial infarction complicated by cardiogenic shock: a report from the SHOCK Trial and Registry. *Am Heart J* 2006;152:686–92.

40. Menon V, Slater JN, White HD, et al. Acute myocardial infarction complicated by systemic hypoperfusion without hypotension: report of the SHOCK Trial Registry. *Am J Med* 2000;108:374–80.

41. Topol EJ, Goldschlager N, Ports TA, et al. Hemodynamic benefit of atrial pacing in right ventricular myocardial infarction. *Ann Intern Med* 1982;96:594–7.

42. Brodie BR, Stuckey TD, Hansen CJ, et al. Timing and mechanism of death determined clinically after primary angioplasty for acute myocardial infarction. *Am J Cardiol* 1997;79:1586–91.

43. LeDoux JF, Tamareille S, Felli PR, et al. Left ventricular unloading with intra-aortic counter pulsation prior to reperfusion reduces myocardial release of endothelin-1 and decreases infarction size in a porcine ischemia-reperfusion model. *Catheter Cardiovasc Interv* 2008;72:513–21.

44. Vogel RA, Shawl F, Tommaso C, et al. Initial report of the National Registry of Elective Cardiopulmonary Bypass Supported Coronary Angioplasty. *J Am Coll Cardiol* 1990;15:23–9.

45. Bartlett RH, Roloff DW, Custer JR, et al. Extracorporeal life support: the University of Michigan experience. *JAMA* 2000;283:904–8.

46. Thiele H, Sick P, Boudriot E, et al. Randomized comparison of intra-aortic balloon support with a percutaneous left ventricular assist device in patients with revascularized acute myocardial infarction complicated by cardiogenic shock. *Eur Heart J* 2005;26:1276–83.

47. De Luca G, Suryapranata H, Stone GW, et al. Abciximab as adjunctive therapy to reperfusion in acute ST-segment elevation myocardial infarction: a meta-analysis of randomized trials. *JAMA* 2005;293:1759–65.

48. Antoniucci D, Valenti R, Migliorini A, et al. Abciximab therapy improves survival in patients with acute myocardial infarction complicated by early cardiogenic shock undergoing coronary artery stent implantation. *Am J Cardiol* 2002;90:353–7.

49. Chan AW, Chew DP, Bhatt DL, et al. Long-term mortality benefit with the combination of stents and abciximab for cardiogenic shock complicating acute myocardial infarction. *Am J Cardiol* 2002;89:132–6.

50. Giri S, Mitchel J, Azar RR, et al. Results of primary percutaneous transluminal coronary angioplasty plus abciximab with or without stenting for acute myocardial infarction complicated by cardiogenic shock. *Am J Cardiol* 2002;89:126–31.

51. Huang R, Sacks J, Thai H, et al. Impact of stents and abciximab on survival from cardiogenic shock treated with percutaneous coronary intervention. *Catheter Cardiovasc Interv* 2005;65:25–33.

52. Hasdai D, Harrington RA, Hochman JS, et al. Platelet glycoprotein IIb/IIIa blockade and outcome of cardiogenic shock complicating acute coronary syndromes without persistent ST-segment elevation. *J Am Coll Cardiol* 2000;36:685–92.

53. Vlaar PJ, Svilaas T, van der Horst IC, et al. Caradiac death and reinfarction after 1 year in the Thrombus Aspiration during Percutaneous Coronary Intervention in Acute Myocardial Infarction Study (TAPAS): a 1-year follow-up study. *Lancet* 2008;371:1915–2053.

54. Klein LW, Shaw RE, Krone RJ, et al. Mortality after emergent percutaneous coronary intervention in cardiogenic shock secondary to acute myocardial infarction and usefulness of a mortality prediction model. *Am J Cardiol* 2005;96:35–41.

55. Zhu MM, Feit A, Chadow H, et al. Primary stent implantation compared with primary balloon angioplasty for acute myocardial infarction: a meta-analysis of randomized clinical trials. *Am J Cardiol* 2001;88:297–301.

56. Antoniucci D, Valenti R, Santoro GM, et al. Systematic direct angioplasty and stent-supported direct angioplasty therapy for cardiogenic shock complicating acute myocardial infarction: in-hospital and long-term survival. *J Am Coll Cardiol* 1998;31:294–300.

57. Yip HK, Wu CJ, Chang HW, et al. Comparison of impact of primary percutaneous transluminal coronary angioplasty and primary stenting on short-term mortality in patients with cardiogenic shock and evaluation of prognostic determinants. *Am J Cardiol* 2001;87:1184–8.

58. Kastrati A, Dibra A, Spaulding C, et al. Meta-analysis of randomized trials on drug-eluting stents vs. bare-metal stents in patients with acute myocardial infarction. *Eur Heart J* 2007;22:2706–13.

59. Mehta RH, Harjai KJ, Boura J, et al. Prognostic significance of transient no-reflow during primary percutaneous coronary intervention for ST-elevation acute myocardial infarction. *Am J Cardiol* 2003;92:1445–7.

60. Stone GW, Ohman EM, Miller MF, et al. Contemporary utilization and outcomes of intra-aortic balloon counterpulsation in acute myocardial infarction. *J Am Coll Cardiol* 2003;41:1940–5.

61. Cohen MG, Kelly RV, Kong DF, et al. Pulmonary artery catheterization in acute coronary syndromes: insights from the GUSTO IIb and GUSTO III trials. *Am J Med* 2005;118:482–8.

62. King SB III, Smith SC Jr, Hirshfeld JW Jr, et al. 2007 focused update of the ACC/AHA/SCAI 2005 guideline update for percutaneous coronary intervention: a report of the American College of Cardiology/American Heart Association Task Force on Practice Guidelines. *J Am Coll Cardiol* 2008;51:172–209.

63. Fincke R, Hochman JS, Lowe A, et al. Cardiac power is the strongest hemodynamic correlate of mortality in cardiogenic shock: a report from the SHOCK trial registry. *J Am Coll Cardiol* 2004;44:340–8.

64. Webb JG, Sanborn TA, Sleeper LA, et al. Percutaneous coronary intervention for cardiogenic shock in the SHOCK Trial Registry. *Am Heart J* 2001;141:964–70.

65. Sleeper LA, Ramanathan K, Picard MH, et al. Functional capacity and quality of life following emergency revascularization for cardiogenic shock complicating acute myocardial infarction. *J Am Coll Cardiol* 2005;46:266–73.

66. Singh M, White J, Hasdai D, et al. Long-term outcome and its predictors among patients with ST-segment elevation myocardial infarction complicated by shock. *J Am Coll Cardiol* 2007;50:1752–8.

# Chapter 11

# Coronary artery bypass grafting

Cheuk-Kit Wong and Harvey D. White

## Introduction

Cardiogenic shock complicating MI is dynamic, often progressive, and associated with very high early mortality. In the 1970s, patients with cardiogenic shock were considered inoperable, and treatment was conservative with administration of fluid, inotrope support, and, in selected patients, intra-aortic balloon pumping [1,2]. However, most patients died by 1 year. Several surgical groups reported results of coronary artery bypass grafting (CABG) in patients who were unable to be weaned from intra-aortic balloon pumping, and the in-hospital mortality was 50% [3].

In the western Washington experience with early surgery, within 16 hours, mortality was around 35% [4]. Other groups reported a hospital mortality of around 30% for patients operated on at an average of 4 days after infarction with a further late mortality at 2 years of around 30% [5]. However, given the unavoidable bias in operating on selected patients, surgery for cardiogenic shock remained controversial until the only randomized prospective study of surgery in patients with cardiogenic shock "Should We Emergently Revascularize Occluded Coronaries for Cardiogenic Shock" (SHOCK) trial was performed [6].

## Role of coronary artery bypass grafting versus percutaneous coronary intervention

Percutaneous coronary intervention (PCI) and coronary artery bypass grafting (CABG) are generally considered complementary revascularization options for most patients with coronary artery disease, but the relative merits of these

*Cardiogenic Shock.* Edited by Judith S. Hochman and E. Magnus Ohman.
© 2009 American Heart Association, ISBN: 978-1-4051-7926-3

procedures may differ among patients with cardiogenic shock. PCI has a lower procedural success rate in patients with cardiogenic shock than in those without shock, and no-reflow or poor flow may occur after stenting [6–8]. Also, many shock patients have left main or complex 3-vessel disease that may be treated better with CABG [7–11]. The potential advantages of CABG over percutaneous coronary intervention (PCI) in patients with cardiogenic shock include better protection of ischemic myocardium with cardioplegia, ventricular unloading during cardiopulmonary bypass, and revascularization of noninfarct zones. Bypass surgery can also be performed on chronically occluded coronary arteries that cannot be treated with PCI, and can achieve more complete revascularization. CABG also has the advantage of allowing additional surgery correcting mechanical abnormalities, such as mitral regurgitation.

## The SHOCK trial

In the international, multicenter SHOCK trial, 30-day survival rates were similar with early revascularization and initial medical stabilization. Over half of the mortality occurred within the first 72 hours of onset of cardiogenic shock. However, at 6 months and 1 year, survival rates were higher with early revascularization. Initial revascularization was performed with PCI in 64% of patients and CABG in 36% of patients who underwent revascularization [6,12]. Most survivors reported good quality of life at 1 year [13]. The group difference in survival of 13 absolute percentage points at 1 year favoring those assigned to early revascularization remained stable at 3 and 6 years [13.1% and 13.2%, respectively; hazard ratio (HR), 0.74; 95% confidence interval (CI), 0.57–0.97; log-rank $P = 0.03$]. At 6 years, overall survival rates were 32.8% and 19.6% in the early revascularization and initial medical stabilization groups, respectively [14].

The design and patient flow of the SHOCK trial are shown in Fig. 11.1. The SHOCK protocol recommended that subjects randomly assigned to emergency revascularization have either PCI or CABG within 6 hours of randomization and within 18 hours of onset of shock. The protocol also recommended that emergency PCI be performed only on the infarct-related stenosis, and only in patients with 1-, 2-, or 3-vessel disease where the stenoses in two noninfarct-related arteries were <90%, or were located in arteries supplying small branch vessels.

Patients with a left main coronary stenosis of ≥50%, ≥2 total or subtotal occlusions, stenoses of >90% in two noninfarct-related major arteries, or stenoses unsuitable for PCI were recommended to undergo CABG, as were patients whose PCI proved unsuccessful. Although recommendations were made regarding selection of revascularization procedures, this decision was left to the individual discretion of site investigators.

In the SHOCK trial, 128 patients with confirmed LV failure causing shock underwent early revascularization (81 with PCI and 47 with CABG) [15]. Mean time elapsed between acute myocardial infarction and achievement of

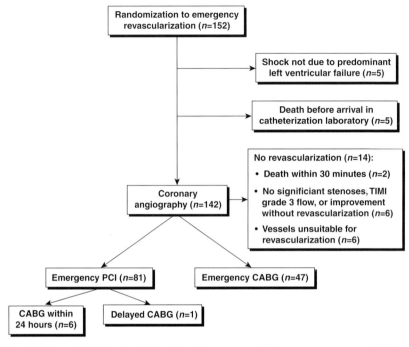

**Fig. 11.1** Flow chart of patients treated with emergency PCI versus emergency CABG in the SHOCK trial. (Reprinted with permission from White HD, Assmann SF, Sanborn TA, et al. *Circulation* 2005;112:1992–2001.)

successful revascularization was 11.0 (6.1–21.4) hours. An intra-aortic balloon pump (IABP) was used in 88.9% of PCI patients and 97.9% of CABG patients [15]. Seven of the 128 patients received both PCI and CABG (6 had CABG performed within 24 hours of PCI) and were included in the PCI group for the purpose of analysis.

Baseline demographics and hemodynamics were similar between the two groups, except that there were more diabetic patients (48.9% vs. 26.9%, $P = 0.02$) and more patients with 3-vessel disease (80.4% vs. 60.3%, $P = 0.03$) or left main disease (41.3% vs. 13.0%, $P = 0.001$) in the CABG group (Table 11.1). In the PCI group, 12.3% of patients had 2-vessel interventions and 2.5% had 3-vessel interventions.

In the CABG group, 84.8% received ≥2 grafts, 52.2% received ≥3 grafts, and 41 of 47 CABG patients (87.2%) were deemed to be completely revascularized by the operating surgeon (Table 11.2).

### Outcome of CABG
Survival at different time points is shown in Fig. 11.2. Survival rates at 30 days were 55.4% with PCI versus 57.4% with CABG ($P = 0.86$), and 51.9% versus

Table 11.1  Extent and severity of coronary disease according to revascularization modality.

| | PCI (*n* = 81) | CABG (*n* = 47) | *P* value |
|---|---|---|---|
| ≥50% stenosis in left main coronary artery (%) | 13.0 | 41.3 | 0.001 |
| Three-vessel disease (%) | 60.3 | 80.4 | 0.03 |
| Either left main or 3-vessel coronary disease (%) | 60.3 | 82.6 | 0.01 |
| Patients with no left main coronary disease | | | |
| Total number of diseased vessels | | | 0.08 |
| 1 vessel (%) | 22.4 | 3.7 | |
| 2 vessels (%) | 23.9 | 25.9 | |
| 3 vessels (%) | 53.7 | 70.4 | |
| Additional occlusions (other than infarct-related artery) | | | 0.41 |
| 0 additional occlusions (%) | 70.3 | 56.0 | |
| 1 additional occlusion (%) | 21.9 | 36.0 | |
| 2 additional occlusions (%) | 7.8 | 8.0 | |
| >90% stenoses in noninfarct-related arteries | | | 0.36 |
| 0 vessels (%) | 64.1 | 48.0 | |
| 1 vessel (%) | 26.6 | 40.0 | |
| 2 vessels (%) | 9.4 | 12.0 | |
| Coronary jeopardy score[*] | | | <0.0001 |
| 2 (%) | 16.7 | 0.0 | |
| 4 (%) | 6.4 | 6.5 | |
| 6 (%) | 28.2 | 6.5 | |
| 8 (%) | 16.7 | 8.7 | |
| 10 (%) | 19.2 | 43.5 | |
| 12 (%) | 12.8 | 34.8 | |
| Mean coronary jeopardy score[†] | 7.1 ± 3.2 | 9.9 ± 2.3 | <0.0001 |

[*]The jeopardy score is a simple method for estimating the amount of myocardium at risk on the basis of the particular location of coronary artery stenoses. The method scores the perfusion territory subtended by the same vessel beyond each significant stenosis, and the summed score of the patient is the jeopardy score for that patient. (Reference: Califf RM, Phillips HR, Hindman MC, et al. Prognostic value of a coronary artery jeopardy score. *J Am Coll Cardiol* 1985;5:1055–63.)

[†]Mean ± SD.

Reprinted with permission from White HD, Assmann SF, Sanborn TA, et al. *Circulation* 2005;112:1992–2001.

**Table 11.2** Details of coronary artery bypass grafting.

| | |
|---|---|
| Complete surgical revascularization (%)* | 87.2 |
| Number of grafts* | |
| 1 (%) | 15.2 |
| 2 (%) | 32.6 |
| 3 (%) | 32.6 |
| 4 (%) | 10.9 |
| 5 (%) | 8.7 |
| Internal mammary arterial graft (%)* | 15.2 |
| Data collected on cardiac surgery form ($n = 36$)† | |
| Median total perfusion time (minutes) | 110 (IQR 88–135) |
| Median total cross-clamp time (minutes) | 62 (IQR 49–78) |
| Concomitant valve procedure (%) | 5.6 |
| Cardioplegia used (%) | 86.1 |
| Cardioplegia delivery (in 31 patients with known cardioplegia use)† | |
| Antegrade only (%) | 58.1 |
| Retrograde only (%) | 6.4 |
| Both (%) | 35.5 |
| Types of cardioplegia (in 31 patients with known cardioplegia use)‡ | |
| Crystalloid (%) | 22.6 |
| Blood (%) | 87.1 |
| Additives (%) | 54.8 |

*These data were collected throughout the trial.
†Data on perfusion time, cross-clamp time, concomitant valve procedures, and cardioplegia were collected in only 36 patients after institution of a cardiac surgery data collection form partway through the trial.
‡More than one type of cardioplegia was used during some procedures.
IQR, inter-quartile range.
Reprinted with permission from White HD, Assmann SF, Sanborn TA, et al. *Circulation* 2005;112:1992–2001.

46.8% at 1 year ($P = 0.71$). Exploratory analysis found no significant interactions between the revascularization modality (PCI vs. CABG) and the anatomic extent of coronary disease (left main disease, 3-vessel disease, left main and/or 3-vessel disease, or disease extent measured with coronary jeopardy score). Likewise, no interactions were noted for age when using a cut point of 75 years, or for diabetes mellitus. Among hospital survivors who were assigned to receive early revascularization, there was no significant difference ($P = 0.51$) in long-term

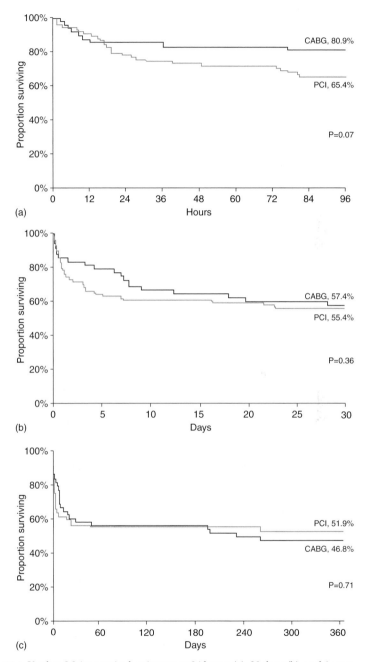

**Fig. 11.2** Kaplan–Meier survival estimates at 96 hours (a), 30 days (b), and 1 year (c) in patients treated with early PCI versus early CABG. PCI, percutaneous coronary intervention; CABG, coronary artery bypass grafting. (Reprinted with permission from White HD, Assmann SF, Sanborn TA, et al. *Circulation* 2005;112:1992–2001.)

survival between PCI and CABG surgery as the primary emergency mode of revascularization (7.0 and 9.3 deaths per 100 patient-years, respectively) [14].

Among subjects receiving surgery, the survival rate at 30 days was 63.4% for the 41 subjects who achieved complete revascularization versus 16.7% in the 6 subjects who did not achieve complete revascularization ($P = 0.07$); the 1-year survival rate for these groups was 51.2% and 16.7% ($P = 0.19$), respectively. Complete revascularization, defined as successful PCI of the proximal half of all major arteries with significant stenoses, was achieved in only 23.1% of PCI patients.

The results of the SHOCK trial suggest that CABG is an excellent complementary treatment option for early revascularization in patients with cardiogenic shock. The similar treatment benefit observed among subjects receiving CABG versus those receiving PCI, despite the greater prevalence of more severe coronary artery disease and diabetes mellitus among the former, may be explained by achievement of more complete revascularization with CABG.

No other randomized trials comparing early revascularization with initial medical stabilization in patients with cardiogenic shock have included CABG as part of the initial revascularization strategy. The Swiss Multicenter Trial of Angioplasty for Shock (SMASH) was terminated early for logistical reasons after 55 subjects had been randomly assigned to receive either PCI or medical treatment; CABG was performed in only one patient [16].

## Surgical techniques

The traditional approach to bypass surgery is to use warm induction, cold cardioplegia, cooling the heart to reduce energy requirements, and warm reperfusion with grafting first of the infarct-related artery (IRA). The heart is usually vented to unload the heart during cardiopulmonary bypass. Cardioprotection is very important in this procedure, and administration of antegrade and retrograde cardioplegia, as well as down the grafts, provides immediate protection of myocardium from further ischemic damage [17].

The internal mammary artery is usually preferred for grafting because of its better long-term patency compared with vein grafting to the left anterior descending artery. There are, however, a number of important considerations in the clinical setting of cardiogenic shock, including the size of the internal mammary artery and whether appropriate blood flow can be achieved in the presence of hypotension. Choice of conduit also depends on issues such as propensity to bleed following administration of adjunctive abciximab or clopidogrel, as harvesting of the internal mammary arteries may be associated with uncontrollable bleeding. Administration of vasoconstrictors, possibly leading to poor flow distal to internal mammary or radial grafts, may also influence a preference for choice of vein grafting. The most important consideration, however, is the longer operative time associated with use of arterial grafts. In the SHOCK trial, the use of left internal mammary arterial grafts in 15.2% of subjects despite the presence of cardiogenic shock is noteworthy.

## Comparison with contemporary percutaneous coronary intervention

The PCI success rate for patients with cardiogenic shock remains lower than for patients without shock. A recent German registry of 1333 patients with cardiogenic shock reported a final TIMI 3 flow rate of 75.2% [18]. Although there have been many advances with PCI, including stenting [11], which reduces reintervention rates, and the use of glycoprotein IIb/IIIa inhibitors [19–22], patients with cardiogenic shock continue to have a lower likelihood of successful PCI than those without cardiogenic shock [6–8]. The use of drug-eluting stents in patients with STEMI (including 23 patients with cardiogenic shock) has been shown to achieve rates of vessel patency and complications at 30 days similar to those seen with bare metal stents, without an increase in risk of stent thrombosis and with less need for reintervention at 300 days of follow-up [23]. Long-term stent thrombosis, however, remains a major concern with drug-eluting stents [24].

Contemporary PCI with stenting is associated with a high rate of periprocedural infarction. Delayed enhancement magnetic resonance imaging (MRI) shows infarction in 23% of cases [25], with distal embolization of plaque material (and occlusive thrombus) being an important mechanism of infarction. Another contributory mechanism is "snow-plowing" of the plaque at the site of the occlusion, which causes periprocedural infarction, as evaluated by MRI in 11% of patients due to a compromise of side branches and collaterals.

Multivessel PCI in shock patients is associated with worse outcomes [11,26]. Whether more complete revascularization with multivessel PCI in the acute phase is superior to the strategy of performing acute PCI to the culprit vessel and leaving nonculprit stenoses for subsequent treatment, as used in most patients in the SHOCK trial, remains unknown.

## Timing of surgery

The timing of performing CABG in the setting of acute myocardial infarction has always been a controversial issue. Some surgeons avoid operating early on these patients because of higher operative mortality based on results in the 1980s (up to 10% for operation within 7 days vs. 2.4% for operation between 8 and 30 days) [27].

Previous observational studies of the effects of CABG were often performed in lower risk patients, and in addition, patients often had revascularization several days after developing shock, introducing a survival bias with these patients having declared themselves as patients likely to do well. However, in the Myocardial Infarction Triage and Intervention (MITI) registry in the period between 1988 and 1994 [28], 1299 of 12,000 consecutive patients with acute infarction underwent CABG, and there was no difference in hospital mortality in high-risk patients operated on during the first 24 hours after admission compared with those operated on later in the hospital course (8.3% vs. 7.2%; $P = 0.60$). Factors that predicted hospital mortality in those who underwent bypass surgery included increased age, prior bypass surgery, infarct extension, and stroke. Long-term outcome in those who underwent bypass surgery was excellent. Three-year survival was better in patients treated with surgery than in those treated medically (83% vs. 66%; $P < 0.0001$), and this difference remained after multivariate adjustment for baseline differences (HR, 0.68; 95% CI, 0.55–0.85).

## Guidelines

In the current European Society of Cardiology and American College of Cardiology/American Heart Association guidelines [29,30], acute myocardial infarction with cardiogenic shock is listed as a Class IA indication (i.e. a condition for which there is evidence for and/or general agreement that a given procedure or treatment is useful and effective) for PCI, and a Class IA indication for CABG if the patient has suitable coronary anatomy.

## Contemporary practice

For a patient whose condition is deteriorating in the catheterization laboratory, many interventionists may opt for emergency PCI on stenoses not ideally suited for that procedure, knowing that, whereas CABG might achieve more complete revascularization, PCI can be performed more promptly. Also, with an occluded infarct-related artery, the status of the distal vessel is usually unknown until coronary guidewire crossing restores some antegrade flow. PCI may therefore be frequently performed on patients with suboptimal anatomy in preference to delayed CABG.

Emergency CABG is not widely considered to be an integral part of contemporary management of patients with cardiogenic shock, as reflected by NRMI registry data [31]. Data from 1995 to 2004 (including the periods before and after publication of the SHOCK trial in 1999) in 7356 patients presenting with cardiogenic shock complicating acute myocardial infarction showed rising rates of revascularization with primary angioplasty, but not with bypass surgery (Fig. 11.3). In centers where expert surgical facilities are available, Table 11.3 shows the major factors that may determine the choice of CABG versus PCI in treating cardiogenic shock from left ventricular dysfunction complicating acute myocardial infarction.

Percutaneous Coronary Intervention

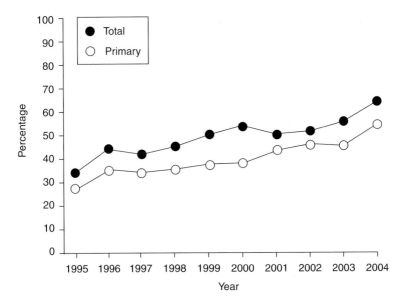

Coronary Artery Bypass Graft Surgery

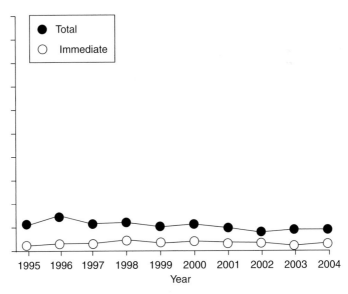

**Fig. 11.3** Revascularization rates in patients with cardiogenic shock at presentation ($n = 7356$). (Reprinted with permission from Babaev A, Frederick PD, Pasta DJ, et al. *JAMA* 2005;294:448–54.)

**Table 11.3** Cardiogenic shock following myocardial infarction.

1. **Timing of shock relative to onset of acute myocardial infarction**
   If the time from onset of acute myocardial infarction is short (<3–6 hours), salvage of myocardium may be achieved; any delay in performing CABG will be associated with more progression of myocardial necrosis, and PCI may be preferred.

2. **Status of infarct-artery antegrade flow and collateral flow to the infarct zone**
   The speed of infarct progression depends on these factors. PCI achieves more timely reperfusion and may be preferable if there is poor antegrade flow or poor collaterals.

3. **Extent of coronary disease in the noninfarct-related artery**
   Hypercontraction of these zones over time will lead to ischemia if these zones are supplied by arteries with severe flow-limiting stenoses. CABG may be performed because of its capacity for providing more complete revascularization.

4. **Bleeding risk**
   Bleeding associated with antiplatelet, antithrombin, and fibrinolytic medications may make PCI the preferred option.

5. **Capacity of CABG for achieving more complete revascularization** may make CABG the preferred option.

6. **The presence of mechanical complications** makes CABG the preferred option.

7. **Age**
   The increasing risk of stroke with age in patients undergoing CABG may make PCI the preferred option in elderly patients.

In the Society of Thoracic Surgeons National Cardiac Database (2002–2005) of 708,593 patients with and without cardiogenic shock undergoing CABG, patients with preoperative cardiogenic shock constituted 14,956 (2.1%) of patients undergoing CABG yet accounted for 14% of all CABG deaths. Operative mortality in cardiogenic shock patients was high and surgery-specific, rising from 20% for isolated CABG to 33% for CABG plus valve surgery and 58% for CABG plus ventricular septal repair. Factors associated with a higher risk of death were identified by multivariable analysis and summarized into a simple bedside risk score (c statistic = 0.74) that accurately stratified those with low (<10%) to very high (>60%) mortality risk in that database [32] (Figures 11.4 and 11.5).

The findings from the SHOCK trial support early revascularization, including CABG as appropriate, as currently recommended in the guidelines. However, numerous factors may hinder hospitals to provide this service, including resources. Also, public reporting systems of operative outcome may deter surgeons taking on high-risk patients, such as those with cardiogenic shock.

Score

| Age | <50 | <55 | 55-59 | 60-64 | 65-69 | 70-74 | 75-79 | 80 + |
|---|---|---|---|---|---|---|---|---|
| Points | 0 | 2 | 4 | 6 | 8 | 10 | 12 | 14 |

☐

| Serum Creatinine | < 1.0 | 1.0 – 1.19 | 1.2 – 1.39 | 1.4 – 1.89 | 1.9 + |
|---|---|---|---|---|---|
| Points | 0 | 3 | 5 | 8 | 12 |

☐

| Ejection Fraction | 40 and above | 30 – 39 | Under 30 |
|---|---|---|---|
| Points | 0 | 2 | 5 |

☐

| Surgery Type | CABG Only | AV + CABG | MV + CABG | VSR Repair + CABG |
|---|---|---|---|---|
| Points | 0 | 6 | 6 | 15 |

☐

| Gender | Male | Female |
|---|---|---|
| Points | 0 | 5 |

☐

| Prior Cardiovascular Surgery | No | Yes |
|---|---|---|
| Points | 0 | 7 |

☐

| MI within last 7 days | No | Yes |
|---|---|---|
| Points | 0 | 2 |

☐

| Immunosuppressive Treatment | No | Yes |
|---|---|---|
| Points | 0 | 5 |

☐

| Resuscitation (CPR <1 hr prior to surgery) | No | Yes |
|---|---|---|
| Points | 0 | 4 |

☐

| Intra-Aortic Balloon Pump Used | No | Yes |
|---|---|---|
| Points | 0 | 5 |

☐

| Operative Status | Emergent/Urgent | Salvage |
|---|---|---|
| Points | 0 | 12 |

☐

Total Score: ☐

**Fig. 11.4** Nomogram to predict postoperative death in patients with cardiogenic shock undergoing CABG. MI = myocardial infarction; CPR = cardiopulmonary resuscitation; AV = aortic valve surgery; MV = mitral valve surgery; VSR = ventricular septal rupture. Reprinted with permission from Mehta RH, Grab JD, O'Brien SM, et al. *Circulation* 2008;117:876–85.

In New York state, where such a score card system is in place, data from the SHOCK registry showed that patients wait significantly longer after onset of cardiogenic shock for CABG than patients outside of New York state (101.2 hours vs. 10.3 hours for non-New York patients, $P < 0.001$) [33].

# Conclusions

Surgery and PCI are complementary procedures for the management of patients with cardiogenic shock. Emergency CABG should be considered the preferred therapy in shock patients for whom PCI is unlikely to achieve complete revascularization, or for whom there are associated left ventricular mechanical complications (including mitral regurgitation), left main, or severe 3-vessel coronary disease. Although some surgeons are unwilling to take these high-risk patients

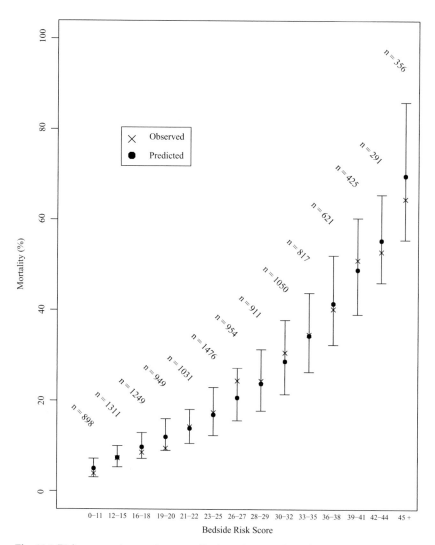

**Fig. 11.5** Risk score and operative mortality in patients with cardiogenic shock undergoing cardiac surgery. Vertical bar extends from 5th to 95th percentiles of the distribution of predicted risk as calculated by original full model. Reprinted with permission from Mehta RH, Grab JD, O'Brien SM, et al. *Circulation* 2008;117:876–85.

to surgery, data from the SHOCK trial showed that appropriately selected patients do well with surgery, and patients should not be denied this potentially life-saving therapy. In the future, advances in cardioplegia, anesthesia, and perioperative support using ventricular assist devices may produce even better surgical results.

# References

1. Scheidt S, Ascheim R, Killip T III. Shock after acute myocardial infarction. A clinical and hemodynamic profile. *Am J Cardiol* 1970;26:556–64.

2. Scheidt S, Wilner G, Mueller H, et al. Intra-aortic balloon counterpulsation in cardiogenic shock. Report of a co-operative clinical trial. *N Engl J Med* 1973;288: 979–84.

3. Sanders CA, Buckley MJ, Leinbach RC, et al. Mechanical circulatory assistance. Current status and experience with combining circulatory assistance, emergency coronary angiography, and acute myocardial revascularization. *Circulation* 1972;45: 1292–313.

4. DeWood MA, Notake RN, Hensley GR, et al. Intraaortic balloon counterpulsation with and without reperfusion for myocardial infarction shock. *Circulation* 1980;61: 1105–12.

5. Laks H, Rosenkranz E, Buckberg GD. Surgical treatment of cardiogenic shock after myocardial infarction. *Circulation* 1986;74:III11–16.

6. Hochman JS, Sleeper LA, Webb JG, et al. Early revascularization in acute myocardial infarction complicated by cardiogenic shock. SHOCK Investigators. Should We Emergently Revascularize Occluded Coronaries for Cardiogenic Shock. *N Engl J Med* 1999;341:625–34.

7. Antoniucci D, Valenti R, Santoro GM, et al. Systematic direct angioplasty and stent-supported direct angioplasty therapy for cardiogenic shock complicating acute myocardial infarction: in-hospital and long-term survival. *J Am Coll Cardiol* 1998;31:294–300.

8. Gacioch GM, Ellis SG, Lee L, et al. Cardiogenic shock complicating acute myocardial infarction: the use of coronary angioplasty and the integration of the new support devices into patient management. *J Am Coll Cardiol* 1992;19:647–53.

9. Moosvi AR, Khaja F, Villanueva L, et al. Early revascularization improves survival in cardiogenic shock complicating acute myocardial infarction. *J Am Coll Cardiol* 1992;19:907–14.

10. Hibbard MD, Holmes DR Jr, Bailey KR, et al. Percutaneous transluminal coronary angioplasty in patients with cardiogenic shock. *J Am Coll Cardiol* 1992;19:639–46.

11. Webb JG, Lowe AM, Sanborn TA, et al. Percutaneous coronary intervention for cardiogenic shock in the SHOCK trial. *J Am Coll Cardiol* 2003;42:1380–6.

12. Hochman JS, Sleeper LA, White HD, et al. One-year survival following early revascularization for cardiogenic shock. *JAMA* 2001;285:190–2.

13. Sleeper LA, Ramanathan K, Picard MH, et al. Functional status and quality of life after emergency revascularization for cardiogenic shock complicating acute myocardial infarction. *J Am Coll Cardiol* 2005; 46:266–73.

14. Hochman JS, Sleeper LA, Webb JG, et al. Early revascularization and long-term survival in cardiogenic shock complicating acute myocardial infarction. *JAMA* 2006;295:2511–15.

15. White HD, Assmann SF, Sanborn TA, et al. Comparison of percutaneous coronary intervention and coronary artery bypass grafting after acute myocardial infarction complicated by cardiogenic shock: results from the Should We Emergently Revascularize Occluded Coronaries for Cardiogenic Shock (SHOCK) trial. *Circulation* 2005;112:1992–2001.

16. Urban P, Stauffer JC, Bleed D, et al. A randomized evaluation of early revascularization to treat shock complicating acute myocardial infarction: the (Swiss) Multicenter Trial of Angioplasty for Shock–(S)MASH. *Eur Heart J* 1999;20:1030–8.

17. Allen BS, Buckberg GD, Fontan FM, et al. Superiority of controlled surgical reperfusion versus percutaneous transluminal coronary angioplasty in acute coronary occlusion. *J Thorac Cardiovasc Surg* 1993;105:864–79.

18. Zeymer U, Vogt A, Zahn R, et al. Predictors of in-hospital mortality in 1333 patients with acute myocardial infarction complicated by cardiogenic shock treated with primary percutaneous coronary intervention (PCI): results of the primary PCI registry of the Arbeitsgemeinschaft Leitende Kardiologische Krankenhausärzte (ALKK). *Eur Heart J* 2004;25:322–8.

19. Chan AW, Chew DP, Bhatt DL, et al. Long-term mortality benefit with the combination of stents and abciximab for cardiogenic shock complicating acute myocardial infarction. *Am J Cardiol* 2002;89:132–6.

20. Giri S, Mitchel J, Azar RR, et al. Results of primary percutaneous transluminal coronary angioplasty plus abciximab with or without stenting for acute myocardial infarction complicated by cardiogenic shock. *Am J Cardiol* 2002;89:126–31.

21. Hasdai D, Harrington RA, Hochman JS, et al. Platelet glycoprotein IIb/IIIa blockade and outcome of cardiogenic shock complicating acute coronary syndromes without persistent ST-segment elevation. *J Am Coll Cardiol* 2000;36:685–92.

22. Stone GW, Grines CL, Cox DA, et al. Comparison of angioplasty with stenting, with or without abciximab, in acute myocardial infarction. *N Engl J Med* 2002;346: 957–66.

23. Lemos PA, Saia F, Hofma SH, et al. Short- and long-term clinical benefit of sirolimus-eluting stents compared to conventional bare stents for patients with acute myocardial infarction. *J Am Coll Cardiol* 2004;43:704–8.

24. Lagerqvist B, James SK, Stenestrand U, Lindback J, Nilsson T, Wallentin L. Long-term outcomes with drug-eluting stents versus bare-metal stents in Sweden. *N Engl J Med* 2007;356:1009–19.

25. Porto I, Selvanayagam JB, Van Gaal WJ, et al. Plaque volume and occurrence and location of periprocedural myocardial necrosis after percutaneous coronary intervention: insights from delayed-enhancement magnetic resonance imaging, thrombolysis in myocardial infarction myocardial perfusion grade analysis, and intravascular ultrasound. *Circulation* 2006;114:662–9.

26. Webb JG, Sleeper LA, Buller CE, et al. Implications of the timing of onset of cardiogenic shock after acute myocardial infarction: a report from the SHOCK trial registry. *J Am Coll Cardiol* 2000;36:1084–90.

27. Kennedy JW, Ivey TD, Misbach G, et al. Coronary artery bypass graft surgery early after acute myocardial infarction. *Circulation* 1989;79:I173–8.

28. Every NR, Maynard C, Cochran RP, Martin J, Weaver WD. Characteristics, management, and outcome of patients with acute myocardial infarction treated with bypass surgery. Myocardial Infarction Triage and Intervention Investigators. *Circulation* 1996;94:II81–6.

29. Antman EM, Anbe DT, Armstrong PW, et al. ACC/AHA guidelines for the management of patients with ST-elevation myocardial infarction–executive summary: a report of the American College of Cardiology/American Heart Association Task Force

on Practice Guidelines (Writing Committee to Revise the 1999 Guidelines for the Management of Patients With Acute Myocardial Infarction). *Circulation* 2004;110:588–636.

30. Van de Werf F, Ardissino D, Betriu A, et al. Management of acute myocardial infarction in patients presenting with ST-segment elevation: the Task Force on the Management of Acute Myocardial Infarction of the European Society of Cardiology. *Eur Heart J* 2003;24:28–66.

31. Babaev A, Frederick PD, Pasta DJ, et al. NRMI Investigators. Trends in management and outcomes of patients with acute myocardial infarction complicated by cardiogenic shock. *JAMA* 2005;294:448–54.

32. Mehta RH, Grab JD, O'Brien SM, et al. Clinical characteristics and in-hospital outcomes of patients with cardiogenic shock undergoing coronary artery bypass surgery: insights from the Society of Thoracic Surgeons National Cardiac Database. *Circulation* 2008;117:876–85.

33. Apolito RA, Greenberg MA, Menegus MA, et al. Impact of the New York State Cardiac Surgery and Percutaneous Coronary Intervention Reporting System on the management of patients with acute myocardial infarction complicated by cardiogenic shock. *Am Heart J* 2008;155:267–73.

# Index

Author Disclosure Table

| Working group member | Employment | Research grant | Other research support | Speakers bureau/honoraria | Expert witness | Ownership interest | Consultant/advisory board | Other |
|---|---|---|---|---|---|---|---|---|
| Ashley | Cleveland Clinic | None | None | None | None | None | None | None |
| Bates | University of Michigan | None | None | None | None | None | None | None |
| Buller | University of British Columbia | None | None | None | None | None | None | None |
| Dzavik | Toronto General Hospital | None | None | None | None | None | None | None |
| Geppert | Wilhelminen Hospital | Austrian Society of Cardiology* | None | GSK, Arginox* | None | None | None | None |
| Ginsberg | Cooper University Hospital | None | None | None | None | None | None | None |
| Goldstein | William Beaumont Hospital | None | None | None | None | None | None | None |
| Hasdai | Rabin Medical Center | None | None | None | None | None | None | None |
| Hochman | New York University School of Medicine | Arginox Pharmaceuticals+ | None | Datascope, Schering-Plough Corporation* | None | None | Millennium Pharmaceuticals, Inc, Schering-Plough Research Institute* | None |

| | | | | | | | |
|---|---|---|---|---|---|---|---|
| Hollenberg | Cooper Hospital | None | None | None | None | None | None |
| Holmes | Mayo Clinic | None | None | None | None | None | None |
| Ohman | Duke University Medical Center | Bristol Myers Squibb, CV Therapeutics, Inc, Daiichi Sankyo, Datascope, Eli Lilly & Company, Sanofi-Aventis, Schering-Plough Corporation, The Medicines Company* | Bristol Myers Squibb, Daiichi Sankyo, Eli Lilly & Company, Sanofi-Aventis, Schering-Plough Corporation, The Medicines Company* | None | None | Inovise+ | CV Therapeutics, Inc, Inovise, Liposcience, Northpoint Domain, Pozen, Inc* Abiomed, Datscope, The Medicines Company, WebMD (theheart.org)+ |
| Iakobishvili | Rabin Medical Center | None | None | None | None | None | None |
| Katz | Duke University Medical Center | None | The Medicines Company* | None | None | None | None |
| Menon | Cleveland Clinic | None | None | None | None | None | None |
| Milano | Duke University | Thoratel* | Thoratel* | None | None | None | None |
| Motiei | Mayo Clinic | None | None | None | None | None | None |
| Parrillo | Cooper University Hospital | Deep Breeze, Robert Wood Johnson/NJ Heath Initiative+ | None | None | Deep Breeze* | None | None |
| Reynolds | NYU Medical Center | None | None | None | None | None | None |
| Rogers | Duke University | Thoratel+ | None | None | None | None | Thoratel+ |

## Author Disclosure Table (*Continued*)

| Working group member | Employment | Research grant | Other research support | Speakers bureau/ honoraria | Expert witness | Ownership interest | Consultant/advisory board | Other |
|---|---|---|---|---|---|---|---|---|
| Sketch | Duke University Medical Center | None | None | None | None | None | None | None |
| White | Auckland City Hospital | None | None | None | None | None | None | None |
| Wong | Dunedin School of Medicine, Otago University | None | None | None | None | None | None | None |

*Modest
+Significant

This table represents the relationships of writing group members that may be perceived as actual or reasonably perceived conflicts of interest as reported on the Disclosure Questionnaire which all writing group members are required to complete and submit. A relationship is considered to be "Significant" if (a) the person receives $10,000 or more during any 12 month period, or 5% or more of the person's gross income; or (b) the person owns 5% or more of the voting stock or share of the entity, or owns $10,000 or more of the fair market value of the entity. A relationship is considered to be "Modest" if it is less than "Significant" under the preceding definition.

# The AHA Clinical Series

## SERIES EDITOR • ELLIOTT ANTMAN

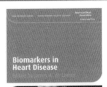

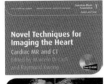
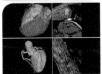

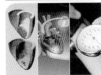

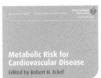
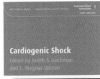

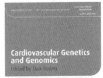

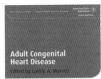

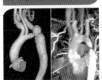
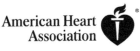